BACK STABILITY

Integrating Science and Therapy

Second Edition

Christopher M. Norris, MSc
Director, Norris Associates
Oxford, United Kingdom

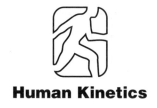

Human Kinetics

Library of Congress Cataloging-in-Publication Data

Norris, Christopher M.
   Back stability : integrating science and therapy / Christopher M.
Norris. -- 2nd ed.
        p. ; cm.
      Includes bibliographical references and index.
      ISBN-13: 978-0-7360-7017-1 (hard cover : alk. paper)
      ISBN-10: 0-7360-7017-6 (hard cover : alk. paper) 1.   Backache--
Treatment. 2. Backache--Prevention. 3. Backache--Exercise therapy.
I. Title.
      [DNLM: 1.   Low Back Pain--therapy. 2.   Exercise Therapy--methods. 3.
Low Back Pain--prevention & control. 4.   Lumbosacral Region--
physiology.   WE 755 N854b 2008]
      RD771.I58N67 2008
      617.5'6406--dc22

                                                                 2008001941

ISBN-10: 0-7360-7017-6
ISBN-13: 978-0-7360-7017-1

The Web addresses cited in this text were current as of August 2007, unless otherwise noted.

Acquisitions Editor: Loarn D. Robertson, PhD; **Managing Editors:** Heather M. Tanner and Melissa J. Zavala; **Copyeditor:** Julie Anderson; **Proofreader:** John Wentworth; **Indexer:** Nancy Ball; **Permission Manager:** Dalene Reeder; **Graphic Designer:** Joe Buck; **Graphic Artist:** Yvonne Griffith; **Cover Designer:** Keith Blomberg; **Photographer (cover):** © Neil Bernstein; **Photographer (interior):** © Human Kinetics; **Photo Office Assistant:** Jason Allen; **Visual Production Assistant:** Joyce Brumfield; **Art Manager:** Kelly Hendren; **Associate Art Manager:** Alan L. Wilborn; **Illustrator:** Mic Greenberg; **Printer:** Thomson-Shore, Inc

We thank Doug Nelson of Bodywork Associates in Champaign, Illinois, for his expertise and assistance during the photo shoot for this book.

Printed in the United States of America   10 9 8 7 6 5 4 3 2 1

Human Kinetics
Web site: www.HumanKinetics.com

United States: Human Kinetics
P.O. Box 5076
Champaign, IL 61825-5076
800-747-4457
e-mail: humank@hkusa.com

Canada: Human Kinetics
475 Devonshire Road Unit 100
Windsor, ON N8Y 2L5
800-465-7301 (in Canada only)
e-mail: info@hkcanada.com

Europe: Human Kinetics
107 Bradford Road
Stanningley
Leeds LS28 6AT, United Kingdom
+44 (0) 113 255 5665
e-mail: hk@hkeurope.com

Australia: Human Kinetics
57A Price Avenue
Lower Mitcham, South Australia 5062
08 8372 0999
e-mail: info@hkaustralia.com

New Zealand: Human Kinetics
Division of Sports Distributors NZ Ltd.
P.O. Box 300 226 Albany
North Shore City
Auckland
0064 9 448 1207
e-mail: info@humankinetics.co.nz

For Hilde, Sophie, Twig, and Max

Contents

Preface   ix

Acknowledgments   x

Exercise Finder   xi

Part I Conceptual Foundation   1

Chapter 1 What Is Back Stability?   3

Scope of the Problem   3

A New Look at the Etiology and Treatment of Back Pain   3

Model Used in This Book: Lumbar Stabilization   9

Summary   12

Chapter 2 Biomechanics of the Lumbar Spine   15

Anatomy of the Vertebral Column   15

Axial Compression   25

Movements of the Lumbar Spine and Pelvis   28

Mechanics of Bending and Lifting   33

Lifting Methods   36

Summary   38

Chapter 3 Stabilization Mechanisms of the Lumbar Spine   39

Posterior Ligamentous System   39

Thoracolumbar Fascia   40

Trunk Muscle Action   44

Intra-Abdominal Pressure Mechanism   55

Summary   58

Chapter 4 Principles of Muscle Imbalance   61

Basic Concepts   61

Muscle Adaptation to Increased and Decreased Usage   65

Training Specificity   67

Changes in Muscle Length   68

Summary   70

Part II Establishing Stability   71

Chapter 5 Posture   73

Optimal Postural Alignment   73
Postural Stability and Body Sway   74
Basic Postural Assessment   74
Principles of Postural Correction   81
Posture Types and How to Correct Them   83
Summary   87

Chapter 6 Muscle Balance Tests   105

Assessing Stretched Muscles—Testing Inner-Range Holding Ability   105
Assessing Shortened Muscles   106
Principles of Muscle Stretching   106
Stretching Target Muscles   108
Assessing Segmental Control   108
Summary   109

Chapter 7 Foundation Movements   129

Teaching Your Clients to Control Pelvic Tilt   129
Teaching Your Clients to Identify and Assume the Neutral Position   131
Teaching Your Clients to Use Abdominal Hollowing   132
Teaching Your Clients to Contract the Multifidus Muscles at Will   137
Summary   137

Part III Progressing Stability Training   163

Chapter 8 Limb Loading   165

Superimposed Limb Movements   165
Summary   167

Chapter 9 Unstable Base   191

Theory of Proprioception   191
Benefits of Training   192
Summary   193

Chapter 10 Gym Ball   203

Gym Ball Exercises   203
Summary   204

Chapter 11 Foam Rollers   219

Principles   219
Summary   219

Part IV Building Back Fitness 225

Chapter 12 Faults With Traditional Abdominal Training 227

Sit-Up 227
Straight-Leg Raise 229
Potentially Dangerous Exercises 230
Summary 232

Chapter 13 Abdominal Training Using Stability Concepts 233

Modifications of the Sit-Up 233
Modifications of the Straight-Leg Raise (SLR) 234
Ab Roller Exercises 234
Testing Midsection Muscle Endurance 234
Summary 235

Chapter 14 Resistance Training for Core Strength 249

Weight Training 249
Summary 254

Chapter 15 Speed and Power in Core Training 271

Theory of Power Through Speed Training 271
Summary 273

Chapter 16 Functional Training 283

Movement Analysis 283
Movement Components 284
Lifting Techniques 285
Summary 289

Part V Clinical Application 299

Chapter 17 Preliminary Client Assessment 301

Assessing Pain 301
Assessing Disability 301
Summary 305

Chapter 18 Designing the Program 309

Needs Analysis 309
Program Aims 312
Training Plan 313
Principles for Designing a Stability Program 314
Summary 316

Chapter 19 Case History Illustrations   **317**

Overweight Client   317

Athlete With Poor Stability   318

Client With Acute Pain   319

Patient Unwilling to Exercise   320

Pregnant Client With Back Pain   321

Summary   322

Glossary   323

Bibliography   325

Index   337

About the Author   347

Preface

The first edition of *Back Stability* presented a new approach to the treatment of low back pain, one that encouraged movement rather than rest and gave patients the opportunity to actively participate in their own health care. Both the approach and the book were well received, and for this second edition I have gone further. I have subtitled the book *Integrating Science and Therapy* to emphasize that I have taken back pain information from around the world and brought it together into a single, readily usable form. My intention is to bring the science from the laboratories and universities and put it firmly where it is most needed: the therapist's treatment room; the local gym, school, and sports club; and the living rooms of the millions of people who experience back pain. Why is this necessary? Isn't *Back Stability* already popular enough?

Let me cite a real-life case history to answer this. A 42-year-old secretary I know complained of low back pain. Her pain was worse with housework and especially prolonged sitting. If she did gardening, the next day she woke with stiffness and required about half an hour for her back to "get going." Because she was busy, she did not seek help but instead started going to the gym to work her pain off. She got steadily worse and began to experience pain into her buttocks and then down her legs. Eventually she saw her physician, who referred her for a magnetic resonance imaging scan. The scan came back showing minimal wear and tear but normal discs and facet joints and no nerve impingement. Her specialist told her to be grateful because the scan showed nothing wrong. When she asked what could be done about her pain, she was told that she would have to put up with it because it was normal for someone who had reached "the wrong side of 40." She left the specialist's clinic with the same pain she had entered with. Is this really the best that we can offer? Have our health care services reached the point where we advise clients to spend large sums of money on tests and specialist fees but are unable to offer any real help? I hope not, and I know that by reading this book you share my vision of a healthy back for life.

This book combines information from several sources. The scientific information that I present comes from fields within both medicine (anatomy, physiology, and pathology) and sport (biomechanics, exercise physiology, and motor skill training). This is combined with practical knowledge gained from nearly 30 years working as a physiotherapist, exercise professional, and teacher. This combination of evidence-based practice pervades *Back Stability*.

In part I (Conceptual Foundation), I present updated information on the mechanisms of stability and discuss stability as part of an overall muscle balance approach. I include scientific findings that have been published since the first edition of the book. The concepts of functional training are introduced, and these run through the whole of the exercise approach featured in *Back Stability*. Part II (Establishing Stability) deals with the basic skills required to develop stability. Assessment of posture and muscle balance is highlighted, and I introduce foundation movements to teach your patients. I describe teaching points in detail so you can accurately prescribe the movements and use a process of clinical decision making when determining which exercise to use with which patient.

Part III (Progressing Stability Training) takes you from the treatment couch to the rehab room and uses progressive exercise and basic equipment to develop greater stability. Again, important teaching points are emphasized, and exercise modifications are used to enhance prescriptive precision. Part IV (Building Back Fitness) takes you from the rehab room to the gym and deals with abdominal training, resistance apparatus, speed and power, and practical functional progressions. In part V (Clinical Application), I use real-life patient examples to illustrate how to structure the full *Back Stability* program stage by stage. I also include tick lists that you can use with patients to make exercise prescription easier.

For the second edition of *Back Stability,* I have included photographs of the exercise techniques. To make these even more useful, where appropriate I have overlaid the photographs to show body alignment. To emphasize "real-life" situations, some models demonstrate poor technique. A teaching point is used where this occurs. Bullet points are used to aid quick reference of exercise technique, and two colors are used throughout for emphasis. The book itself is larger to make it easier to "dip into." I sincerely hope that this book will not stay on your bookshelf but will become heavily thumbed as it travels with you into the treatment room, rehab room, and gym.

Acknowledgments

To the patients I have treated over a 25-year period, thank you for placing your faith in me.

To the more than 400 therapists to whom I have taught these techniques during a 15-year period—I have learned from you more than I have given.

Exercise Finder

Abdominal Hollowing: Standing 154
Abdominal Machine 263
Abdominal Slide 205
Active Knee Extension, Holding Thigh 121
Active Knee Extension, Pushing Against Thigh 122
Assessing Muscle Balance in the Gluteus Maximus 111
Assessing Muscle Balance in the Gluteus Medius 112
Assessing Muscle Balance in the Iliopsoas 110
Axial Loading 306
Back Extension (Frame) 258
Back Extension (Machine) 257
Back Extensor Endurance Test (Biering-Sorensen Test) 246
Back Flattening 92
Balance Beam Walk 220
Barbell Lunge 270
Basic Crunch 243
Basic Superman 207
Bench Curl 238
Bent-Knee Sit-Up 236
Bent-Knee Sit-Up Endurance Test 247
Bilateral Straight Leg Lowering 240
Bridge 208
Bridge From Crook Lying (Shoulder Bridge) 173
Bridge With Heel Raise on Roller 223
Bridge With Leg Lift 173
Bridge With Leg Lift and Extension 210
Bridge With Leg Lift on Gym Ball 209
Bridge With Pelvic Tilt 209
Bridge With Therapist Pressure 210
Cable Crossover 256
Cat Stretch 124
Chest–Pelvis Stacking 93
Controlled Forward Bending 148
Controlled Sit-Down 296
Crook-Lying Assisted Pelvic Tilt 145
Deadlift 281
Deadlift From Bench 294
Door Frame Stretch 102
Double Crunch 245
Dumbbell Row 266
Forward Bending 127

Forward Lean With Pulley 298
Forward Lean With Step and Push 297
Forward Stride (Walk) Standing Multifidus Contraction 161
Four-Point Kneeling Abdominal Hollowing 153
Four-Point Kneeling Arm Lift 217
Four-Point Kneeling Arm and Leg Lift (Full Birddog) 177
Four-Point Kneeling Arm and Leg Lift on Foam Roller 222
Four-Point Kneeling Body Sway 174
Four-Point Kneeling Leg Lift (Birddog) 176
Four-Point Kneeling Leg Movement 175
Four-Point Kneeling Pelvic Shift 174
Free Squat 216
Full Heel Slide 239
Gluteus Maximus Inner-Range Exercise 89
Good Morning 268
Gym Ball Bridge on Roller 224
Half Lunge 119
Half Lunge Without Chair 91
Half-Sitting Arm and Leg Movements 206
Hang Clean 279
Heel Bridge 212
Heel Slide—Basic Movement 168
Heel Slide Maneuver Using Pressure Biofeedback 113
High (Two-Point) Kneeling (Assisted) Hip Hinge Action 146
Hip Abduction Test 116
Hip Hinge With Stick (Revision) 291
Hip Hinge With Table Support 147
Hip Hitch 184
Kneeling Rock-Back 126
Lateral Pulldown 255
Leg Lowering 169
Leg-Raise Throw 278
Lying Barbell Row 265
Low Pulley Spinal Rotation 261
Lying Passive Back Extension 98
Lying Pelvic Raise 241
Lying Trunk Curl Over Ball 206
Lying Trunk Curl With Leg Lift 207
Medicine Ball Trunk Curl 277
Modified Trunk Curl 88

Monkey Squat 293

Muscle Reaction Speed Using a Mobile Platform 195

Neutral Position Maintenance 200

Ober Test 115

Ober Test Stretch 120

One-Arm Pulley Row 260

One-Leg Lift 126

One-Leg Heel Bridge 212

One-Hand Dumbbell Side Flexion 267

Pelvic Motion Control in the Frontal Plane: The Trendelenburg Sign 141

Pelvic Motion Control in the Sagittal Plane: Standing Hip Scissor 142

Pelvic Rock on Rocker Board 198

Pelvic Rock on Wobble Board 199

Pelvic Shift With Leg Lift 185

Pelvic Shift With Unloading 183

Plyometric Flexion and Extension Using a Punching Bag 275

Plyometric Side Bend Using a Punching Bag 274

Power Clean 280

Prone Abdominal Hollowing Test Using Pressure Biofeedback 113

Prone Kneeling Lumbar–Pelvic Rhythm 140

Prone-Lying Abdominal Hollowing 156

Prone-Lying Bent-Leg Lift 172

Prone-Lying Gluteal Brace 171

Prone-Lying Multifidus Contraction 158

Prone Fall 213

Prone Fall With Arm Lift 213

Prone Fall With One-Leg Lift 214

Prone Tuck on Roller 224

Rapid Displacement in Sitting 194

Reproduction of Active Positioning 152

Reproduction of Passive Positioning 151

Reverse Bridge 211

Reverse Bridge and Roll 211

Reverse Crunch 244

Rotary Torso Machine 262

Scapula Repositioning 101

Seated Rowing 259

Self-Monitored Hip Hinge 292

Side Crunch 245

Side Bridge Endurance Test 248

Side Flexion Test 118

Side-Lying Body Lift (Side Bridge) 181

Side-Lying Hip Abduction 143

Side-Lying Hip Lift 180

Side-Lying Knee Lift (Clamshell) 178

Side-Lying Leg Abduction 179

Side-Lying Leg Rotation 179

Side-Lying Multifidus Contraction Using Femoral Pressure 162

Side-Lying Multifidus Contraction Using Rhythmic Stabilization 159

Side-Lying Spine Lengthening 180

Single Bent-Leg Raise 170

Sitting Abdominal Hollowing 155

Sitting Assisted Pelvic Tilt 144

Sitting Bilateral Hip Adductor Stretch 94

Sitting Hamstring Stretch 188

Sitting Hip Flexor Shortening 97

Sitting Hip Hinge 201

Sitting Hip Hinge and Stand-Up 295

Sitting Knee Raise 190

Sitting Knee Raise on Gym Ball 205

Sitting Lateral Tilt Using Gym Ball 150

Sitting Pelvic Tilt, Progressing to Balance Board 197

Sitting Pelvic Tilt Reeducation 99

Sitting Pelvic Tilt Using Gym Ball 149

Sitting Multifidus Contraction 160

Sitting Sternal Lift 189

Sitting Trunk Flexion With Overpressure 124

Sitting Wide Splits 95

Spinal Lengthening 96

Squat 269

Standing Hip Abduction 186

Standing Hip Hinge 140

Standing Hip Hinge With Table 187

Standing Knee Raising 138

Standing Passive Pelvic Tilt 139

Standing Sternal Lift 182

Standing Squat 220

Sternal Lift 103

Straight-Leg Raise 307

Straight-Leg Raise Test 117

Superman With Arms 208

Supine-Lying Abdominal Hollowing 157

Supine-Lying Leg Lift 221

Thomas Test 114

Thomas Test Stretch 118

Thoracic Joint Mobilization 100

Throwing and Catching on a Mobile Surface 196

Tripod Position 125

Trunk Curl 237

Trunk Flexion With High Pulley (Pulley Crunch) 264

Trunk Rotation 306

Trunk Side Flexor Stretch 123

Twist and Throw With Medicine Ball 276

Two-Leg Raise 218

Two-Point Kneeling Balance 223

Wall Bar–Hanging Leg Raise 242

Wall Sit 215

Weight Bag Passive Stretch 102

Part I
Conceptual Foundation

Because the approach used in this book differs somewhat from what you may have seen in the past, it is important to understand the theoretical basis for what you read. I begin in chapter 1 with an introduction to back pain and back instability. People who suffer from back pain may be subjected to manipulation, instructed to perform exercises, or told to work out; they may be given chemicals to relax their muscles and may be poked with electric needles—all intended to alleviate their pain. But surprisingly few professionals understand that a great deal of low back pain occurs for one simple reason: instability. Instability occurs when the spine is not supported by the tissues surrounding it and therefore wobbles in ways that cause tissue swelling or impinge on nerves. Traditional approaches are often quite helpful but for some clients simply do not address the cause of back pain completely. Such approaches often stop short of restoring full function and instead leave clients with slightly less pain but still guarding their back when they try to do simple everyday actions.

The purpose of this book is to teach you how to deal with back pain by helping your clients stabilize their spines. From discussion of the basic etiology of pain in chapter 1, I proceed in chapter 2 to explain how the spine works: its anatomy, its movements, and even the physics of lifting.

In chapter 3, I show you how the anatomical lessons of the first two chapters lead logically to certain specific, but frequently ignored, treatments. Chapter 4 puts the back stability approach into the context of the wider muscle imbalance approach.

I hope you will digest these chapters thoroughly; without the conceptual foundation that they provide, the rest of the book will appear to be little more than one more listing of exercises. If you appreciate the theoretical underpinnings of the following chapters, however, you will see that the how-to chapters open for your clients a world of new possibilities that traditional programs cannot provide.

Chapter 1
What Is Back Stability?

Back pain is a universal problem, one that is particularly important in the largely sedentary Western world. New information about this condition is stimulating new ways to manage it, focusing particularly on innovative approaches to exercise.

SCOPE OF THE PROBLEM

As many as 80% of people in the Western world will suffer at least one disabling episode of low back pain during their lives; at any time, as many as 35% of the population suffers from some kind of back pain (Frymoyer and Cats-Baril 1991). The cost is tremendous, both financially and in terms of personal suffering. Most people with low back pain recover within 6 weeks, but 5% to 15% of subjects progress to permanent disability, accounting for up to 90% of total expenditures for this condition (Liebenson 1996). Unfortunately, recurrence of back pain after an acute episode is common. More than 60% of those suffering an acute episode of low back pain will experience another bout within a year, and 45% of these will have a second recurrence within the following 4 years (Liebenson 1996).

Key point: As many as 15% of people with low back pain progress to permanent disability, and 60% suffer from a recurrence of pain within 1 year.

Back pain is universal. Sufferers in the United States spend $60 billion per year treating it (Frymoyer and Gordon 1989) and receive $27 billion for permanent disability. The rate of increase in back pain is 14 times greater than the population growth, and during a period when disability awards for all conditions rose by 347%, awards for back pain increased by 2,680% (Frymoyer and Cats-Baril 1991).

In the United Kingdom, 46.5 million working days were lost through back pain in 1989—representing a cost to the National Health Service of £0.5 billion ($840 million) per year and an even larger cost to industry of £5.1 billion ($8.59 billion) in lost production (CSP 1998; Tye and Brown 1990). In 1994 to 1995, 14 million people in the United Kingdom visited their doctors for back pain and lost 116 million working days.

A massive 7% of physician time is spent treating back pain, but the success rate is very poor. Only 50% of people actually return to work within 6 weeks, and 60% of sufferers experience a second bout of back pain within 1 year of the onset of the original condition (Airaksinen et al. 2005).

More worrying for parents is a poll in the United Kingdom (CSP 2004) showing that back pain prevalence in schoolchildren now approaches that of adults. A combination of nonergonomic school furniture, poor posture, and rapidly decreasing activity levels is producing a time bomb for our health services.

A NEW LOOK AT THE ETIOLOGY AND TREATMENT OF BACK PAIN

Despite the tremendous increase in the number of back pain sufferers in the past 2 decades, popular understanding about the nature of back pain has remained somewhat static. It is commonly believed that back pain results from a structural injury or fault that must be corrected to reduce pain and restore full function. According to this viewpoint, normal function is impossible—or even dangerous—until the defective structure has changed (Zusman 1998).

Although it is true that many people with low back pain exhibit structural changes, computed tomography scans reveal positive findings in up to 50% of normal, asymptomatic subjects (Boden et al. 1990; Jensel et al. 1994)! It is the same with radiographic changes in the lumbar spine: As many people without pain show evidence of disc degeneration as do those with pain (Nachemson 1992).

The purpose of an X ray is to identify an abnormality, or a structural change or pathology of bone. Studies have shown that more than 75% of spinal X rays present no useful clinical information. In a study of 1,095 lumbar X rays, 46% were normal or had "incidental findings," and a further 32% had "radiological findings of questionable clinical significance" (Scavone et al. 1981). Typical changes on lumbar radiographs often associated with long-standing back pain are largely unrelated to eventual outcome.

Degenerative changes, disc narrowing, and the presence of osteophytes are all common diagnoses given out freely to worried clients, but these do not correlate with the presence of low back pain (LBP) at all (Bigos et al. 1994, Craton 2006). X rays have little place in the diagnosis of long-term (chronic) back pain, to the extent that the European Guidelines for the Management of Chronic Non-specific Low Back Pain (Airaksinen et al. 2005) state, "We do not recommend radiographic imaging for chronic non-specific low back clients."

Studies with cadavers have shown no correlation between structural changes in the lumbar spine and a history of low back pain (Videman et al. 1990), and large disc lesions with nerve compression (often a common diagnosis) may be totally asymptomatic (Saal 1995).

Key point: Structural changes in the spine are as likely in asymptomatic people as in those with low back pain and loss of function.

Nonorganic Causes of Back Pain

At least three sources of back pain do not originate in the sufferer's body: iatrogenic, forensic, and behavioral (cf. Zusman 1998).

• Iatrogenic factors (brought on by the practitioner) include labels of disability and the consequences of deconditioning through prolonged

(bed) rest. For example, a label such as *prolapsed disc* is far more threatening to a client than *simple back pain,* even though the total amount of pain experienced by the client may be the same in both cases. Labels that imply disease or disability, such as *arthritis,* also suggest severe conditions even though a mild form of the pathology may be present. Alternatives such as *slight roughening* or *normal wear and tear* are less threatening. Although avoiding activities that place stress on the back is important and limited rest has its place, prolonged bed rest has been shown to be counterproductive. Deyo and colleagues (1986) compared 2 days of bed rest with 2 weeks of bed rest. They found both periods to be equally effective in terms of pain reduction, but the 2-week period led to significant negative effects attributable to immobilization (such as weakening and stiffness around the spine) that were not present in the 2-day period.

• Forensic factors (associated with legal proceedings) contribute significantly to chronic back pain. In a study of 2,000 back pain clients (Long 1995), involvement in litigation was the only factor that accurately predicted that a person would not rapidly return to work.

• Two important behavioral factors are perceived disability and anticipation of pain.

1. Perceived disability. Clients often fail to take part in daily activities because they believe they are physically incapable of doing the task—although structural changes in their spines do not bear out this belief (Zusman 1998). Perceived disability is often associated with a mistaken fear of reinjury (Vlaeyen et al. 1995).

2. Anticipation of pain. Often the anticipation of pain rather than pain itself is enough to limit activity and create protective behaviors (Zusman 1998). The physical changes brought about by the fear of pain can be measured on surface electromyograph (sEMG). Main and Waddell (1996) applied experimental noxious stimuli to the upper trapezius of normal subjects and those with back pain. Normal subjects showed the expected reflex increase in sEMG activity in the trapezius muscles. Those with back pain, however, showed the reaction

not in the upper trapezius but rather in the lumbar region—suggesting that the subjects viewed any pain as an inherent part of their back condition even when the pain was occurring in another part of their bodies.

Key point: Perceived disability and the anticipation of pain contribute significantly to loss of function.

Psychology of Low Back Pain

Let's look at the psychological factors involved in back pain. Pain and disability are not the same thing; pain is simply a client symptom, whereas disability results from restricted activity. Pain has three aspects (Loeser 1980): **nociception,** pain itself, and suffering.

Generally, in chronic low back pain (CLBP), nociception and pain have less effect than do suffering and pain behavior. The effect of pain is therefore greater than the pain itself. This may not have been the case when the back pain originally occurred, but over time the effect of the injury and pain itself have become secondary to the suffering and physical changes that the injury has caused. In CLBP, then, if we focus all of our treatment on pain reduction, we will fail to address a very large part of the client's condition.

Aspects of Pain

Nociception—process by which stimuli act on pain sensors (mainly in the skin and superficial tissues) to produce nerve impulses. Nociceptive pain acts as a protective mechanism in normal individuals.

Pain—perception of a pain sensation by the brain. This may occur even when there is no tissue damage.

Suffering—an emotional response to pain. This same response may be caused by features other than pain, however, such as anxiety and grief.

Key point: Focusing treatment on pain reduction alone fails to address the whole of the client's condition.

Pain is both a sensory and an emotional experience. It is more than an indication of simple tissue damage, and if treatment focuses on tissues alone, the emotional aspect of pain may go unaltered. Pain signals pass from receptors in the body tissues to the brain, where the signals are experienced or felt. However, in their journey from sensor to brain, the signals are always modulated or changed slightly by the nervous system before they reach conscious awareness and are felt. It is impossible to separate pain sensation, then, from the emotional effect of pain: The two are permanently intertwined. The International Association for the Study of Pain (IASP) has defined pain as

> an unpleasant sensory and emotional experience associated with actual or potential tissue damage, or described in terms of such damage. (Merskey and Bogduk 1994)

Pain is seen here as a mental state rather than simply a stimulus. Even if tissue damage is not present, pain may still be experienced. Additionally, pain is very much a personal experience, and the IASP definition emphasizes the belief that tissue damage may occur. This is especially important to the concept of fear of movement.

Why Is Chronic Low Back Pain Disabling?

Disability is simply a restriction of activity. The World Health Organization (WHO) defines disability as

> any restriction or lack (resulting from an impairment) of ability to perform an activity in the manner or within the range considered normal for a human being. (WHO 1980)

What is of interest is how CLBP leads to disability. It is often assumed that pain lasting for a prolonged period will inevitably lead to disability purely as a result of time. However, clinically this is not what we see. It is common to see clients who demonstrate high levels of disability with very little pain as well as clients who have high levels of pain with very little disability. The combination of pain with lack of activity over time can lead to a preoccupation with physical symptoms and a change in the client's belief about the meaning of her pain (Main and Waddell 2004). Clients learn to avoid activities that they belief will cause or exacerbate pain and to rely on passive coping strategies rather than active ones.

Key point: Clients learn to avoid activities that they believe will increase their pain and rely on passive (not doing) coping strategies rather than active (doing) strategies.

Passive coping strategies see clients handing over responsibility for their care to a therapist with the attitude that there is nothing they personally can do to help themselves. They often engage in negative self-talk, using phrases like "I can't get comfortable with this back" or "I couldn't do that because of my back." They tend to avoid activities and situations that they believe will cause or exacerbate pain, even if they have not tried the activities. When using active coping strategies, clients take part in their own care. They often use exercise, seek treatment, and adapt their lifestyle to continue with daily activities.

In chapter 17 we look at methods to assess disability at the outset of our treatment, and in chapter 16 we will see how functional exercise targets disability attributable to back pain.

New Model for Low Back Pain Management

Most people traditionally have perceived back pain as a structural condition that requires rest. New information is challenging this approach, however, viewing back pain at least in part as a functional change that requires functional management. Exercise is at the forefront of this new approach.

Traditional Model

Rest is still the most common treatment for back pain, despite the fact that prolonged bed rest has been shown to be harmful. Controlled exercises restore function, reduce distress and perceived disability, diminish pain, and promote a return to work (Waddell 1987). Rest has little effect on the natural history of back pain and may actually increase its severity (Twomey and Taylor 1994). For back pain without significant radiation, bed rest probably should be limited to a maximum of 2 days. Longer periods are almost certainly counterproductive because of the negative effects of whole-body immobilization (Spitzer et al. 1987).

Surgery is effective in only a small group of low back pain clients. Waddell (1987) argued that surgical intervention can help only 1% of clients. Comparing surgically and conservatively treated clients suffering from disc prolapse, Weber (1983) found no difference in outcome after 2 years. Intensive conservative management can successfully treat more than 80% of clients with clinically diagnosed sciatica and radiological evidence of nerve root entrapment (Bush et al. 1992). According to Allan and Waddell (1989), "disc surgery . . . [has left] more tragic human wreckage in its wake than any other operation in history."

Two studies warrant closer observation, because they strengthen the argument against general back surgery. Brox and colleagues (2003) investigated 64 clients with low back pain lasting longer than 1 year who had radiographic evidence of disc degeneration in the lower lumbar spine. The clients were divided into two groups; the first received lumbar fusion (screws) and postoperative physiotherapy, and the second underwent three exercise sessions per week for 3 weeks together with cognitive education. At 1-year follow-up, improvements in back pain, use of analgesics, emotional distress, life satisfaction, and return to work were no different between the surgery and rehabilitation groups. The success rate according to an independent observer was 70% after surgery and 76% after rehabilitation. In addition, 18% of those in the surgical group suffered complications.

In a further study, Keller and colleagues (2004) assessed physical performance indicators for the two groups. The exercise group performed significantly better in muscle strength than did the lumbar fusion group. The bone density at L3-L4 (the third and fourth lumbar vertebrae) decreased in the lumbar fusion group but remained unchanged in the exercise group. Clearly, surgery for this condition is unwarranted.

Key point: Most long-term back pain should be viewed as a functional change requiring functional management.

New Model

In proposing a new model for the treatment of low back pain, Waddell (1987) recommended that the client's role change from one of resting and passively receiving treatment to taking action and sharing responsibility for restoration of function. Rehabilitation professionals increasingly are adopting this philosophy, using exercise programs to enhance lumbar stabilization (Jull and Richardson 1994b; Norris 1995a; O'Sullivan et al. 1997). Following are some examples:

• For a herniated lumbar disc. A rehabilitation program that emphasized skill-based exercise therapy for the spine effectively treated herniated lumbar discs (Saal and Saal 1989) and rehabilitated football players with back injury (Saal 1988). The program aimed to restore automatic control of muscular stabilization of the trunk by teaching subjects to maintain a correct lumbar pelvic position (i.e., neutral position—see following discussion) while performing progressively more complex tasks. In a study by Skall and colleagues (1994), intensive exercise when pain was not a limiting factor was more effective than mild mobilizing exercise 5 weeks following disc surgery. A 1-year follow-up showed a trend favoring the intensive exercise group. Even when the diagnosis is uncertain, progressive exercise—consisting of strengthening, proprioceptive training, and aerobic training—may restore pain-free function (Deutsch 1996). Pain, physical dysfunction, and psychosocial dysfunction improved following a 10-week exercise program for clients with chronic low back pain studied by Risch and colleagues (1993), whereas all three factors worsened for those who remained inactive.

• For spondylolysis or spondylolisthesis. A back stability program targeting the anterolateral abdominals and multifidus was more effective than conventional rehabilitation in clients with radiographic diagnosis of spondylolysis or spondylolisthesis (O'Sullivan et al. 1997). In this study, one group of clients underwent a 10-week program of gym work (including trunk curl exercises), general exercises such as swimming, and

pain-relieving modalities. A second group, which engaged only in back stability exercises, showed a statistically significant reduction in pain intensity, pain descriptor scale, and functional disability that was maintained at a 30-month follow-up (figure 1.1). This trial provides strong evidence for the effectiveness of stabilization programs for the lumbar spine. I have expanded some of these techniques for use in this book.

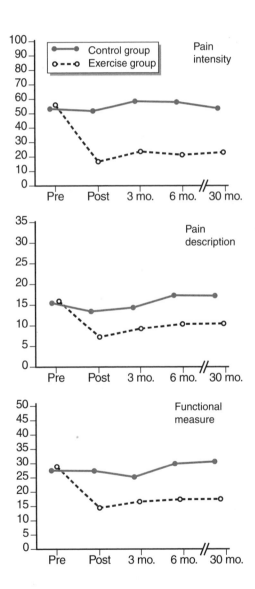

Figure 1.1 A comparison of conventional exercise and stability exercise effects on spondylolysis/spondylolisthesis.

Data from P.B. O'Sullivan, L. Twomey, and G.T. Allison, 1998, "Altered abdominal muscle recruitment in patients with chronic back pain following a specific exercise intervention," *Journal of Orthopedic and Sports Physical Therapy* 27: 114-124.

- For stabilization of the spine. A back stability program has been shown to be superior to surgery. Fairbank and colleagues (2005) found no significant difference in outcome measures at 2-year follow-up between surgical stabilization of the lumbar spine and an intensive exercise-based stabilization program. Complications occurred in 19 participants in the surgical group, but no complications were seen in the rehabilitation group. The cost of surgery was, of course, higher; the mean total cost for surgery was £7,830 (US $15,560), whereas that for rehabilitation was £3,304 (US $6,566) (Rivero-Arias et al. 2005). So, for safety, effectiveness, and cost, exercise wins out against surgery for the treatment of CLBP.

- For chronic low back disorder. Goldby and colleagues (2006) compared a spinal stabilization program with manual therapy or education only in the treatment of 346 subjects with CLBP. Their results showed the lowest scores for pain measured on a numerical rating scale for the stabilization group. When the researchers measured quality of life (Nottingham Health Profile score), the stabilization group scored 56.8% at 12-month follow-up compared with 36.5% and 37.3% for the manual therapy and education groups, respectively. These authors stated that

> spinal stabilization rehabilitation is more effective over time than manual therapy or . . . education . . . at reducing pain, disability, dysfunction, medication intake and improving the quality of life in patients with chronic low back disorder.

The integrated back stability (IBS) approach used in this book has been evaluated in a pilot study during the treatment of CLBP (Norris and Mathews 2006). Twenty-seven subjects were given the IBS program over a six-week period. Significant improvements were shown on scores for pain, disability, fear of movement, and patient experience.

Further Evidence Supporting the New Model

When the scientific literature in general is reviewed, the picture is the same: Support for rehabilitation is unequivocal. Assessing 31 randomized controlled trials (RCTs) on all forms of

surgical treatment for back pain, Gibson and Waddell (2005) found only limited evidence to support surgery, there is, however, strong evidence for the need for intensive exercise programs following any surgery for back pain (Ostelo et al. 2003).

Best practice now focuses on making rehabilitation integral to clinical management rather than a secondary intervention, an approach predicted to reduce sickness absence and incapacity attributable to LBP by 30% to 50% (Waddell and Burton 2005).

Two Cochrane reviews have supported the use of exercise in the management of LBP. Looking at 61 RCTs, Hayden and colleagues (2005) concluded that exercise therapy was effective at decreasing pain and improving function in adults with chronic low back pain. Graded activity programs were shown to improve absenteeism in people with subacute low back pain.

Addressing functional restoration for workers with back pain, Schonstein and colleagues (2003) looked at 18 RCTs and found that functional restoration programs supervised by a physiotherapist reduced sick days for workers with chronic back pain. These authors concluded that successful rehabilitation for this condition should consist of three components: (1) a physical conditional program, (2) close association with work-related goals and outcomes, and (3) correction of dysfunctional beliefs using a cognitive behavioral intervention.

Muscle Isolation or Movement Integration?

Back stability works. But we must be cautious, because some studies cast doubt on reliance on muscle isolation techniques alone. Outcome measures for stability training using muscle isolation have shown stability training to be no more effective than standard physiotherapy rehabilitation. Cairns and colleagues (2000) looked at 97 clients with recurrent LBP and compared conventional physical therapy alone with conventional physical therapy plus muscle isolation exercises. The authors assessed treatment outcome using a standard Roland and Morris Disability Questionnaire. Both groups showed significant clinical improvement, but the addition of muscle isolation exercise did not give any further benefit. Koumantakis and colleagues (2005a) compared rehabilitation using a general trunk muscle endurance program with muscle isolation exercise in a population of 55 clients with recurrent LBP. After the 8-week trial, the researchers found no difference in paraspinal muscle tests between the two groups. Interestingly, in a later study by this group (Koumantakis et al. 2005b), stability exercises were used in both exercise groups, but only one group had muscle isolation actions as well. The authors concluded that stabilization exercises (isolation actions) provided no additional benefit to subjects who had *no clinical signs of instability*.

The approach that this book takes is an integrated one. We progress from muscle isolation to the enhancement of functional movements to give the client the best chance of complete recovery and return to a fully healthy lifestyle.

Key point: Take an integrated approach to back stability, progressing from muscle isolation to functional movements.

MODEL USED IN THIS BOOK: LUMBAR STABILIZATION

This book presents a program of back treatment based on the new model of active client participation. The most important concept underlying the program is that of lumbar back stability versus lumbar back instability.

Instability of the lumbar spine is not the same as hypermobility. In both conditions, the range of motion is greater than normal. However, instability is present when there is "an excessive range of abnormal movement for which there is no protective muscular control." There is no instability in hypermobility, however, because the "excessive range of movement . . . has complete muscular control" (Maitland 1986). The essential feature of stability is therefore the ability of the body to control the whole range of motion of a joint, in this case the lumbar spine.

Key point: Stability of a joint implies the body's ability to control the entire range of motion around that joint.

An unstable lumbar spine cannot maintain correct vertebral alignment. Because the unstable segment is less stiff (less resistant to movement), movement within the spinal column increases even under minor loads—thereby altering both the quality and quantity of motion. Unstable lumbar spines often reveal no clinical damage to the spinal cord or nerve roots and no incapacitating deformity. If untreated, however, an unstable spine may irritate or damage neural tissue, leading to positive neurological signs on clinical examination. Positive neurological examination, therefore, does not preclude prescription of stabilization exercise, because instability may indeed cause the positive findings.

The excessive movement in an unstable spine may either stretch or compress pain-sensitive structures, leading to inflammation (Kirkaldy-Willis 1990; Panjabi 1992). A number of physical signs can suggest instability in a clinical assessment, as outlined in Physical Signs of Instability, as follows. See also chapter 17.

Why do we not simply stiffen the spine completely? Because too much stiffness will prevent free motion of the spine. Ultimately, a stiffer spine has less movement, until eventually complete stiffness becomes *rigidity*. This is nonfunctional. The job of the stability system is to monitor spinal motion and modulate muscle action to vary spinal stiffness depending on the loads imposed on the spine. Lower loads require less stability and lower

---

Physical Signs of Instability

Step deformity (spondylolisthesis) or rotation deformity (spondylolysis) on standing, which decreases when the patient is lying down

Transverse band of muscle spasm, which decreases when the patient is lying down

Localized muscle twitching while shifting weight from one leg to the other

Juddering or shaking during forward bending

Alteration to passive intervertebral motion testing, suggesting excessive mobility in the sagittal plane

Paris 1985; Maitland 1986

...s through reduced muscle contrac-
...ds require the opposite.

...: The stability system monitors spinal motions and modulates muscle action. This varies spinal stiffness to match the load imposed on the spine.

Stable Movement and Position of the Lumbar Spine

Both the gross and fine positions of the lumbar spine are vital to back stability and may be described in terms of neutral zone and neutral position. Control of these positions requires an interplay among several body systems and forms the basis of the back stability program.

Movement in the Neutral Zone

We have defined lumbar instability as an excessive range of motion without muscular control. Another way to visualize instability is as a loss of stiffness (Pope and Panjabi 1985)—not the negative condition we refer to when we speak of a stiff back but rather a positive factor referring to the amount of resistance that a structure (in this case, the spine) provides to move against a force. Less stiffness leads to more movement from application of the same force. If a back is not stiff enough, it will buckle and move under very little force, resulting in compression or stretching of sensitive structures. Pain is the consequence.

Key point: Stiffness is the ratio of change in force to change in length of a material. Material that is more stiff (a metal bar) takes more force to bend it; tissue that is less stiff (a rope) takes less force.

Panjabi and colleagues (1989) proposed the concept of the neutral zone—the zone in which movement occurs at the beginning of the range of motion before any effective resistance is offered from either the muscular system or the spinal column. The neutral zone is the range of motion that lacks effective restraint (stiffness), either active or passive. It is the vertebral displacement that occurs before resistance is offered. A grossly unstable spinal segment has quite a large neutral zone (figure 1,2). Physiotherapists use this concept when they assess lumbar joint movements by palpation—they note the onset either of motion resistance or of pain as they move the joint. In the case of the lumbar spine in the prone position, movement of this type is usually in a posteroanterior direction.

The passive stability system (ligaments and bone contour) reduces motion toward the end of the neutral zone. Our strategy, however, is to reduce the size of the neutral zone by increasing stiffness offered by **muscle stability**. Exercise that increases muscle stability may reduce motion within the neutral zone before the passive elements even come into play. Neutral zone motion is different from the total range of motion; even though stabilizing exercise increases muscle stiffness, it does not reduce the total range of motion. Panjabi

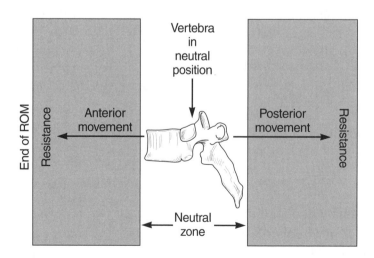

Figure 1.2 The neutral zone. ROM = range of motion.

(1992), who investigated the relationship between total range and neutral zone range by studying the effect of external fixation on the cervical spine in cadavers, noted that neutral zone motion declined more than 70% in association with a decrease of only 40% in total range of motion. In reducing the size of the neutral zone, the back stability program decreases the amount of motion that occurs when minimal forces are imposed on the spine (i.e., those same forces that, when experienced hour after hour, can produce the compression and stretching that lead to back pain). A stable back is not constantly buffeted by minor stresses related to mere sitting or standing, such as those that occur in people with unstable spines.

Key point: Instability alters both the quality and quantity of lumbar motion.

Neutral Position of the Lumbar Spine

The neutral position of the lumbar spine is different from the neutral zone. Lumbar neutral position refers to an overall movement of the lumbar spine rather than to individual movements between vertebrae. Lumbar neutral position is midway between full flexion and full extension as brought about by posterior and anterior tilting of the pelvis. Teaching your client to identify and maintain the neutral position of his lumbar spine is a key component of each stage of the back stability program, because the neutral position places minimal stress on body tissues. Also, because postural alignment is optimal, the neutral position is generally the most effective position from which trunk muscles can work.

Key point: The neutral position of the lumbar spine is important in all stages of the back stability program because it minimizes stress.

Achieving and Maintaining Spinal Stability

Three interrelated systems maintain spinal stability (figure 1.3). Inert tissues (in particular, ligaments) provide passive support; contractile tissues give active support; and neural control centers

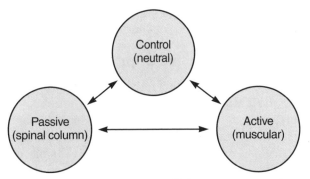

Figure 1.3 The spinal stabilizing system consists of three interrelating subsystems.
Reprinted, by permission, from M.M. Panjabi, 1992, "The stabilization of the spine. Part 1. Function, dysfunction, adaptation, and enhancement," *Journal of Spinal Disorders* 5(4): 383-389.

coordinate sensory feedback from both systems (Panjabi 1992). Because one or two systems may compensate for reduced stability in another, the active system may sometimes increase its contribution to stability to minimize stress on the passive system (Tropp et al. 1993). When the goal of rehabilitation is to heal the spine, appropriate exercise—by enabling the active system to take more of the total load placed on the back—can permit the passive system to repair itself. The net results are decreased pain and increased function. Conversely, continually loading the passive system without proper support from the active system can increase the time to recovery and lead to further tissue damage.

Simply developing muscle strength, however, is insufficient. To provide maximum relief to the passive system, one must augment both of the other systems (i.e., the active and neural control systems). Yet many popular strength exercises for the trunk actually increase mobility in this region to dangerously high levels (Norris 1993, 1994b). Rather than improving stability, exercises of this type may reduce stability and therefore exacerbate symptoms—especially those associated with inflammation. An example is the bilateral straight-leg-raise movement, where both legs are lifted simultaneously from a supine lying position. Although people performing this exercise may indeed strengthen their abdominal muscles, they often fail to maintain pelvic alignment. Anterior tilting of the pelvis leads to lumbar facet compression and overstretches the anterior spinal tissues. In this case, the anterior longitudinal ligament of the spine may be overstretched, reducing the effect of an important passive stabilizing structure (see chapter 12).

Passive Support

Passive support of the lumbar region is provided by stretching (especially of ligaments) and compression of soft tissues. A compressed ligament is more relaxed and offers less support through stiffness. In full lumbar extension, for example, as may occur when one is standing with an anteriorly tilted pelvis, the lumbar facet joints are loaded and compressed. The anterior structures, including the anterior longitudinal ligament, are stretched: Stability is provided (passively) through elastic recoil of this ligament and because facet joints of the spine are forcibly closed.

Developing Active Lumbar Stability

Poor postural control can leave the spine vulnerable to injury by placing excessive stress on the body tissues (Kendall et al. 1993). In the lumbar spine, the trunk muscles protect spinal tissues from excessive motion. To do this, however, the muscles surrounding the trunk must be able to co-contract isometrically when appropriate (Richardson et al. 1990). The synergistic interaction between various trunk muscles is complex; some muscles act as prime movers to create the gross movements of the trunk, whereas others function as stabilizers (fixators) and neutralizers to support the spinal structures and control unwanted movements. Rehabilitation through active lumbar stabilization not only deals with the torque-producing capacity of muscles, as is true of many traditional programs, but also seeks to enable a person to unconsciously and consistently coordinate an optimal pattern of muscle activity (Jull and Richardson 1994a).

Developing the Neural System

The neural system links the passive and active systems. On detecting movement within the neutral zone, the neural system relays information to the active system (muscles) about the position and direction of movement. The muscles' ability to contract and maintain stability (i.e., to increase stiffness and reduce the size of the neutral zone) depends on the speed and accuracy with which the information is relayed. The vital aspects of neural system development are therefore accuracy of movement and speed of reaction. Thus, the stability program emphasizes accuracy of movement early on; speed comes later.

Key point: The back stability program emphasizes movement accuracy early in the program. Speed comes later.

Motor Control

The active, passive, and neural systems are linked together through the process of motor control. At any time, the central nervous system monitors the stability of the spine to provide the right amount of tissue stiffness for optimal function. If there is too little stiffness, stress will be imposed on the delicate discs, joints, and nerves of the spine. Too much stiffness, and movement will be compromised.

The central nervous system uses two processes to monitor and change spinal stability: feedforward and feedback. *Feedforward* is a process that predicts what forces will be imposed on the spine and provide enough stability before movement occurs. *Feedback* means that motion occurs, and when stress builds, stability is changed as a result. More detail is given on motor control strategies in back stability in chapter 3.

SUMMARY

- Low back pain is a massive challenge to health care professionals and a major financial drain on Western economies.

- Low back pain produces alterations in behavior patterns that can exacerbate the condition.

- The traditional structural approach to treating back pain must be balanced with restoration of function.

- New approaches to treating back pain emphasize the use of exercise rather than rest.

- Back stability consists of three inter-relating control systems: active, passive, and neural.

- Although traditional exercise systems that work the trunk may strengthen muscle, they also may reduce total back stability.

- The integrated back stability (IBS) approach progresses from muscle isolation and correc-tion of movement dysfunction to enhance-ment of functional actions.

- Enhancing the active and neural systems can partially compensate for decrements in the passive system.

- Enhanced movement accuracy and muscle reaction speed are vital to full rehabilitation of the back.

Chapter 2
Biomechanics of the Lumbar Spine

To explain how the back is stabilized, I must briefly review some important aspects of spinal anatomy. Chapter 1 introduced the concept of the passive stability system—the brakes provided by inert tissues that will stretch only a certain amount (both individually and as systems of tissues) before they restrict further movement. In this chapter, I describe this passive system for each of the major physiological movements of the lumbar spine and then use the example of bending and lifting to illustrate the importance of stability.

ANATOMY OF THE VERTEBRAL COLUMN

The gross anatomy of the lumbar spine includes vertebral bones and joints, ligaments, spinal discs, facet joints, and the sacroiliac joint. Although none of these structures moves in isolation, it is clearer to describe them individually.

Vertebral Bones and Joints

The adult human vertebral column contains 33 vertebrae. Five vertebrae are fused to form the sacrum and four are fused to form the coccyx. The remaining 24 movable vertebrae are divided among the cervical (7), thoracic (12), and lumbar (5) regions (figure 2.1). Any two neighboring vertebrae make up a spinal segment (figure 2.2). To understand how the vertebrae fit together in the spine, one must know the parts of the typical vertebra.

The two vertebrae within a spinal segment are attached (**articulated**) by both joints and ligaments. There are three joints—the articulating triad—consisting of the disc, which forms the joint between the bodies of adjacent vertebrae, and the two facet joints (also called zygapophyseal or apophyseal joints), where the inferior articular processes on either side of the upper vertebra come together with the superior articular processes on either side of the lower vertebra.

Key point: A spinal segment contains two adjacent vertebrae, articulating with each other through the intervertebral disc and two facet joints. The articulations form a triad.

The disk and its associated facet joints are intimately linked both structurally and functionally. Degeneration of the intervertebral disc as a result of injury can lead to degeneration of the neighboring facet joints (Vernon-Roberts 1992); as we shall see later, the ligamentous support to both structures is continuous.

We can compare the spinal segment to a simple leverage system (Kapandji 1974), with the facet joints forming a fulcrum. The posterior tissues (ligamentous and muscular) and the anteriorly placed disc resist both compressive and tensile forces. The ligaments themselves may be categorized into three interrelating functional groups as shown in table 2.1.

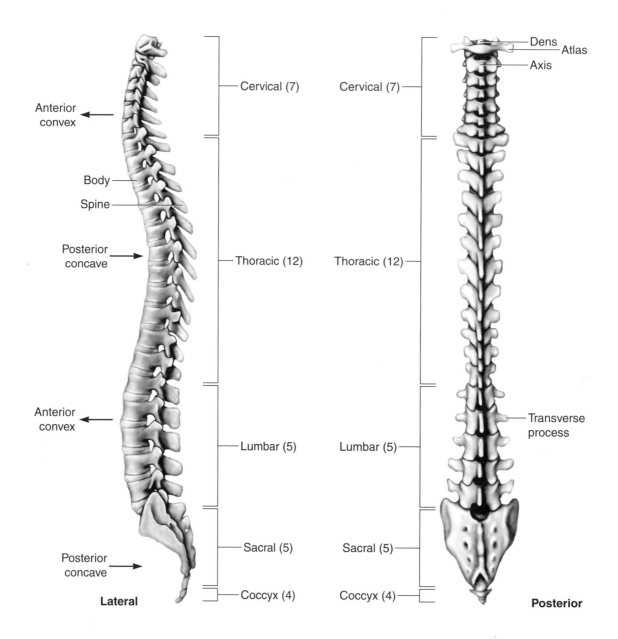

Figure 2.1 The vertebral column.

Reprinted from R. Behnke, 2006, *Kinetic Anatomy*, 2nd ed. (Champaign, IL: Human Kinetics), 120.

Ligaments

The neural arch ligaments consist mainly of the ligamentum flavum and the interspinous ligament, with the supraspinous and intertransverse ligaments providing additional support (figure 2.3). Although these four ligaments are traditionally described as separate structures, they are actually merged at their edges and act functionally as a single unit. This point bears significantly on the question of how one stabilizes the back.

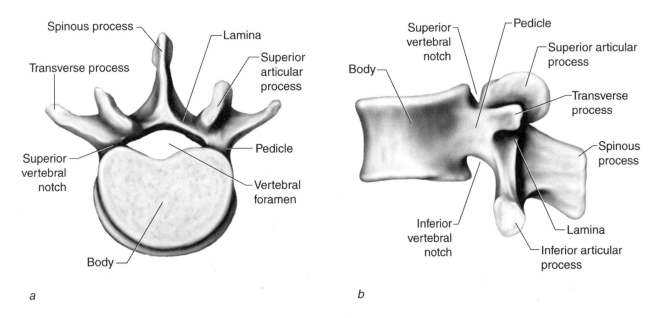

a   b

Figure 2.2 A typical spinal segment: *(a)* superior view, *(b)* lateral view.
Reprinted from R. Behnke, 2006, *Kinetic Anatomy*, 2nd ed. (Champaign, IL: Human Kinetics), 122.

Table 2.1   Ligaments of the Spinal Segment

Neural arch	Capsular	Ventral
Ligamentum flavum Interspinous ligament Supraspinous ligament Intertransverse ligament	Facet joint capsule (reinforced by the ligamentum flavum)	Anterior longitudinal ligament Posterior longitudinal ligament

Based on F.H. Willard, 1997, The muscular, ligamentous and neural structure of the low back and its relation to back pain. In *Movement stability and low back pain*, edited by A. Vleeming et al. (Edinburgh, United Kingdom: Churchill Livingstone).

On dissection, when the bony components of the neural arch are removed, the neural arch ligaments can be seen to maintain their continuity (Willard 1997). The lateral fibers of the ligamentum flavum are continuous with the facet joint capsule (Yong-Hing et al. 1976) and form the rear wall of the spinal canal. The anterior border of the interspinous ligament is a continuation of the ligamentum flavum, whereas the posterior border of this ligament is thickened into the supraspinous ligament. If the boundary joining the interspinous and supraspinous ligaments is cut, the tensile stiffness is reduced by 40% (Dumas et al. 1987), illustrating the importance of their dual structure. The supraspinous ligament merges with the thoracolumbar fascia (TLF) (figure 2.4), which in turn connects with the deep abdominal muscles (see p. 51). The force generated by the deep abdominal muscles therefore can be transmitted through the TLF, via the supraspinous ligament, directly into

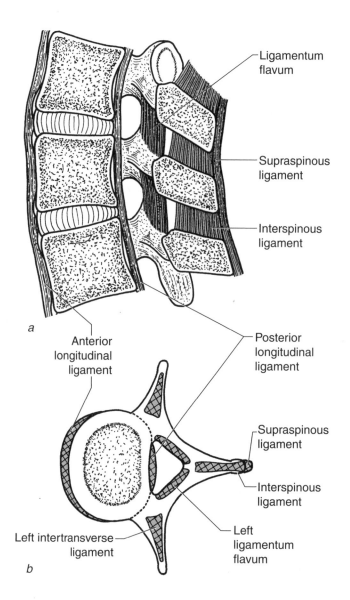

a

Ligamentum flavum

Supraspinous ligament

Interspinous ligament

Anterior longitudinal ligament

Posterior longitudinal ligament

Supraspinous ligament

Interspinous ligament

Left intertransverse ligament

Left ligamentum flavum

b

Figure 2.3 Ligaments of the spinal segment: *(a)* side view, *(b)* superior view.

Reprinted from R. Behnke, 2006, *Kinetic Anatomy*, 2nd ed. (Champaign, IL: Human Kinetics), 127.

the ligamentum flavum—preventing this ligament from buckling toward the spinal cord. This is one way the deep abdominals assist in spinal stabilization.

Not only abdominal muscles affect the spine. The interspinous ligament merges with the supraspinous ligament and then with the TLF, forming the interspinous–supraspinous–thoracolumbar (IST) ligamentous complex (Willard 1997). The IST complex attaches the **fascia** of the back to the lumbar spine. The importance of this system is that tension developed in the extremities is transmitted to the vertebral column, making the seemingly distant limb musculature essential to the rehabilitation of spinal function. The intertransverse ligament, although small, becomes more important **caudally** as it expands into the iliolumbar ligament, the importance of which I discuss later.

Key point: Tension from the deep abdominal muscles is transmitted through the fascia directly to the spine.

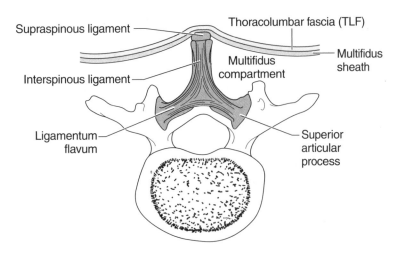

Figure 2.4 Interspinous–supraspinous–thoracolumbar (IST) ligamentous complex. The IST complex supports the lumbar spine by anchoring the thoracolumbar fascia and multifidus sheath to the facet joint capsules.

The capsule of the facet joint is reinforced posteriorly by the multifidus muscle and anteriorly by the ligamentum flavum. It is surrounded by fascia, which itself is continuous with that covering the ligamentum flavum and the **investing fascia** of the vertebral body. The facet joint capsule therefore can be seen as a bridge of connective tissue between the ligaments of the neural arch and those of the vertebral body (Willard 1997) (figure 2.5).

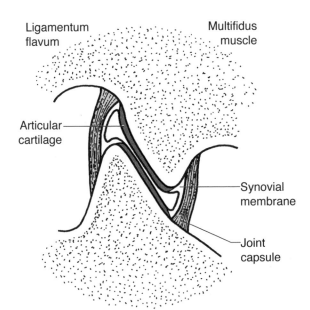

Figure 2.5 Facet joint capsule.

Reprinted, by permission, from J. Watkins, 1999, *Structure and function of the musculoskeletal system* (Champaign, IL: Human Kinetics), 142.

The anterior longitudinal ligament (ALL) and posterior longitudinal ligament (PLL) lie **ventrally** within the spinal segment. The ALL is the stronger of the two and extends from the **occiput** to the sacrum, where it merges with the sacroiliac joint capsule. The ALL has two sets of fibers (Bogduk and Twomey 1991). The superficial fibers span several vertebral segments, whereas the deep fibers attach loosely to the annulus of the spinal disc (figure 2.6). The PLL exists in the cervical spine as the tectorial membrane and extends caudally to the **periosteum** of the sacrum. The PLL expands as it passes the intervertebral discs and narrows around the vertebral body. Because the PLL is considerably weaker than the ALL, the main ligamentous restriction to **flexion** is not from the PLL but from the ligamentum flavum and the facet joint capsule into which it merges. The ligamentum flavum and facet joint capsules combine to offer 52% of the resistance to flexion in the lumbar spine (Bogduk and Twomey 1991). The structural pairing of the PLL and the ligamentum flavum is functionally obvious as well. Load-deformation (stress–strain) curves plotted for the two ligaments are similar (Panjabi and White 1990), suggesting in this case that the two ligaments may have a similar purpose.

The longitudinal ligaments are viscoelastic, meaning that they stiffen when loaded rapidly. They do not store all the energy used to stretch them because they lose some energy as heat, a feature known as hysteresis. When loaded repeatedly,

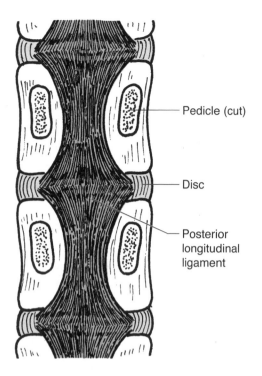

Figure 2.6 Vertical section through pedicles in lumbar region: posterior aspect of vertebral bodies showing attachment of posterior longitudinal ligament to spinal discs.

Reprinted, by permission, from J. Watkins, 1999, *Structure and function of the musculoskeletal system* (Champaign, IL: Human Kinetics), 147.

these ligaments become even stiffer, and the hysteresis is less marked, making them more prone to fatigue failure (Hukins 1987). The supraspinous and interspinous ligaments are farther from the flexion axis and therefore need to stretch more than the posterior longitudinal ligament when they resist flexion.

With age, all ligaments gradually lose their ability to absorb energy (Tkaczuk 1968). The stiffest ligament in the spine is the posterior longitudinal ligament; the most flexible is the supraspinous (Panjabi et al. 1987). The ligamentum flavum in the lumbar spine is pretensioned (possesses tension at rest) when the spine is in its neutral position, a situation that compresses the spinal disc. This ligament has the highest percentage of elastic fibers of any tissue in the body (Nachemson and Evans 1968) and contains nearly twice as much elastin as collagen. The anterior longitudinal ligament and joint capsules are among the strongest ligamentous tissues in the body, whereas the interspinous and posterior longitudinal ligaments are the weakest (Panjabi et al. 1987).

Key point: The ligamentum flavum is the most elastic ligament in the body and the main ligament limiting flexion. It forms the anterior portion of the facet joint capsule.

Spinal Discs

Twenty-four intervertebral discs lie between successive vertebrae, making the spine an alternatively rigid and then elastic column. The amount of flexibility in a particular spinal segment is determined by the size and shape of the disc and by the resistance to motion of the soft tissue that supports the spinal joints. The discs increase in size as they descend the column, the lumbar discs having an average thickness of 10 mm, twice that of the cervical discs. The disc shapes are accommodated to the curvatures of the spine and to the shapes of the vertebrae. The greater anterior widths of the discs in the cervical and lumbar regions reflect the curvatures of these areas. Each disc has three closely related components—the annulus fibrosis, nucleus pulposus, and cartilage end plates (figure 2.7).

The annulus contains layers of fibrous tissue arranged in concentric bands—about 20—like those in an onion. The fibers within each band are parallel, with the various bands angled at 45° to each other. The bands are more closely packed anteriorly and posteriorly than they are laterally, and those innermost are the thinnest. Fiber orientation, although partially determined at birth, is influenced by torsional stresses in the adult (Palastanga et al. 1994). The posterolateral regions have a more irregular makeup—possibly one reason why they become weaker with age and more predisposed to injury.

Key point: The spinal discs have fewer concentric bands posterolaterally than in other regions, and these are irregular—making this region of the disc more susceptible to injury.

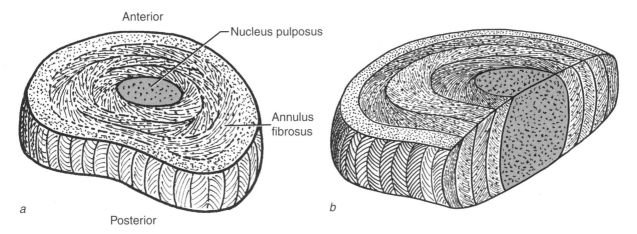

Anterior

Nucleus pulposus

Annulus fibrosus

a

Posterior

b

Figure 2.7 *(a)* Concentric bands of annular fibers. *(b)* Horizontal section through a disc.

Reprinted, by permission, from J. Watkins, 1999, *Structure and function of the musculoskeletal system* (Champaign, IL: Human Kinetics), 142.

The annular fibers pass over the edge of the cartilage end plate of the disc and are anchored to the bony rim of the vertebra and to its periosteum and body. The attaching fibers are actually interwoven with the fibers of the bony **trabeculae** of the vertebral body. The outer layer of fibers blend with the posterior longitudinal ligament; some authors claim that the anterior longitudinal ligament has no such attachment (Vernon-Roberts 1987).

Resting on the surface of the vertebra, the hyaline cartilage end plate is approximately 1 mm thick at its outer edge and becomes thinner toward its center. The central portion of the end plate acts as a semipermeable membrane to facilitate fluid exchange into and out of the disc; it also protects the vertebral body from excessive pressure. In a person's early life, canals from the vertebral body penetrate the end plate, but these disappear after the age of 20 to 30. The end plate then starts to ossify and become more brittle, whereas the central portion thins and, in some cases, is completely destroyed.

The nucleus pulposus is a soft hydrophilic (water-attracting) substance taking up about 25% of the total disc area. It is continuous with the annulus, but the nuclear fibers are far less dense than those of the annulus. Mucopolysaccharides called proteoglycans fill the spaces between the collagen fibers of the nucleus, giving the nucleus its water-retaining capacity and making it mechanically plastic. Metabolically very active, the area between the nucleus and annulus is sensitive both to physical force and to chemical and hormonal influences (Palastanga et al. 1994). Although the collagen volume of the nucleus remains unchanged, the proteoglycan content decreases with age—leading to a net reduction in water content. Early in a person's life, the water content may be as high as 80% to 90%, but this decreases to about 70% by middle age.

The lumbar discs are the largest avascular structures in the body. The nucleus obtains fluids by passive diffusion from the margins of the vertebral body and across the cartilage end plate—particularly across the center of the end plate, which is more permeable than the periphery. Intense anaerobic activity within the nucleus (Holm et al. 1981) can lead to lactate buildup and low oxygen concentration, placing the nuclear cells at risk. Inadequate adenosine triphosphate levels may lead to cell death. Some researchers hypothesize that regular exercise involving movement of the spine may improve the nutrition of the disc—and over the years might not only improve the general health of discs but even slow the loss of height attributable to water loss from discs.

Key point: The lumbar spinal discs are avascular and depend on fluid exchange by passive diffusion. Regular movement and activity are vital to this process.

Facet Joints

The facet joints are synovial joints (i.e., they contain synovial fluid, a viscous fluid) between the inferior articular process of one vertebra and the superior articular process of its neighbor. As with other typical synovial joints, the facet joints have articular cartilage, a synovial membrane to contain the fluid, and a joint capsule, but they also have a number of unique features.

The facet joint capsule holds about 2 ml of synovial fluid. Its anterior wall is formed by the ligamentum flavum; posteriorly, the capsule is reinforced by the deep fibers of the multifidus muscle. At its superior and inferior poles, the joint leaves a small gap, creating the subscapular pockets. These are filled with fat, contained within the synovial membrane. Within the subscapular pocket lies a small foramen for passage of the fat in and out of the joint as the spine moves.

The capsule contains three structures of interest. The first is the connective tissue rim, a thickened wedge-shaped area that makes up for the curved shape of the articular cartilage in much the same way as the menisci of the knee do. The second structure is an adipose tissue pad, a 2 mm fold of synovium filled with fat and blood vessels. The third structure is the fibroadipose meniscoid, a 5 mm leaflike fold that projects from the inner surfaces of the superior and inferior capsules. The last two structures have a protective function. Flexion leaves some of the articular facets' cartilage exposed—both the adipose tissue pad and the fibroadipose meniscus cover the exposed regions (Bogduk and Engel 1984).

With aging, cartilage of the facet joint can split parallel to the joint surface, pulling a portion of joint capsule with it. The split cartilage, with its attached piece of capsule, forms a false intra-articular meniscoid (Taylor and Twomey 1986). Flexion normally draws the fibroadipose meniscus out from the joint, and it moves back in with **extension.** If the meniscus fails to move back, it will buckle and remain under the capsule, causing pain (Bogduk and Jull 1985). A mobilization or manipulation that combines flexion and rotation may relieve pain by allowing the meniscoid to move back to its original position.

Many of the structures described here are capable of producing pain when placed under stress caused by the presence of nociceptors (pain receptors) and mechanoreceptors within their tissue. The pain supply of spinal tissues is listed in table 2.2.

Effects of Aging

The length of the spinal column reduces with aging but not generally because of reducing disc height, as is usually suggested. The reduction in general body height occurs initially through the loss of horizontal trabeculae within the vertebra itself. These horizontal fibers form ties across the vertebra a little like the rafters in a house roof. When the horizontal trabeculae degenerate, the vertical trabeculae buckle through weight

Table 2.2   Pain (Nociceptor) Supply of Spinal Tissue

Structure	Nerve supply
Vertebra	No nociceptors are found in periosteum or blood vessels of cancellous bone.
Intervertebral disc	Peripheral annulus is innervated. Granulation and scar tissue may grow into degenerative disc, and this tissue may contain nociceptors.
Dura and nerve root sleeve	Direct stimulation will give rise to pain.
Facet joint capsule	Rich supply of nociceptors is present.
Ligament and fascia	Structures are richly innervated.
Muscle	Mechanoreceptors are found in muscle, nociceptors in muscle fascia.

Adams et al. 2002; Waddell 2004.

bearing and in some cases may actually fracture (Twomey and Taylor 2000). Eventually, the end plate becomes concave, a process that occurs earlier in females because of estrogen loss during menopause. Measurement of discal thickness shows no loss of height as part of the natural aging process. The vertebral height changes that do occur are accompanied by horizontal expansion of the disc, causing the discal "waist" (center section) to thicken.

Over the years, the collagen makeup of the disc changes, and the water content of the disc decreases. Fissures occur initially in the circumference of the disc , and in time these spread into radially directed fissures. Blood vessels and even nerve fibers grow through the fissures toward the center of the disc (Adams et al. 2002). The appearance of radial fissures may at first sight suggest an increased tendency for nuclear migration through the fissure, causing disc **prolapse.** However, the loss of the fluid nature of the nucleus by this time actually prevents significant nuclear migration. The loss of fluidity in the disc also generally reduces range of motion over time.

Key point: Fissures throughout the disc annulus associated with aging do not lead to disc prolapse because there is a parallel loss of fluid within the disc nucleus.

Changes to the facet joints occur differentially between the anteromedial third and the posterior two thirds of the joint. The anteromedial aspect of the joint is stressed during lumbar flexion movements (discussed subsequently), and as a result the subchondral bone in the area hypertrophies by age 40 and begins to show vertical splitting. The posterior aspect of the joint ages more slowly because of its reduced weight-bearing function in comparison with the rest of the joint.

The proteoglycan of the disc's nucleus makes it hydrophilic, and its ability to transmit load relies on high water content, yet proteoglycan content declines from about 65% in early life to about 30% by middle age (Bogduk and Twomey 1987). When the proteoglycan content of the disc is high (up to age 30 in most subjects), the nucleus pulposus is gelatinous, producing a uniform fluid pressure.

After this age, the lower water content of the disc leaves the nucleus unable to build as much fluid pressure. Less central pressure is produced, and the load is distributed more peripherally, eventually causing the annular fibers to become fibrillated and to crack (Hirsch and Schajowicz 1952). The net result is that a disc's reaction to compressive stress declines with age (figure 2.8).

The age-related changes in discs cause greater susceptibility to injury. This fact—combined with a general reduction in fitness and changes in trunk movement patterns related to activities of daily living—greatly increases the risk of injury in older people. Previously inactive persons over the age of 40 should engage in trunk exercises, under the supervision of a physical therapist, before attending fitness classes.

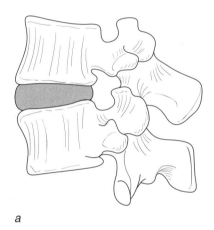

a

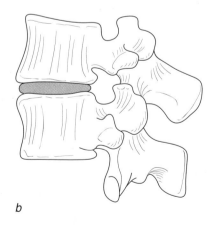

b

Figure 2.8 Age-related changes in lumbar discs. *(a)* Maximal disc height and end plate length of youth. *(b)* Reduced measurements through aging.

Sacroiliac Joint

As with the lumbar spine, the sacroiliac joint (SIJ)—the rather large surface where the sacrum (the five fused bottom vertebrae of the spine) fits into the pelvis (figure 2.9)—is stabilized by several ligaments that connect to muscles within the region. The iliolumbar ligament attaches to the transverse process of L5, and in some subjects to those of L4 as well (Willard 1997), and passes anteromedially to the iliac crest and the surface of the ilium. The iliolumbar ligament resists movement between the sacrum and lumbar spine, particularly that of **lateral flexion.** When the ligament is cut, movement of the lumbar spine (L5) on the sacrum increases significantly—lateral flexion by nearly 30%, and flexion, extension, and rotation by 18% to 23% (Yamamoto et al. 1990). The superior aspect of the SIJ capsule is an extension of the iliolumbar ligament, whereas the anterior portion of the capsule merges into the sacrotuberous ligament.

The sacrotuberous ligament has a triangular shape extending between the posterior iliac spines, SIJ capsule, and coccyx (figure 2.9). The tendon of biceps femoris (the large muscle at the back of the upper leg) extends over the ischial tuberosity to attach to the sacrotuberous ligament (Vleeming et al. 1989); the ligament also attaches to some of the deepest fibers of the multifidus muscle (the multifidus runs vertically down the entire length of the back, on either side of the spine) (Willard 1997). Movement at the sacroiliac joint is described as nutation and counternutation (table 2.3). The sacrotuberous ligament resists nutation of the sacrum, whereas the long dorsal sacroiliac ligament resists counternutation.

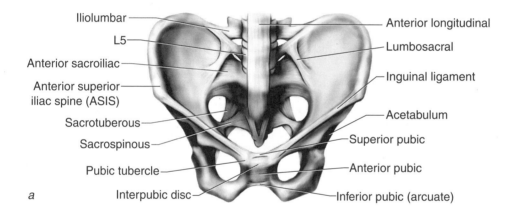

Iliolumbar —
L5 —
Anterior sacroiliac —
Anterior superior iliac spine (ASIS) —
Sacrotuberous —
Sacrospinous —
Pubic tubercle —
Interpubic disc —
— Anterior longitudinal
— Lumbosacral
— Inguinal ligament
— Acetabulum
— Superior pubic
— Anterior pubic
— Inferior pubic (arcuate)

a

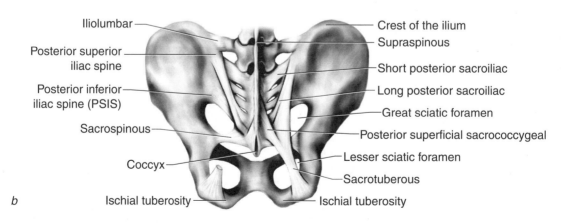

Iliolumbar —
Posterior superior iliac spine —
Posterior inferior iliac spine (PSIS) —
Sacrospinous —
Coccyx —
Ischial tuberosity —
— Crest of the ilium
— Supraspinous
— Short posterior sacroiliac
— Long posterior sacroiliac
— Great sciatic foramen
— Posterior superficial sacrococcygeal
— Lesser sciatic foramen
— Sacrotuberous
— Ischial tuberosity

b

Figure 2.9 The sacroiliac joint and its supporting ligaments: *(a)* anterior aspect and *(b)* posterior aspect.

Reprinted from R. Behnke, 2006, *Kinetic anatomy*, 2nd ed. (Champaign, IL: Human Kinetics), 139.

Table 2.3 Movement of the Sacroiliac Joint (SIJ)

Nutation	Counternutation
Sacrum tilts anteriorly.	Sacrum tilts posteriorly.
Sacral base moves down and forward, and apex moves up.	Sacral base moves up and back, and apex moves down.
Size of pelvic outlet increases and pelvic inlet decreases.	Size of pelvic inlet increases and pelvic outlet decreases.
Movement occurs in standing.	Movement occurs in non-weight-bearing position such as lying.
Movement increases as lumbar lordosis increases.	Movement increases as lumbar lordosis decreases (flat-back posture).
Iliac bones are pulled together, and SIJ is impacted.	Iliac bones move apart, and SIJ is distracted.
Superior aspect of pubis is compressed.	Inferior aspect of pubis is compressed.

Even though it is difficult to see this from observing anatomical diagrams, the sacrum is not fused with the pelvis—so when I speak of movement of the sacrum, I mean motion within the pelvis as opposed to motion of the pelvis, where the entire structure is moving on the hip. Greater movement ranges have been reported in non-weight-bearing than weight-bearing movements. Non-weight-bearing movements have exhibited as much as 12° innominate rotation during flexion, together with 8 mm of translation during extension (Lavignolle et al. 1983); weight-bearing movements were reduced to 2.5° rotation and 1.6 mm maximal translation (Sturesson et al. 1989). In a study of healthy people aged 20 to 50 years, Jacob and Kissling (1995) found average rotational motion at the SIJ to be 2°, whereas symptomatic patients averaged 6°.

Nutation of the SIJ is an anterior tilting of the sacrum on the fixed **innominate bones.** The sacral base moves down and forward, whereas the sacral apex moves up, increasing the **pelvic outlet.** Nutation occurs in standing and increases as **lordosis** deepens. By pulling the iliac bones together, nutation compresses the SIJ as well as the superior portion of the pubic symphysis. Counternutation is the opposite movement, with the sacral base moving up and back and the apex moving downward. This movement occurs in non-weight-bearing situations, such as lying prone, and increases as the lordosis is reduced and the low back is flattened. During counternutation, the iliac bones move apart, the **pelvic inlet** increases, and the pelvic outlet reduces (Kesson and Atkins 1998).

A variety of movements occur about the SIJ during trunk actions (Lee 1994). During forward bending of the trunk, the pelvis tilts anteriorly and the sacrum moves into extension (coccyx moving backward; i.e., nutation around an oblique axis), causing the iliac crests and posterior superior iliac spines to **approximate** (i.e., press toward each other) and the ischial tuberosities and the anterior superior iliac spines to separate. During side bending, the trunk laterally flexes and the pelvis shifts to the opposite direction to maintain balance. With left lateral flexion and right pelvic shift, the right innominate bone rotates posteriorly, and the left innominate rotates anteriorly. The sacrum rotates to the right. During trunk rotation, the pelvis rotates in the same direction; therefore, with left trunk rotation, the right innominate anteriorly rotates and the left posteriorly rotates. The sacrum is driven into left rotation.

AXIAL COMPRESSION

Vertical loading of the lumbar spine (axial compression) occurs during upright (standing or sitting) postures, exacerbating certain forms of back pain. Knowledge of loading can help us to design safer exercise programs for people with back pain.

Compression of the Vertebral Bodies

Within the vertebra itself, compressive force is transmitted by both the cancellous (spongy) bone of the vertebral body and its cortical bone shell. Until about the age of 40, the cancellous bone contributes about 25% to 55% of the vertebra's strength. As aging-related decreases in bone density lead to a decline in the proportion of cancellous bone, the cortical bone shell carries a greater proportion of load (Rockoff et al. 1969). As the vertebral body is compressed, a net flow of blood out of it (Crock and Yoshizawa 1976) reduces bone volume and dissipates energy (Roaf 1960). Blood returns slowly as the force is reduced—leaving a latent period after the initial compression and diminishing the shock-absorbing properties of the bone. Exercises that involve prolonged periods of repeated shock to the spine (e.g., jumping on a hard surface) are therefore more likely to damage vertebrae than those that load the spine for short periods and allow recovery of the vertebral blood flow before repeating a movement.

Key point: Blood flows out of the vertebral body with loading, decreasing its shock-absorbing properties. Exercises that repeatedly load the spine without allowing recovery can therefore lead to accumulated stress.

Compression of Intervertebral Discs

During standing, 12% to 25% of axial compression forces are transmitted between adjacent vertebrae by the facet joints (see discussion on p. 27); the intervertebral disc absorbs the rest of the force (Miller et al. 1983). The annulus fibrosis of a healthy disc resists buckling; even if a disc's nucleus pulposus has been removed, its annulus alone can exhibit a load-bearing capacity similar to that of the fully intact disc for a brief period (Markolf and Morris 1974). When exposed to prolonged loading, however, the collagen lamellae of the annulus eventually buckle (see figure 2.7).

Throughout the waking day, discal loading diminishes a person's height until the forces inside the disc equal the load forces (Twomey and Taylor 1994). By reducing axial loading, lying down permits restoration of the former spinal length. Lying in a flexed position speeds the regain of lost height as the lumbar discs are distracted (unloaded) during flexion (Tyrrell et al. 1985). Application of an axial load compresses the fluid nucleus of the disc, causing it to expand laterally. This lateral expansion stretches the annular fibers, preventing them from buckling. The degree of discal compression depends on the weight imposed and the rate of loading. A 100 kg axial load can compress a disc by 1.4 mm and cause a lateral expansion of 0.75 mm (Hirsch and Nachemson 1954). The stretch in the annular fibers stores energy, which is released when the compression stress is removed. The stored energy gives the disc a certain springiness, which helps to offset any deformation that occurred in the nucleus. A force applied rapidly is not lessened by this mechanism, but its rate of application is slowed, giving the spinal tissues time to adapt.

Deformation of the disc occurs more rapidly at the onset of axial load application, the majority of its deformation occurring within 10 min of onset. After this time, deformation continues but slows to a rate of about 1 mm/hr (Markolf and Morris 1974), leading to loss of height throughout the day. Under constant loading, the discs exhibit *creep* (i.e., they continue to deform even though the load is not increasing). Because compression causes an increase in fluid pressure, fluid is actually lost from both the nucleus and the annulus. About 10% of the water within the disc can be squeezed out by this method (Kraemer et al. 1985), the exact amount dependent on the size and duration of the applied force. When the compressive force is reduced, the fluid is absorbed back through pores in the cartilage end plates of the vertebra. Exercises that axially load the spine reduce a person's height through discal compression—squat exercises in weight training, for example, can create compression loads in the L3-L4 segment of 6 to 10 times body weight (Cappozzo et al. 1985). Researchers have observed average height losses of 5.4 mm over a 25 min period of general weight training and 3.25 mm after a 6 km run (Leatt et

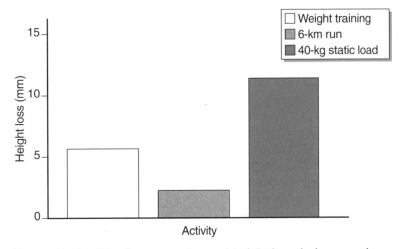

Figure 2.10 Discal compression and height loss during exercise.

al. 1986) (figure 2.10). Static axial loading of the spine with a 40 kg barbell over a 20 min period can reduce a subject's height by as much as 11.2 mm (Tyrrell et al. 1985). Clearly, exercises that involve this degree of spinal loading are unsuitable for people with discal pathology.

Key point: Exercises that compress (axially load) the spine for a prolonged period result in loss of height of more than 1 cm through fluid loss from the disc nucleus. This type of exercise is contraindicated in a client with discal pathology.

The vertebral end plates of the discs are compressed centrally and are able to undergo less deformation than either the annulus or the cancellous bone. The end plates are therefore likely to fail (fracture) under high compression (Norkin and Levangie 1992). Discs subjected to very high compressive loads can show permanent deformation without herniation (Farfan et al. 1976; Markolf and Morris 1974). However, such compression forces may lead to formation (Bernhardt et al. 1992): The disc end plate (which joins the disc to the vertebral body) ruptures, and nuclear material from the disc passes through to the vertebral body itself. Bending and torsional stresses on the spine, when combined with compression, are more damaging than compression alone, and

degenerated discs are particularly at risk. Average failure torques for normal discs are 25% higher than for degenerative discs (Farfan et al. 1976). Degenerative discs also demonstrate poorer viscoelastic properties and therefore a reduced ability to attenuate shock.

Compression of Facet Joints

The orientations of facet joints differ among various regions of the spine, thereby altering the available motion. In the mid- and lower cervical spine, for example, rotation and lateral flexion are limited but flexion and extension are possible. In the thoracic spine, flexion and extension are limited but lateral flexion and rotation are free. At the thoracolumbar junction (T12-L1), rotation is the only movement that is limited; in the lumbar spine, both rotation and lateral flexion are limited.

The superior and inferior alignment of the facet joints in the lumbar spine means that during axial loading in the neutral position, the joint surfaces slide past each other. However, anywhere between T9 and T12, the orientation of the facet joints may change from those characteristic of the thoracic spine to those characteristic of the lumbar spine. Therefore, the level at which particular movements will occur can vary considerably among subjects. During lumbar movements, displacement of the facet joint surfaces causes them to impact, or press together. Because the sacrum is inclined and the body and disc of L5 are wedge-shaped, during axial loading L5 is subjected to a shearing force. This force is resisted by the more anterior orientation of the L5 inferior articular processes. As the lordosis increases, moreover, the anterior longitudinal ligament and the anterior portion of the annulus fibrosis are stretched, providing tension to resist the bending force. Additional stabilization is provided for the L5 vertebra by the iliolumbar ligament, attached to the L5 transverse process. This ligament, together with the facet joint capsules, stretches to resist the **distraction force.**

Once the axial compression force stops, release of the stored elastic energy in the spinal ligaments reestablishes the neutral lordosis. With compression of the lordotic lumbar spine, or in cases where gross disc narrowing has occurred, the inferior articular processes may actually contact the **lamina of the vertebra** below (see figure 2.11). In this case, the lower joints (L3-L4, L4-L5, L5-S1) may bear as much as 19% of the compression force, whereas the upper joints (L1-L2, L2-L3) bear only 11% (Adams et al. 1980).

MOVEMENTS OF THE LUMBAR SPINE AND PELVIS

Much of the material for this section comes from Norris (1995a; 1998), to which I refer you for further reading.

Flexion and Extension

Both disc height and the horizontal length of the vertebral end plate affect the range of motion attainable during **sagittal plane** movement of the lumbar spine. Greatest range of motion occurs with a combination of maximum disc height and maximum end plate length (figure 2.8). Because this alignment most often occurs in young females, they possess the greatest ranges of motion at the lumbar spine. With aging, disc height and end plate length become more similar between the sexes, equalizing the available range of motion for males and females in old age (Twomey and Taylor 1994).

During flexion movements, the anterior annulus of a lumbar disc is compressed, whereas the posterior fibers are stretched. Similarly, the nucleus pulposus of the disc is compressed anteriorly, whereas pressure is relieved over its posterior surface. Because the total volume of the disc remains unchanged, however, its pressure should not increase. The increases in pressure seen with posture changes are attributable not to the bending motion of the bones within the vertebral joint itself but to the soft tissue tension created to control the bending. If the pressure at the L3 disc for a 70 kg standing subject is 100%, supine lying reduces the pressure to 25%. The pressure variations increase dramatically as soon as the lumbar spine is flexed and tissue tension increases (figure 2.12). The sitting posture increases intradiscal pressure to

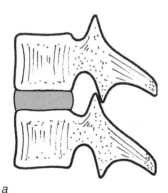
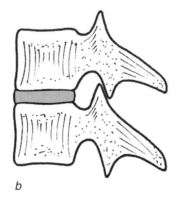
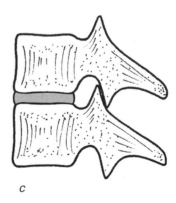

a   b   c

Figure 2.11   Results of compression on discs and facet joints. *(a)* Normal disc thickness and alignment of superior and inferior articular processes. *(b)* Reduced disc thickness resulting in increased compression load on facet joint. *(c)* Extra-articular impingement of facet joint.

Reprinted, by permission, from J. Watkins, 1999, *Structure and function of the musculoskeletal system* (Champaign, IL: Human Kinetics), 146.

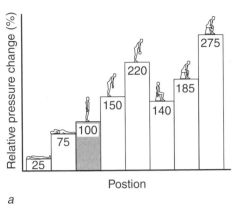

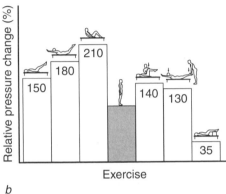

Figure 2.12 Pressure changes in the third lumbar disc: *(a)* in different positions; *(b)* in different muscle-strengthening exercises.

Reprinted from *Sports injuries: Diagnosis and management,* 2nd ed., C.M. Norris, page 344. Copyright 1998, with permission from Elsevier.

140%, whereas sitting and leaning forward with a 10 kg weight in each hand increase pressure to 275% (Nachemson 1992). The selection of an appropriate starting position for trunk exercises is therefore of great importance. Spinal exercise from a slumped sitting posture, for example, places considerably more stress on spinal discs than the same movement beginning from crook-lying position (lying on the back with the knees and hips flexed, feet flat on the floor).

The posterior annulus stretches during flexion, whereas the nucleus is compressed onto the posterior wall. Because the posterior portion of the annulus is the thinnest part, the combination of stretch and pressure to this area may result in discal bulging or herniation. Because layers of annular fibers alternate in direction, rotation movements stretch only half of the fibers at any given time. The disc is more easily injured during

a combination of rotation and flexion, which stretches all the fibers at the same time.

Key point: The lumbar discs are more easily injured in movements that combine rotation and flexion. Avoid these actions when prescribing exercise to susceptible clients.

As the lumbar spine flexes, the lordosis flattens and then reverses at its upper levels. Reversal of lordosis does not occur at L5-S1 (Pearcy et al. 1984). Flexion of the lumbar spine involves a combination of anterior **sagittal rotation** and anterior translation. As sagittal rotation occurs, the articular facets move apart, permitting the translation movement to occur. Translation is limited by impaction of the inferior facet of one vertebra on the superior facet of the vertebra below. As flexion increases, or if the spine is angled forward on the hip, the surface (i.e., the top) of the vertebral body faces more vertically, increasing the shearing force attributable to gravity. The forces involved in facet impaction therefore increase to limit translation of the vertebra and stabilize the lumbar spine. Because the facet joint has a curved articular facet, the load is not concentrated evenly across the whole surface but is focused on the anteromedial portion of the facets (figure 2.13).

The sagittal rotation movement of the facet joint causes the joint to open and is therefore limited by the stretch of the joint capsule. The posteriorly placed spinal ligaments are also tightened. Adams and colleagues (1980) used mathematical modeling to analyze the forces that limit sagittal rotation within the lumbar spine. These investigators found that the disc contributes 29% of the limit to movement, the supraspinous and interspinous ligaments 19%, and the facet joint capsules 39%. In one experiment, the researchers cut (and thereby released) various posterior tissues in cadavers to measure the effects of those tissues on flexion range. Range of motion increased about 4° when the posterior ligaments were released and 9° when the capsule was released. Releasing the **pedicles** increased the flexion range by 24° in young (14-22 years) subjects. Cutting all the posterior elements increased the flexion range by 100% in the young subjects but by only 60% in the elderly (61-78 years) subjects.

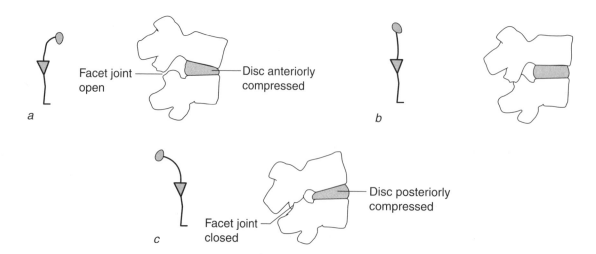

Figure 2.13 Lumbar vertebral orientation in *(a)* flexion, *(b)* standing (neutral position), and *(c)* extension.
Reprinted, by permission, from J. Watkins, 1999, *Structure and function of the musculoskeletal system* (Champaign, IL: Human Kinetics), 147.

During sustained flexion, tissue overstretch results in creep—gradually increasing the range of motion as tissues elongate over time. With aging, the amount of creep is greater, but recovery takes longer (Twomey and Taylor 1994). Occupations that involve prolonged flexion with little recovery (e.g., bricklaying or sitting with poor posture) provide little chance for the overstretched tissue to recover, leading to chronic adaptation of both soft tissue and bone. Such people suffer from a high incidence of chronic postural back pain with many acute episodes (Twomey et al. 1988).

Key point: Sustained flexion results in creep of the lumbar tissues (i.e., a gradual increase in range of motion over time). Prolonged flexion with inadequate tissue recovery can lead to chronic adaptation and consequent pain.

During extension, anterior structures are under tension, whereas posterior structures are first taken off stretch and then compressed (depending on the range of motion). Extension movements subject the vertebral bodies to posterior sagittal rotation. The inferior articular processes move downward, causing them to press against the lamina of the vertebra below. Once the bony block has occurred, if further load is applied, the upper vertebra will axially rotate by pivoting on the impacted inferior articular process. The inferior articular process will move backward, overstretching and possibly damaging the joint capsule (Yang and King 1984). Repeated movements of this type eventually can lead to erosion of the laminal periosteum (Oliver and Middleditch 1991). At the site of impaction, the joint capsule may catch between the opposing bones, creating another source of pain (Adams and Hutton 1983). Because structural abnormalities can alter a vertebra's axis of rotation, considerable variation exists among subjects (Klein and Hukins 1983).

Rotation and Lateral Flexion

During rotation, torsional stiffness is provided by the outer layers of the annulus, by the orientation of the facet joints, and by the cortical bone shell of the vertebral bodies themselves. Moreover, the annular fibers of the disc are stretched as their orientation permits; because alternating layers of fibers are angled obliquely to each other, some fibers will be stretched whereas others relax. A maximum range of 3° of rotation can occur before the annular fibers will be microscopically damaged and a maximum of 12° before tissue failure (Bogduk and Twomey 1987). The spinous processes separate during rotation, stretching the supraspinous and interspinous ligaments.

Impaction occurs between the opposing articular facets on one side, causing the articular cartilage to compress by 0.5 mm for each 1° of rotation and providing a substantial buffer mechanism (Bogduk and Twomey 1987). If rotation continues beyond this point, the vertebra pivots around the impacted facet joint, causing posterior and lateral movement. The combination of movements and forces places stress on the impacted facet joint by compression, the spinal disc by torsion and shear, and the capsule of the opposite facet joint by traction. The disc provides only 35% of the total resistance (Farfan et al. 1976).

Key point: The passive anchor to rotation comes from (a) facet joint impaction, (b) torsion and shear of the disc, and (c) stretch of both ligaments and the facet capsule.

When the lumbar spine is laterally flexed, the annular fibers toward the concavity of the curve are compressed and begin to bulge, whereas those on the convexity of the curve are stretched. The **contralateral fibers** of the outer annulus and the contralateral intertransverse ligaments help to resist extremes of motion (Norkin and Levangie 1992). Lateral flexion and rotation occur as coupled movements. In the neutral position, rotation of the upper four lumbar segments is accompanied by lateral flexion to the opposite side; rotation of the L5-S1 joint, however, occurs with lateral flexion to the same side. The nature of the coupling varies with the degree of flexion and extension. In the neutral position, rotation and lateral flexion occur to the opposite side, called type I movement (i.e., right rotation is coupled with left lateral flexion). But when the lumbar spine is in flexion or extension, rotation and lateral flexion occur in the same direction, called type II movement (i.e., right rotation is coupled with right lateral flexion). In the concavity of lateral flexion, the inferior facet of the upper vertebra slides downward on the superior facet of the vertebra below, reducing the area of the intervertebral foramen on that side. On the convexity of the laterally flexed spine, the inferior facet slides upward on the superior facet of the vertebra below, increasing the diameter of the intervertebral foramen.

Key point: When the lumbar spine is in the neutral position, right rotation of the spine occurs simultaneously (is coupled) with left lateral flexion. When the lumbar spine is not in neutral position, right rotation is coupled with right lateral flexion, and vice versa.

Lumbar–Pelvic Rhythm

When people bend forward as though to touch their toes, the movement comes from both the pelvis and the lumbar spine. The pelvis anteriorly tilts on the femur, whereas the lumbar spine flexes on the pelvis. The combined movement of both lumbar and pelvic motion is called lumbar–pelvic rhythm. With the lumbar spine held immobile and the knees locked, the pelvis can tilt only to roughly 90° hip flexion (hamstring tightness limits further movement). To touch the floor, one must also flex the lumbar spine. Similarly, with the pelvis held immobile, lumbar flexion is limited to about 30° to 40°, with most movement occurring at the lower lumbar segments. Therefore, to achieve full forward bending, one must move both body segments. When flexing to midrange levels during daily living, people can significantly reduce their lumbar flexion by using anterior pelvic tilt. Reduced ability to anteriorly tilt the pelvis increases the need to flex the lumbar spine, opening the possibility of postural pain through repetitive loading of the lumbar tissues.

When a person bends forward from a standing position, the pelvis and lumbar spine rotate in the same direction. Lumbar flexion accompanies anterior tilt of the pelvis (figure 2.14a). In the upright posture, the feet and shoulders are static, and the pelvis and lumbar spine move in opposite directions (figure 2.14b)—lumbar extension compensates for an anteriorly tilted pelvis to maintain the head and shoulders in an upright orientation. Table 2.4 describes the relationship between various pelvic movements and the corresponding hip joint action.

Controlling Spinal Range of Motion

If the trunk is moving slowly, a subject feels tissue tension at the end range and is able to stop a movement short of the full end range—thereby

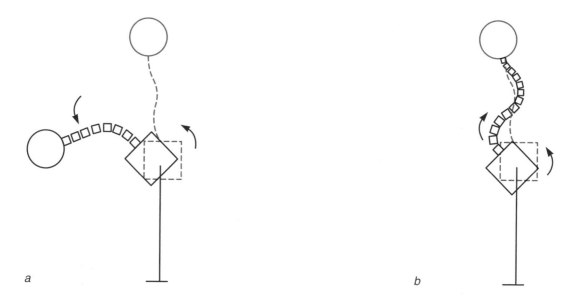

Figure 2.14 *(a)* Lumbar–pelvic rhythm in open chain formation occurs in the same direction. Anterior pelvic tilt accompanies lumbar flexion. *(b)* Lumbar–pelvic rhythm in closed kinetic chain formation occurs in opposite directions. Anterior pelvic tilt is compensated by lumbar extension.

Reprinted from *Sports injuries: Diagnosis and management,* 2nd ed., C.M. Norris, page 165. Copyright 1998, with permission from Elsevier.

Table 2.4   Relationship of Pelvis, Hip Joint, and Lumbar Spine During Right Lower-Extremity Weight Bearing and Upright Posture

Pelvic motion	Accompanying hip joint motion	Compensatory lumbar motion
Anterior pelvic tilt	Hip flexion	Lumbar extension
Posterior pelvic tilt	Hip extension	Lumbar flexion
Lateral pelvic tilt (pelvic drop)	Right hip adduction	Right lateral flexion
Lateral pelvic tilt (hip hitch)	Right hip abduction	Left lateral flexion
Forward rotation	Right hip medial rotation	Rotation to the left
Backward rotation	Right hip lateral rotation	Rotation to the right

Reprinted, by permission, from C.C. Norkin and P.K. Levangie, 1992, *Joint structure and function: A comprehensive analysis,* 2nd ed. (Philadelphia, PA: Davis), 317

protecting the spinal tissues from overstretching. However, rapid trunk movements can build up sufficient momentum to push the spine to the full end range, thereby stressing the spinal tissues. Many amateur and even professional sports directors, teachers, and coaches have their charges engage in rapid and ballistic warm-up exercises, performed with high numbers of repetitions. These activities can lead to excessive flexibility and a reduction in passive stability of the spine.

MECHANICS OF BENDING AND LIFTING

Most people bend regularly throughout the day, and many engage in lifting actions either at work or in their home. This section briefly describes the mechanical factors and the muscle work involved in lifting and bending. See chapter 16 for proper lifting techniques.

Lifting as a Set of Torques

Lifting an object from the ground is actually a rather complex mechanical problem. One must create a set of torques (technically, torque = force × distance to axis of rotation), involving both the body and the object to be lifted, that will produce the desired outcome (figure 2.15). The forces created during flexion by leverage, body weight, and muscle force—plus those created by the weight being lifted—must be overcome by an opposing extension force created by the hip extensor muscles as they contract on the spine.

- If the spine is not stable, posterior pelvic tilting brought about by the hip extensors (gluteus maximus and the hamstrings) merely increases the flexion of the spine.

- If the spine is stable, the power created when the hip extensors posteriorly tilt the pelvis is transmitted by the erector spinae along the length of the spine to the upper limb, which then delivers the force to the object being lifted.

The hip extensor muscles are better suited than the erector spinae to initiate a lift from a flexed position. A 150 lb (68 kg) pound athlete develops a torque of about 10,000 inch-pounds (1,130 N·m) in lifting a 450 lb (204 kg) weight. Although the hip extensors can generate a torque of about 15,000 inch-pounds (1,695 N·m), the erector spinae can generate only 3,000 (339 N·m), or 30% of that required to perform the lift (Farfan 1988). Note that the bulk of the muscles creating the force (gluteus maximus) are some distance from the limb controlling the movement (compare this arrangement with the fingers: The muscles that flex and extend the fingers are located not right above the fingers, where they would be in the way, but in the

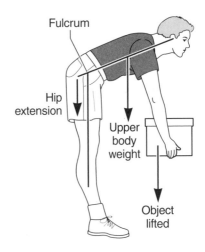

Figure 2.15 The mechanics of lifting.

forearm). When prescribing exercises within the back stability program to help reeducate a person in correct lifting habits, emphasize use of the hip extensors (spinal extensors are far less important in this case), working with a stable spine. The hip hinge action, which emphasizes the gluteals, is effective (see p. 140).

Modeling the spine as a cantilever system according to standard mechanical principles, one can calculate the torques of various forces acting on the spine during lifting. Where the leverage is in equilibrium, the sum of the torques is zero, with flexion forces exactly balancing extension forces. It is possible to calculate both the force needed to lift an object and the resulting compression force on the lumbar spine (Sullivan 1997). To lift a weight, the muscles and connective tissues in the lumbar spine must counteract the flexion caused by the weight by providing an equal amount of extension (figure 2.15). However, because the weight is far from the fulcrum whereas the lower back muscles and tissues are very near to it, the muscles and tissues have much less leverage and must therefore exert much more force than just the weight of the object being lifted. Meanwhile, the vertebral joints experience a compression that is the sum of this force and the weight of the object. That sum is much greater than the weight alone and can be very large indeed! More than 50 years ago, Percy (1957) used postmortem measurements of actual vertebral strength to estimate that lifting a weight heavier than 110 kg (242.5

lb) would exceed the compressive strength of vertebrae. Such calculations clearly indicate that the spinal column alone cannot bear excessively large weights without undergoing severe damage. To reduce the compressive force acting on the spinal column when lifting large amounts of weight (e.g., in Olympic weightlifting), an individual must substantially strengthen all the vertebral reinforcing mechanisms reviewed in chapter 3.

Key point: The spinal column itself is not strong enough to bear the compression force from lifting heavy weights. The force created by the torque of lifting heavy weights can be many times the force of the weight itself—the muscles and connective tissues of the lumbar spine must bear the large majority of the forces involved. If these soft tissues are not sufficiently trained, severe injury can result.

Flexion Relaxation Response in Lifting

When a subject flexes her spine during a lift, the erector spinae are electrically silent just short of full flexion (Kippers and Parker 1984). This phenomenon, called the flexion relaxation response or critical point, is the result of elastic recoil (rebound) of the posterior ligaments and musculature. This point does not occur in all people (discussed later) and occurs later in the range of motion when weights are carried (Bogduk and Twomey 1991). During the final stages of flexion and from 2° to 10° extension (Sullivan 1997), movement occurs by recoil of the stretched tissues rather than by active muscle work.

Key point: During bending, the erector spinae are electrically silent just short of full flexion. This phenomenon is the flexion relaxation response.

If the erector spinae are in spasm, chronic low back pain often obliterates the flexion relaxation response. Failure of the muscles to relax prevents adequate perfusion with fresh blood and can lead to local **ischemic** muscle pain. Interestingly,

during a squat lift with the back perfectly straight, the latissimus dorsi contracts powerfully at the beginning of the lift—perhaps to initiate extension by pulling on the thoracolumbar fascia (McGill and Norman 1986; Sullivan 1997). With extremely heavy lifts of any type, as subjects flex forward to the point of electrical silence, the positions of the vertebrae suggest that they do not reach the point at which the ligaments would be loaded (i.e., stretched or tensioned greater than at rest) (Cholewicki and McGill 1992).

The electrical silence of the muscles and the anatomical alignment of the vertebral segments suggest that the final degrees of flexion as well as the first degrees of extension occur through elastic recoil of the spinal extensor muscles. The length–tension relationship in muscles (figure 2.16) shows that a muscle loses active tension as it is stretched—but even toward the end of the range of movement, there is little decrease in total tension because an increase in passive force (recoil, as happens with a stretched rubber band) largely makes up for the decrease in active contraction. As the spine returns from a fully flexed position, the ligaments may produce some 50 N·m of tension while the recoiling muscles produce 200 N·m. The combined extensor forces of the two passive systems are the major component of the posterior ligamentous system supporting the spine (Bogduk and Twomey 1991).

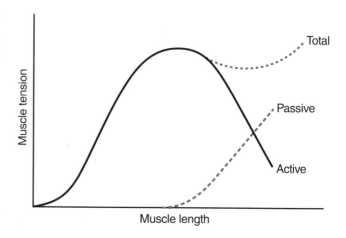

Figure 2.16   The length–tension relationship in muscles.

Reprinted from *Sports injuries: Diagnosis and management*, 2nd ed., C.M. Norris, page 18. Copyright 1998, with permission from Elsevier.

Hamstring Muscle Activity During Bending

Bending incorporates movement at both the hip and lumbar spine. Activity of the gluteals and hamstrings controls pelvic tilt, whereas the extension force from the erector spinae muscles powers lumbar extension. Alteration in the sequencing (timing of movement of one body part relative to another) of hip and lumbar spine movement patterns during forward bending has been proposed as a risk factor for the development of low back pain (Esola et al. 1996). Changes in both lumbar motion range and motion velocity have been noted in people with low back pain (McClure et al. 1997). People with low back pain demonstrate reduced hip mobility during forward bending (Porter and Wilkinson 1997), but other motions of the hip remain largely unaltered. Changes in the activity level of the hamstrings may be responsible for this movement dysfunction (Wong and Lee 2004). Interestingly, alteration in stretch tolerance rather than stiffness of the hamstrings has been shown to determine this range of motion change in people with nonspecific low back pain (Halbertsma et al. 2001).

Hamstring tightness is a common finding in the patient with low back pain (Nourbakhsh and Arab 2002), and it has been argued that lengthening the hamstrings may allow greater motion to occur at the hips and therefore reduce stress on the lumbar spine (Cailliet 1994). However, hamstring tightness is not related to pelvic tilt position during the standing static posture (Gajdosik et al. 1992) or total pelvic motion range during bending (Norris and Matthews 2006).

Investigation into the timing of the hip extensors and erector spinae muscle activity in forward bending may answer this conundrum. It has been shown that the erector spinae and hamstrings are activated before the gluteus maximus in people without low back pain. In those with low back pain, the muscle activation sequence is unchanged, but the duration of gluteus maximus contraction is shortened (Leinonen et al. 2000). In parallel with the flexion–relaxation phenomenon previously described for the erector spinae, activity of the hamstrings also ceases near end range (97% flexion), and the final angle of pelvic tilt is limited by elastic resistance of these muscles and tension of other posteriorly placed soft tissues (Sihvonen 1997).

Movement of the lumbar spine relative to that of the pelvis has been shown to change during the forward bending movement (Esola et al. 1996). Lumbar spine to hip flexion ratios for early (0-30°), middle (30-60°), and late (60-90°) forward bending have been given at 2:1, 1:1, and 1:2, respectively (Esola et al. 1996), showing an increase in the contribution by the pelvis as forward bending proceeds. Subjects with a history of low back pain tend to have a changed pattern of forward bending compared with normal subjects, although the total range of motion for both groups is generally the same. In people with low back pain, hamstring flexibility is reduced (Esola et al. 1996; Rose et al. 1988) and greater electrical activity in the hamstring muscles is seen (Mooney and Robertson 1976).

Key point: The pattern of forward bending motion is changed in those with low back pain. Additionally, these subjects demonstrate greater electrical activity in the hamstring muscles.

Earlier lumbar motion in the activities of daily living will increase the repetitive stress imposed on the low back and could be an important factor in the recurrence of low back pain, particularly because activities of daily living require only partial forward bending. Hamstring stretching using an active knee extension exercise (pp. 121-122) may be used to safely lengthen short hamstrings, and lumbar–pelvic motion may be improved by using the hip hinge group of exercises progressing to functional lifting actions (see chapter 15).

Arch Model of the Spine

Instead of representing the spine as a cantilever system as just described, one can use the model of an arch (Aspden 1987, 1989). The ends (abutments) of the arch are provided caudally by the sacrum and cranially by a combination of body weight and muscular and ligamentous forces. The principle difference between a lever and an arch is that the lever is externally supported, whereas the arch is intrinsically stable. Any load positioned on the convex surface of the arch will create an internal thrust line that runs in a straight line to the arch abutments (figure 2.17*a*). For the arch

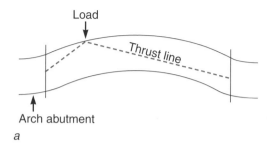

Load

Thrust line

Arch abutment

a

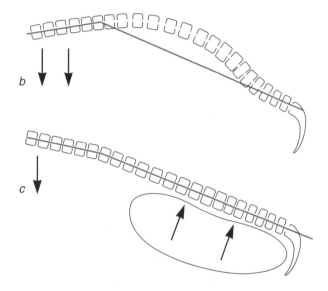

b

c

Figure 2.17 *(a)* General mechanics of an arch. A load on the convex surface of an arch creates an internal thrust line. For stability, the thrust line must stay within the depth of the arch ring. *(b)* Applying the arch model to the spine. Lifting a heavy weight in a stooped position creates a thrust line that moves outside the arch of the spine, making the spine unstable. *(c)* Intra-abdominal pressure acting on the anterior surface of the spine and adjustment of lordosis move the thrust line back within the vertebral bodies.

Reprinted from *Physiotherapy Journal*, C.M. Norris, vol. 181, number 3, "Spinal stabilization," pages 4-12. Copyright 1995, with permission from Elsevier.

can create intra-abdominal pressure that moves the thrust line back into the spine and increases spinal stability (figure 2.17*c*). Moreover, a person can use the spinal muscles (which are intrinsic to the arch) to adjust the lordosis, so that the thrust line continually remains within the arch of the spine. The stiffness of the spine (resistance to bending) also is increased through the TLF and hydraulic amplifier mechanisms.

Some writers believe that the arch model of the spine seriously underestimates the compressive forces on the spine (Adams 1989). For further discussion of intra-abdominal pressure and other stabilizing mechanisms, see chapter 3.

LIFTING METHODS

There are two basic ways to lift something: in the squat lift, a person bends the knees and back; in the stoop lift, the legs remain straight and the back alone bends. Because the legs are apart and bent with the squat lift, an individual can hold the object closer to the body's line of gravity—thereby reducing the length of the lever arm from the body's line of gravity to the center of gravity of the object. The disadvantage of the squat lift is that people are lifting more of their bodies (the legs and trunk as opposed to the trunk alone) and therefore must expend more energy than with a stoop lift. The erector spinae are more active in positions where lordosis is maintained (Delitto et al. 1987); after people have attained a fully erect position when lifting a heavy weight, they tend to lean back to balance the weight and to use their hip flexor muscles to resist further spinal extension and to stabilize their spines.

Key point: In a squat lift, a person can hold a weight closer to the body's center of gravity, thereby reducing the torque on the spine.

In addition to differentiating between the squat lift and stoop lift, we must also examine the difference between using a squat lift with the back lordotic (lumbar spine minimally extended) and with the back flat (lumbar spine minimally flexed). Lumbar curvature is calculated as the angle formed between the surface of the vertebral body of L1 and that of the sacrum (figure 2.18). The population mean value of this angle is 50°,

to remain stable, the thrust line must stay within the physical boundaries of the arch. The deeper within the arch the thrust line stays, the more stable the arch will be. In the case of the spine, the thrust line is positioned within the vertebral bodies.

Because a 100 kg weight lifted in a stooped position (in which lordosis is lost) creates a thrust line outside the spine (figure 2.17*b*), the arch is unstable. By tensing the back extensor and abdominal muscles at the same time, however, one although in children it is increased to 67° and in young males to as much as 74° (Bogduk and Twomey 1991) depending on posture type. The lordosis naturally results from the shapes of the vertebrae and disks of the lumbar spine. The L5-S1 vertebral disc is wedge-shaped, its posterior height typically about 7 mm less than its anterior. The L5 vertebral body also is wedge-shaped, its posterior height typically 3 mm less than its anterior. The remainder of the lordosis occurs because the discs

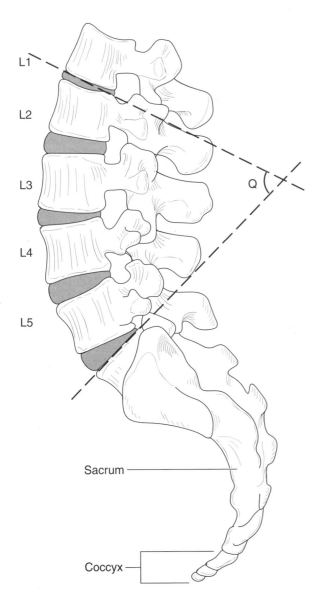

Figure 2.18 The curvature of the lumbar spine can be designated by the angle (Q) formed between lines through the surface of L1 and the sacrum.

Adapted, by permission, from J.K. Loudon, S.L. Bell, and J.M. Johnston, 1998, *The clinical orthopedic assessment guide* (Champaign, IL: Human Kinetics), 54.

themselves (not the vertebral bodies) are wedge-shaped. The sacrum is angled at about 30° to the horizontal, and changes to this angle affect the sacroiliac joint.

Because the orientations of the vertebrae differ between the squat and stoop lifts, the load distribution is affected. The lengths of various trunk muscles also differ between the two lifts. Because the depth of the lumbar discs (6-12 mm) is considerably smaller than the vertical height of the lumbar vertebrae (30-45 mm), even minimal changes in vertebral angles can greatly deform the discs. A flexion angle of 10° to 12°, for example, stretches the posterior annulus by more than 50% (Adams and Dolan 1997). Repeated loading in a lordotic posture can cause compressive stress within the posterior annulus of a disc and load the adjacent facet joints.

Maximal flexion (up to the elastic limit) can thin the posterior annulus and cause posterior prolapse. Recovery from this type of tissue stress is by no means immediate. Only 50% of intervertebral stiffness is regained after a 2 min rest period following a 20 min flexion period (McGill and Brown 1992). Minimal flexion (flat back), however, which brings the vertebral bodies into vertical alignment, equalizes compressive stress across the whole disc and unloads the facets (Adams et al. 1994). At 60% to 80% of maximum flexion, the posterior tissues exert a substantial extensor torque, yet there is only a small compression effect on the lumbar discs. Moreover, tension in the thoracolumbar fascia helps to stabilize the sacroiliac joint, and contractions of the gluteal muscles, the abdominals, and latissimus dorsi increase the TLF tension in a flat-back posture.

To lift a heavy object optimally, one should use a squat lift while maintaining the neutral position of the spine. The spine is likely to flatten as the weight is taken, and this technique should prevent hyperflexion as long as the object is pulled toward the pelvis.

Key point: Have your client perform squat lifts when lifting an object, bringing the object in toward the pelvis. As your client begins to raise the weight, her lumbar spine flattens to minimally compress the lumbar discs and unload the facet joints. In this position, tissue recoil provides substantial extension power.

SUMMARY

- A spinal segment, consisting of two adjacent vertebrae, is comparable to a simple leverage system, connected and held together by ligaments.

- Because spinal ligaments are interconnected with fasciae surrounding back muscles, which in turn eventually merge with ligaments and muscles as distant as the extremities of limbs, movements of most parts of the body can affect the stability of the spine.

- The deep abdominal muscles in particular are very important in keeping the spine stable (i.e., keeping vertebrae in line even during heavy lifting).

- Spinal discs, between each pair of vertebrae, absorb stress through stretching of the elastic fibers in the outer annulus and through cushioning by the highly plastic, hydrophilic nucleus pulposus. With age, the nucleus loses water content and the fibers lose elasticity.

- The facet joints are synovial joints between the inferior articular process of one vertebra and the superior articular process of its neighbor. Their articular cartilage can become brittle with age.

- Within the vertebra itself, compressive force is transmitted by both the cancellous (spongy) bone of the vertebral body and its cortical bone shell. Cancellous tissue declines with age. The vertebrae themselves, however, can bear only a small fraction of the load placed on the spine by heavy weights without experiencing serious injury.

- The muscle sequence in forward bending is changed with those suffering low back pain.

- To successfully bear heavy weight, the spine must be stabilized by muscles and ligaments.

- Coordinated activity of the erector spinae, gluteals, and hamstrings provides the extension force for lifting.

- Movement dysfunction of the bending action often exists in people with low back pain.

Chapter 3
Stabilization Mechanisms of the Lumbar Spine

Devoid of its musculature, the human spine is inherently unstable. The spine of a fresh cadaver stripped of muscle can sustain a load of only 4 to 5 lb (1.8-2.3 kg) before it buckles into flexion (Panjabi et al. 1989). Moreover, the center of gravity of the upper body (when one is standing upright) lies at sternal level (Norkin and Levangie 1992). This combination of flexibility and weight distribution is approximately comparable to balancing a 75 lb (34 kg) weight at the end of a 14 in. (35.5 cm) flexible rod (Farfan 1988).

From a strictly mechanical standpoint, discs don't contribute as much as one might think to the spine's strength: Lifting heavy objects imposes on the lower lumbar spine a compressive force that greatly exceeds the failure load of the vertebral discs unless additional support is present (Bartelink 1957; Morris et al. 1961). Moreover, if compressive and shear forces are not attenuated by muscle contraction, they place considerable stress on the facet joints of the lumbar spine, leading to inflammation of joint structures and eventually joint damage through erosion.

By reducing these forces acting on the lumbar spine, several mechanisms help stabilize the spine (Norris 1995a). These mechanisms, on which this chapter focuses, include the posterior ligamentous system, several processes involving the thoracolumbar fascia, actions of trunk muscles, and intra-abdominal pressure.

Key point: The spinal column by itself is inherently unstable. Without muscle action, severe stress is imposed on the delicate joints and discs. Stability training aims to reduce these forces using muscle action.

POSTERIOR LIGAMENTOUS SYSTEM

The interspinous and supraspinous ligaments, facet joint capsules, and thoracolumbar fascia (TLF) together provide passive support for the spine said to be sufficient to balance between 24% and 55% of imposed flexion stress (Adams et al. 1980). However, the cadaveric experiments on which these figures are based have been questioned (discussed later).

In the unstretched position, collagen fibers within the anterior and posterior longitudinal ligaments and the ligamentum flavum (see figure 2.3) are aligned haphazardly. When the ligaments are stretched as the spine flexes or extends, however, the collagen fibers become aligned and the ligament becomes stiffer (Hukins et al. 1990; Kirby et al. 1989). Stressed by 10% to 13% at rest, the ligaments retract when cut (Hukins et al. 1990). The longitudinal ligaments therefore maintain a compressive force along the axis of the spine, causing it to act somewhat like a stressed beam (Aspden 1992). The ligaments are viscoelastic (i.e., they stiffen when loaded rapidly). Rapid loading therefore increases the thrust within the spine and tends to approximate (bring closer together) the vertebrae, enhancing spinal stability.

Power created by the hip extensors posteriorly tilts the pelvis and is transmitted through the spine to the thorax and upper limbs via the ligamentous system. Some authors have maintained that for this passive mechanism to work, the spine must remain flexed. They argued that if the spine extends, tightness of the posterior ligaments will decrease and their ability to stabilize the spine will be lost (McGill and Norman 1986). More recently, however, it has been shown that the spine need not become **kyphotic** before it can create tension by stretching the tissues (Gracovetsky et al. 1990).

The posterior ligamentous system alone can sustain a maximum torque of only about 50 N·m (Bogduk and Twomey 1991), less than 25% that of the contracting erector spinae. However, two passive systems are at work here (see p. 34). While the posterior ligamentous system is recoiling, the erector spinae are also recoiling. At the point of full flexion, these muscles no longer contract (they are electrically silent), but they do exert a force through recoil much like that of a giant elastic band. The force that the erector spinae create through recoil is about 200 N·m, equal to their potential contractile force. The combined posterior musculoligamentous system therefore provides a substantial stabilizing mechanism in full flexion.

Key point: The posterior ligaments of the spine can sustain 50 N·m of torque and resist more than 50% of the flexion stress imposed on the spine. The passive tension (elastic recoil) in the stretched erector spinae can create 200 N·m of torque, equal to their maximum contraction.

Many of the original studies on spinal ligaments were conducted on cadavers. When a person dies, however, the active systems of the disc stop, and because the disc material naturally absorbs water (it is hydrophilic), the disc actually expands slightly after death. Tissue changes after death are quite common, incidentally; for example, both facial and head hair continue to grow for a short while after death. Because the disc absorbs water in this way (and consequently becomes taller), the ligaments that surround the spinal segment are stretched slightly, making some of the results obtained from cadaveric tests inaccurate (McGill 2002). It has been demonstrated (Sharma et al. 1995) that of the posterior ligaments, the supraspinous ligament, rather than the posterior longitudinal ligament or ligamentum flavum, is the passive structure that most contributes to passive spinal stability.

THORACOLUMBAR FASCIA

The thoracolumbar fascia performs a number of important functions during back stability, which I briefly review here. Note that the fascia also stabilizes the sacroiliac joints.

Structure of the Thoracolumbar Fascia

The thoracolumbar (lumbodorsal) fascia (TLF) has three layers that cover the muscles of the back (figure 3.1). The anterior layer derives from fascia

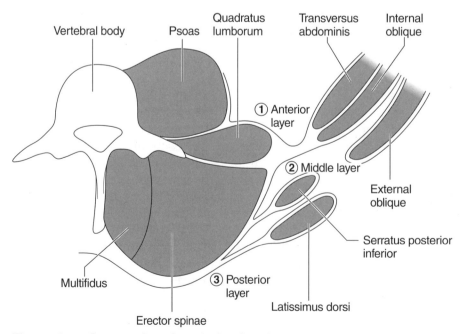

Figure 3.1   Cross section of trunk showing thoracolumbar fascia.

covering the quadratus lumborum and attaches to the transverse processes (Bogduk and Twomey 1991). The middle layer, behind the quadratus lumborum, attaches both to the transverse processes and to the intertransverse ligaments. Laterally, it extends to cover transversus abdominis. The posterior layer, which envelops the erector spinae, attaches from the spinous processes and wraps around the back muscles to blend with the rest of the TLF laterally to the iliocostalis. The point at which the layers blend is the **lateral raphe**.

The superficial layer of the TLF is continuous with the latissimus dorsi and gluteus maximus. Sometimes a few fibers attach to parts of the external oblique and trapezius, and some cross the body midline (Vleeming et al. 1995). At L4-L5 level, fibers from latissimus dorsi and gluteus maximus differ in orientation, giving the superficial layer of the TLF a crosshatched appearance. This appearance may even extend down to the L5-S2 level (Vleeming et al. 1997). The fibers of the deep layer are continuous with the sacrotuberous ligament (and through it to the biceps femoris muscle of the upper leg), and they attach to the posterior superior iliac spines, the iliac crests, and the sacroiliac ligaments (see figure 2.9). In the thoracic region, fibers of the serratus posterior inferior are continuous with the TLF (figure 3.2).

Key point: The TLF is a tough fibrous sheet covering the back. It is tensioned by muscles from above, the side, and below. Through it, these muscles transmit their power across the whole spine.

Thoracolumbar Fascia Mechanism

In addition to its passive role, the TLF has two further capacities that involve muscle contraction. The transversus abdominis, through its attachment to the lateral raphe, pulls on the TLF. Although both attach to the lateral raphe (figure 3.3), the deep **laminae** of the TLF angle upward, whereas the superficial laminae angle downward. As the transversus abdominis contracts and pulls on the lateral raphe, the deep and superficial fibers of the TLF pull laterally for the most part, although some force is transmitted along the length of the TLF.

Originally, this approximating force was calculated as 57% of the force applied to the lateral raphe (Macintosh and Bogduk 1987), an increase in force termed the *gain* of the TLF (Gracovetsky et al. 1985). However, more detailed anatomical investigation has revealed that the torque created by contraction of transversus abdominis onto the TLF is between 3.9 and 5.9 N·m—compared

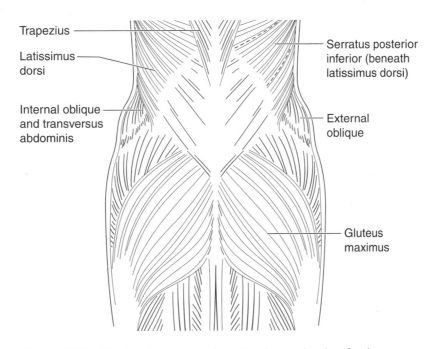

Trapezius

Latissimus dorsi

Internal oblique and transversus abdominis

Serratus posterior inferior (beneath latissimus dorsi)

External oblique

Gluteus maximus

Figure 3.2   Muscle attachments into the thoracolumbar fascia.

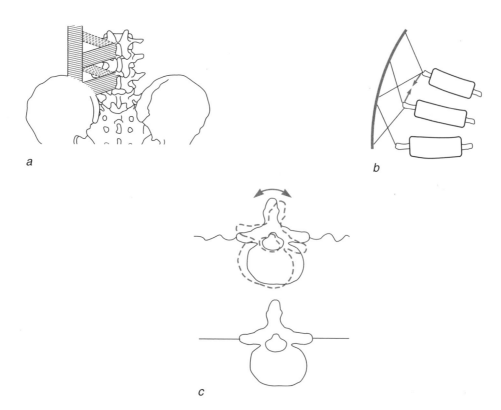

Figure 3.3   *(a)* The thoracolumbar fascia (TLF) mechanism. *(b)* Through its attachment to the lateral raphe, the transversus abdominis pulls on the TLF. *(c)* The lateral tension of the TLF controls intersegmental motion.
(b, c) Based on Hodges et al. 2003; Tesh, Shaw-Dunn, and Evans 1987.

with that from the back extensors of 250 to 280 N·m (Macintosh et al. 1987). Rather than actively extending the spine through the approximating force represented by gain, then, the primary importance of the TLF mechanism described seems to be providing passive resistance to flexion by stiffening the lumbar spine.

Attachment of the TLF to the transverse processes of the lumbar vertebrae may control intervertebral motion to a certain extent (Hodges et al. 2003). Contraction force from the transversus abdominis muscle will be passed onto the TLF and indirectly affect the transverse processes. Approximation of the transverse processes (or more realistically limitation of distraction) may also occur during lateral flexion of the lumbar spine. Resistance to lateral flexion of this type has been calculated to create a force of 14.5 N (Tesh et al. 1987).

Tensioning the TLF through contraction of the transversus abdominis (TrA) muscle has been shown to increase resistance to flexion loads by 9.5 N but to reduce resistance to extension loading by 6.6 N (Barker et al. 2006). Barker and

colleagues showed fascial tension to affect cyclic loading during flexion by reducing vertebral displacement by 26% at the start of loading, reducing to 2% as loading continued. Fascial tension during cyclic loading in extension increased vertebral displacement by 23% at onset, reducing to 1% as loading reached 450 N.

Key point: Tensioning of the TLF using contraction of the TrA muscle reduces vertebral displacement when the spine is loaded in flexion but increases displacement when the spine is loaded in extension.

Thoracolumbar Fascia as Hydraulic Amplifier

The TLF exerts an even greater stabilizing effect through its role in the so-called hydraulic amplifier effect (Gracovetsky et al. 1977). The posterior layer of the TLF is retinacular tissue (i.e., very strong reinforcing connective tissue) that envelops the erector spinae. As the erector spinae contract, the TLF resists the expansion of the bellies of the shortening muscles by increasing tension in the fascia. Some believe that the predominant antiflexion effect of the TLF occurs via this hydraulic amplifier effect rather than by its pull on the transversus abdominis (Macintosh et al. 1987). Restriction of the radial expansion of the erector spinae by the TLF has been shown to increase the stress generated by these muscles by as much as 30% (Hukins et al. 1990).

Thoracolumbar Fascia Coupling and the Sacroiliac Joint

A combination of form closure and force closure stabilizes the sacroiliac joint (SIJ) (Vleeming et al. 1990). Form closure arises from the anatomical alignment of the bones of the ilium and sacrum, where the sacrum forms a kind of keystone between the wings of the pelvis (Norris 1998). Force closure results from muscles pulling laterally onto fascia and ligaments that pass over the joint. The combination of form and force closure creates a very useful self-locking mechanism within the SIJ. Any activity that weakens these forms of closure can create pathological symptoms in the SIJ.

Nutation (see table 2.3) tensions the SIJ ligaments, pulling the posterior parts of the iliac bones together and increasing SIJ compression. Two ligaments are of special importance to self-locking—the sacrotuberous ligament connecting the sacrum to the ischial tuberosity, and the long dorsal sacroiliac ligament from the third and fourth sacral segments to the posterior superior iliac spines. Both ligaments blend over the posterolateral aspect of the sacrum to form an expansion approximately 20 mm wide and 60 mm long. The ligaments attach to the posterior layer of the TLF and to the **aponeurosis** of the erector spinae. Nutation tensions the sacrotuberous ligament, whereas counternutation tensions the long dorsal sacroiliac (SI) ligament. The SI ligament is tensioned by contraction of the biceps femoris and of the gluteus maximus.

Key point: The sacrotuberous ligament and the long dorsal sacroiliac ligament blend to form the sacroiliac expansion.

Forced closure of the SIJ opens the possibility of treating SIJ lesions with exercise therapy either passively (automobilization) or actively through contraction of the biceps femoris, gluteus maximus, latissimus dorsi, or erector spine. Clearly, if muscle affects the SIJ, as has been shown by Vleeming's work (Vleeming et al. 1995), training these muscles could improve SIJ functions. Moreover, any muscle that tensions the TLF should also affect force closure of the SIJ.

When the erector spinae contract, they pull the sacrum forward—inducing nutation of the SIJ and tensing the interosseous and sacrotuberous ligaments. The iliac portion of the muscle tends to pull the cranial aspect of the SIJ together, whereas nutation pulls the caudal aspect apart. The gluteus maximus can compress the SIJ directly and indirectly through its attachment to the sacrotuberous ligament. This occurs particularly when the gluteus maximus contracts with the contralateral latissimus dorsi and both muscles tension the TLF, whose fibers join the two muscles. Tension in the sacrotuberous ligament is increased by tensioning of the long head of the biceps femoris muscle. This occurs most noticeably in a flexed trunk or stooped position, in which the sacrotuberous ligament is also tensioned by the sacral portion of the erector spinae and the gluteus maximus.

Key point: Tension generated by contraction of biceps femoris and gluteus maximus is transmitted via ligaments to the sacroiliac joint itself.

SIJ pain frequently occurs during and after pregnancy, when laxness of the SIJ ligaments reduces form closure of the joints. Female gymnasts experience similar problems: The hyperflexibility developed through gymnastics generally increases the laxity of the pelvic ligaments, reducing the form closure that they produce. The increased muscular stability resulting from the muscular demands of the sport compensates for the laxness, as long as the women continue their activity. When their muscle strength declines after they stop practicing the sport, the SIJ is left unstable and open to pathology. SIJ pain of this type is often helped by using a pelvic belt. Improving force closure of the SIJ by using stabilization techniques for the lumbar spine and enhancing gluteal muscle strength using the hip hinge action can also reduce pain (see p. 140).

Key point: Specific exercise can improve stability of the sacroiliac joint by restoring the natural mechanisms of form closure and force closure.

Stability exercise has been used successfully to treat SIJ conditions. Mooney and colleagues (2001) found changes in muscle balance tests for those suffering SIJ pain. These patients had higher levels of gluteal and latissimus dorsi muscle activity through actively "splinting" the joint. Their core stabilizing muscles were not working properly, so the gluteal and latissimus muscles had to act to compensate for this. By using rotary strengthening, these authors were able to return the patients' muscle activity to normal. Richardson and colleagues (2002) used Doppler imaging to assess SIJ laxity on patients while at the same time studying trunk muscle activity using electromyography (EMG). These authors were able to demonstrate a reduction in joint laxity (i.e., increased SIJ stability) by using transversus abdominis contraction. Reduced general back stability has also been found in people with SIJ dysfunction. Hungerford and colleagues (2003) found changes in internal oblique, multifidus, and gluteus maximus recruitment in the weight-bearing leg of those with SIJ pain. This is significant clinically, because patients with SIJ pain often present with pain that is worsened when standing in a swayback posture (see p. 84) where they favor one leg. Clearly, integrated back stability exercise is vital for the treatment of SIJ dysfunction.

TRUNK MUSCLE ACTION

Facilitating co-contraction of the muscles surrounding the lumbar spine—including the erector spinae, quadratus lumborum, transversus abdominis, multifidus, and the oblique abdominals—in particular is the method chosen to enhance spinal stability. Lumbar spine dissection (Jemmett et al. 2004) has shown individual segmental attachments to the lumbar spine for transversus, psoas, quadratus lumborum, and multifidus (the so-called local or primary stabilizers; see p. 162). The other muscles pass over

the lumbar region without segmental attachment and so are considered global or secondary stabilizers. Let's look at these muscles individually to see their importance.

Spinal Extensor Muscles

The spinal extensors may be broadly categorized as superficial muscles (the erector spinae) that travel the length of the lumbar spine and attach to the sacrum and pelvis and as deep, or intersegmental (unisegmental) muscles (multifidi, interspinales, and intertransversarii) that span the spaces between the individual lumbar segments.

The intersegmental muscles, being more deeply placed, are closer to the center of rotation of the spine and have a shorter lever arm than the superficial muscles. However, their closeness to the center of rotation means that the change in length of intersegmental muscles is less for any given change in the spine's angular position, and the muscles' shorter length gives them a faster reaction time, creating a smoother and more efficient stabilizing control system (Panjabi et al. 1989). The intersegmental nature of these muscles also means that they are able to fine-tune the spinal movements by acting on individual lumbar segments rather than the whole spine (Aspden 1992).

Being larger in size and farther from the center of rotation, the superficial muscles are better placed to create gross sagittal rotation movements, whereas the intersegmental muscles are of greater importance to spinal stability (Panjabi et al. 1989). Furthermore, because the smaller intersegmental muscles have about seven times the number of muscle spindles (Bastide et al. 1989) than the larger muscles have, the smaller muscles have a greater proprioceptive role (see following discussion).

Deep (Intersegmental) Muscles

These muscles lie below the erector spinae, at the level of the spinous process and transverse processes of the vertebra.

Of the deeply placed intersegmental muscles, the multifidus is said to be most important for lumbar stability. The fibers of the multifidus are arranged segmentally, and each **fascicle** of a given vertebra has a separate innervation by the medial branch of the dorsal ramus of the vertebra below (Macintosh and Bogduk 1986).

Studies have also been able to differentiate between deep and superficial portions of this muscle (Moseley et al. 2002). Using arm movements, Moseley and colleagues showed that the superficial multifidus worked with the erector spinae and varied depending on the direction of arm movement. The deep multifidus worked with the transversus abdominis, and these muscles were active to the same degree whatever the arm movement direction. In addition, it seems that the action of individual components of the multifidus is different depending on the body's preparedness for the task, that is, whether the subject is expecting the movement, as though the body was trying to fine-tune its stability response (Moseley et al. 2003).

The primary function of each multifidus fascicle may be to control lordosis at its particular vertebral level and to independently counteract any imposed loading (Aspden 1992). The action of the multifidus can be resolved into a small horizontal and much larger vertical component (figure 3.4),

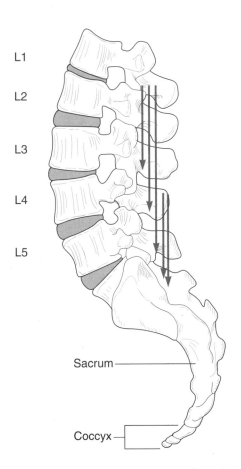

L1

L2

L3

L4

L5

Sacrum

Coccyx

Figure 3.4   Lateral view showing the line of action of the multifidus, with its vertical alignment.

Adapted, by permission, from J.K. Loudon, S.L. Bell, and J.M. Johnston, 1998, *The clinical orthopedic assessment guide* (Champaign, IL: Human Kinetics), 54.

which (as is clear when viewed from the side) acts at 90° to the spinous processes. This configuration enables the multifidus to produce posterior sagittal rotation (rocking) of the lumbar vertebrae (Macintosh and Bogduk 1986). This action neutralizes spinal flexion caused as a secondary action when the oblique abdominals produce spinal rotation. Because the line of action of the long fascicles of the multifidus lies behind the lumbar spine, the muscle also increases lumbar lordosis. The multifidus is active through the whole range of flexion, during rotation in either direction, and during extension movements of the hip (Valencia and Munro 1985). Posterior sagittal rotation occurs during all flexion movements in order to resist the anterior sagittal rotation that naturally accompanies flexion. The role of the multifidus in producing this action is therefore essential to stability of the lumbar spine in normal movements.

Panjabi's (1992) description of instability (as a reduction in stiffness within the neutral zone of the lumbar spine) is particularly relevant to multifidus function. The multifidus is a muscle well positioned to enhance segmental stiffness in the neutral zone and contributes nearly 70% of the stiffness resulting from muscle contraction (Wilke et al. 1995).

Key point: The multifidus contributes nearly 70% of the stiffness imposed on the lumbar spine by muscle contraction.

Real-time ultrasound imaging has revealed marked asymmetry of the multifidus in patients with low back pain (Hides et al. 1994). Cross-sectional area (CSA) of the multifidus was markedly reduced on the **ipsilateral** side to symptoms, the site of reduction corresponding to the level of lumbar lesion as assessed by manual therapy palpation. The muscle also showed a rounder shape, suggesting muscle spasm. The suggested mechanism for the CSA reduction was by inhibition through perceived pain via a long loop reflex. The level of vertebral pathology may have been targeted to protect the damaged tissues from movement. The authors suggested that the rapid muscle wasting (less than 14 days in 20 of the 26 patients studied) may have resulted from spasm-induced reduction in circulation to the muscle.

In addition to noting changes in muscle bulk, Biedermann and colleagues (1991) observed altered fiber types in the multifidus of patients with low back pain (LBP); patients who tended to decrease their physical and social activities as a result of LBP showed a reduced ratio of slow-twitch to fast-twitch muscle fibers. This could be the muscle's adaptive response to changes in functional demand placed on it, or the injury may have caused a shift in recruitment patterns of motor units of the paraspinal muscles, with the fast-twitch motor units being recruited before the slow-twitch units. Pathologic changes in the multifidus following low back pain include a moth-eaten appearance of type I fibers (Hides et al. 1996) and an increase in fatty deposits (Parkkola et al. 1993).

Recovery of multifidus function following low back pain does not occur automatically following the resolution of pain and resumption of normal daily activity. In a study comparing medical treatment alone (1-3 days of bed rest, analgesics, and anti-inflammatory medication) with medical treatment plus specific exercise therapy to the multifidus, Hides and colleagues (1996) showed that multifidus activity could be retrained. Subjects who had experienced first-episode acute low back pain showed an average of 24% reduction in CSA to the multifidus on the painful side. The difference between painful and painless sides changed from nearly 17% after 4 weeks to 14% after 10 weeks in those subjects receiving medical treatment alone. For those who received additional exercise therapy, however, the mean values were 0.7% at 4 weeks, decreasing to 0.24% after 10 weeks (figure 3.5).

Key point: Low back pain leads to reduced cross-sectional area in the multifidus muscle. As the pain reduces, recovery is not automatic—rehabilitation is required.

By injecting an irritant chemical (hypertonic saline) directly into the muscle, researchers have proven that the multifidus can be a source of pain (Cornwall et al. 2006). Using 15 subjects, Cornwall and colleagues found that all experienced local pain, and 13 of the 15 had referred pain. Hypertonic saline is similar to the fluid

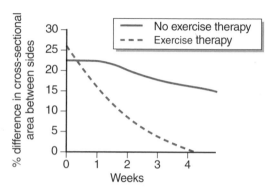

Figure 3.5   Ultrasound imaging results of multifidus muscle recovery.

Reprinted, by permission, from J.A. Hides, C.A. Richardson, and G.A. Jull, 1966, "Multifidus muscle recovery is not automatic after resolution of acute, first-episode low back pain," *Spine* 21: 2763-2769.

produced by swelling, so if the multifidus muscles become inflamed and swollen, they can cause back pain.

Pain can occur in a muscle as a result of spasm. Spasm restricts the blood flow through a muscle and can allow swelling to build up, producing what is known as ischemic pain. Certain activities (e.g., bending over a bench or incorrectly lifting) produce prolonged lumbar flexion in humans. Prolonged lumbar flexion has been shown to produce spasm in the multifidus in cats used as a model for the human spine (Williams et al. 2000). The multifidus goes into spasm in an effort to protect and stabilize the spine, taking stress away from the ligaments, nerves, and delicate joints. However, Williams and colleagues showed that the initial multifidus spasm reduced dramatically, by more than 90% after only 3 min, leaving the spine open to injury.

How long is the multifidus affected in this way after prolonged flexion? This was answered in a study by Jackson and colleagues (2001), who subjected the spine to 20 min of prolonged flexion to produce multifidus spasm followed by fatigue. It took an incredible 7 hr for the affected tissues to recover fully! Thus, if a subject uses prolonged flexion when lifting either in a gym or at work, the detrimental effect this has on the spine will not be undone simply through rest. To prevent serious damage to the spine, athletes and employees must avoid prolonged flexion: In this case, prevention is definitely better than cure.

Key point: Prolonged flexion postures impose serious strain on the spine, which can take many hours to recover. Avoid prolonged flexion!

Isolated rehabilitation of the multifidus alone is not enough for complete rehabilitation. With the plethora of research concerning the multifidus, it is tempting to believe that this muscle is the key to the lumbar spine and to use it in isolation to retrain the spine. Indeed, whole books have been written on this single muscle alone (Johnson 2002). However, many of the exercises used when retraining the multifidus also target other muscles, and in addition many subjects find isolated multifidus contractions extremely difficult. I have taught stabilization techniques to fully qualified physical therapists for 20 years. During that time, most physical therapists on the courses were unable to perform a multifidus contraction without substantial training. If the therapists themselves find the action virtually impossible, what chance do the clients have?

Some interesting studies highlight the problem of muscle isolation techniques when used alone. Using computed tomography, Choi and colleagues (2005) measured the CSA of the multifidus and longissimus muscles (L4-L5 level) following a 12-week rehabilitation program in patients who had undergone surgery for lumbar disc herniation. Resisted back extension was used rather than selective muscle isolation. Both muscles showed significant increases following the program, the CSA of longissimus increasing by 7.2% and that of the multifidus by 29.2%. Danneels and colleagues (2003) used computed tomography to measure the CSA of the multifidus after either (a) stability training alone, (b) stability combined with dynamic resistance training, or (c) stability with static–dynamic training. Their results demonstrated significant increases in CSA only in the group using stabilization combined with static–dynamic training.

The back extensor muscles including the multifidus have been trained in normal subjects using both resistance training alone (San Juan et al. 2005) and resistance training on unstable surfaces (Behm et al. 2005).

The conclusion of these studies and clinical experience is that the multifidus is an important muscle, but it is only one piece in the puzzle that is spinal rehabilitation. To limit exercise therapy to multifidus contraction alone is to deny the patient even the most basic rehabilitation.

Key point: Training the multifidus alone is not enough for full rehabilitation.

Superficial Muscles

These muscles lie on top of the deep muscles, above the level of the spinous process and transverse processes.

Erector Spinae The lumbar erector spinae consists of two muscles: the iliocostalis and the longissimus (figure 3.6). Each of these muscles has two components arising from both the thoracic and lumbar spine. Functionally, therefore, the erector spinae can be considered in four distinct

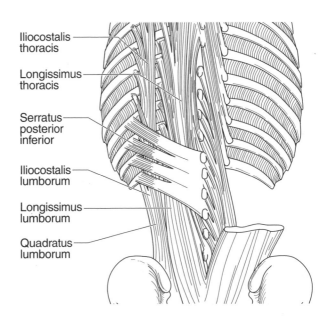

Iliocostalis thoracis

Longissimus thoracis

Serratus posterior inferior

Iliocostalis lumborum

Longissimus lumborum

Quadratus lumborum

Figure 3.6 Muscles of the back.

groups: lumbar longissimus, lumbar iliocostalis, thoracic longissimus, and thoracic iliocostalis (Macintosh and Bogduk 1987).

The force produced by the lumbar longissimus can be resolved into a large vertical vector and a smaller horizontal vector (figure 3.7). However, the fascicle attachments are closer to the axis of sagittal rotation than those of the multifidus, so their effect on posterior sagittal rotation is less. Because the horizontal vectors of lumbar longissimus are directed backward, the muscle is able to draw the vertebrae backward into posterior translation and restore the anterior translation that occurs with lumbar flexion. The upper lumbar fascicles are better equipped to facilitate posterior sagittal rotation, whereas the lower levels are better suited to resist anterior translation.

The lumbar iliocostalis has an action similar to that of the lumbar longissimus. In addition, the muscle cooperates with the multifidus to neutralize flexion caused when the abdominals rotate the trunk.

The thoracic longissimus can indirectly increase lumbar lordosis via its effect on the aponeurosis of the erector spinae. It also indirectly laterally flexes the lumbar spine through its lateral flexion of the thoracic spine.

The thoracic iliocostalis attaches not to the lumbar vertebrae but to the iliac crest. On contraction, these fascicles increase lordosis; through their additional leverage from the ribs, they indirectly laterally flex the lumbar spine. During **contralateral** rotation, the ribs separate, stretching the thoracic iliocostalis, which can therefore limit this movement. On contraction, the thoracic iliocostalis will resist rotation of the rib cage and lumbar spine from a position of contralateral rotation.

Probably the endurance rather than the strength of the erector spinae is important to LBP rehabilitation. Endurance has been used to predict susceptibility to LBP (Biering-Sorensen 1984) and to predict chronicity following injury (Enthoven et al. 2003). The classic Biering-Sorensen test, described on page 246, has been shown to be a reliable measure of spinal endurance in several clinical populations, including both symptomatic (Moffroid et al. 1994) and asymptomatic people (Latimer et al. 1999).

Subjects with a history of LBP may have reduced endurance of the back extensors compared with normal subjects, but they have similar strength (Jorgensen and Nicolaisen 1987). As fatigue increases, subjects with LBP show reduced precision and control of trunk movements. Loss of torque from the trunk muscles in these subjects is relatively less than the loss of control and precision (Parnianpour et al. 1988), indicating that a rehabilitation program should restore endurance for the spinal extensors. Selective recruitment of the torque-producing superficial muscles from the stabilizing deep muscles is also important for rehabilitation of active lumbar stabilization (Ng and Richardson 1994). The test for endurance of the erector spinae muscles is shown in chapter 13.

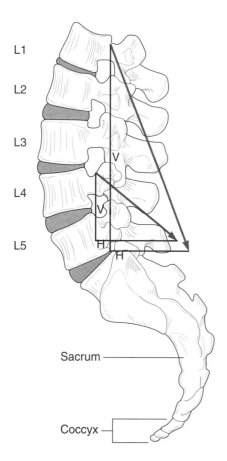

Figure 3.7 Lateral view of the lumbar spine, showing the line of the lumbar iliocostalis and lumbar longissimus and their more oblique orientation. Note the greater horizontal force vector (H) and smaller vertical force vector (V) of the lower fibers of these muscles.

Adapted, by permission, from J.K. Loudon, S.L. Bell, and J.M. Johnston, 1998, *The clinical orthopedic assessment guide* (Champaign, IL: Human Kinetics), 54.

Key point: Endurance of the erector spinae muscles is a vital component of back rehabilitation.

Quadratus Lumborum The quadratus lumborum (QL) (figure 3.6) can be an important back stabilizer in certain circumstances (McGill et al. 1996). The muscle lies deeper than the erector spinae and has medial and lateral fibers. The medial fibers connect the lumbar transverse processes to the ilium and iliolumbar ligament or the 12th rib, whereas the lateral fibers directly connect the ilium and iliolumbar ligament and 12th rib (Bogduk and Twomey 1991). The QL has a small extensor torque and a larger lateral flexion torque and is able to stabilize the lumbar spine via its segmental attachments (McGill et al. 1996). EMG with fine wire electrodes has shown the muscle to be more active during lateral bending than during extension and especially active in upright standing and unilateral carrying (McGill et al. 1996). Side-support actions shift some of the loading of the muscles from the discs and facet joints of the lumbar spine to the side (McGill 1998). This role of the quadratus lumborum as a potential stabilizer of the lumbar spine expands the traditionally recognized role of the muscle as a prime mover of side flexion and as an auxiliary muscle of respiration.

McGill (2002) advocated retraining the QL using the horizontal side-support exercise in various guises (see p. 180) and wrote that the normal value for an endurance hold of this action is 86 s (mean value, combined male and female scores). This compares with endurance values of the trunk extensors of 173 s and trunk flexors of 134 s (McGill et al. 1999). Following chronic low back pain, there is a marked reduction in endurance of the trunk extensors, which is greater than the reduction of either the trunk flexors or trunk lateral flexors including the QL (McGill 2002). Comparative tests for these three muscle groups are shown in chapter 13.

Iliopsoas

The iliopsoas (figure 3.8) consists of the separate psoas and iliacus muscles. The psoas major arises from the vertebral bodies and discs of the lumbar and 12th thoracic vertebrae and from their trans-

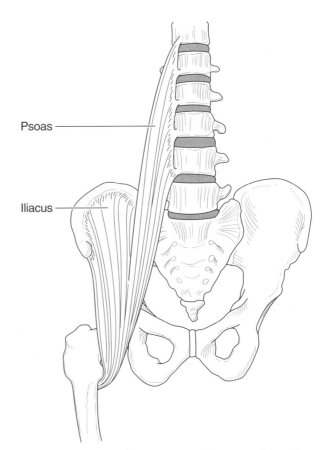

Psoas

Iliacus

Figure 3.8 The iliopsoas muscle, comprising the psoas and the iliacus, anterior view.

verse processes. The muscle passes downward and laterally, beneath the inguinal ligament, to blend with the fibers of iliacus and then to attach onto the posterior aspect of the lesser trochanter of the femur. The iliacus is a large triangular muscle on the anterior aspect of the pelvis. It arises primarily from the upper and posterior portions of the iliac fossa, but some fibers have been found on the sacrum and anterior sacroiliac ligament (Palastanga et al. 1994). The fibers from the iliacus pass downward and medially to blend with those of the psoas major and attach to the lesser trochanter, with a few fibers merging with the joint capsule.

The iliopsoas flexes the hip, anteriorly tilting the pelvis and flexing the lumbar spine. Although these actions are minimal, the psoas major extends the upper lumbar spine and flexes the lower lumbar spine (Bogduk et al. 1992); far more important is the psoas major's production of compression and shear forces over the lumbar spine. The individual fascicles of psoas spiral anteromedially and are all of similar lengths. The lines of action of these fascicles run very close to the axis of rotation of the lumbar spine, giving the muscle fascicles very small torque arms and reducing the muscle's ability to flex the trunk on the stationary hip. However, the compression and shear forces created by the psoas on the lumbar spine are considerable and may even equal full trunk weight. The shearing force exerted on L5-S1 by maximum contraction of a single psoas muscle is nearly twice that exerted on this joint by trunk weight in normal upright standing position (Bogduk et al. 1992).

Key point: The shearing force exerted by the psoas on the lower lumbar spine is nearly double that exerted by trunk weight during normal standing.

Because the two components of iliopsoas have a separate innervation (psoas from the anterior rami and L1-L3, and iliacus from the femoral nerve), they can be activated separately. In a study using fine-wire electrodes guided by high-resolution ultrasound, Andersson and colleagues (1995) showed selective recruitment of the iliacus during contralateral leg extension from single-leg standing. No postural activity was seen in either muscle during relaxed standing or with the whole trunk flexed to 30°. When the contralateral hand was loaded (34 kg weight), the psoas was active but the iliacus was electrically silent. During sitting with a straight back, the psoas was active but the iliacus relatively silent; in relaxed sitting, both muscles were inactive. Both muscles showed moderate activity when subjects sat with an anteriorly tilted pelvis and an increased lordosis. During abdominal exercise, both muscles were active during straight-leg sit-ups—with even higher activity during sit-ups with the knees and hips flexed to 90° (crunch position). However, little activity was seen when subjects performed trunk curls from the crunch position. During straight-leg raising, both muscles were active when the ipsilateral leg was lifted; both were inactive when the contralateral leg was lifted (table 3.1).

Table 3.1   Psoas and Iliacus Activity Measured on Electromyogram as a Percentage of Maximum

Starting position	Psoas %	Iliacus %
Single-leg standing	0	0
Same-leg flexion (90°)	99	99
Opposite-leg extension (30°)	0	26
Same-leg abduction	36	56
Standing	0	0
Standing with trunk flexed to 30°	0	0
Standing with opposite hand holding weight	11	0
Sitting with straight back	9	4
Relaxed sitting	0	0
Sitting, hyperlordosis and pelvic tilt	17	22
Sit-up, straight legs	52	42
Sit-up, legs 45° to floor	88	60
Trunk curl, legs straight	0	0
Trunk curl, legs 90° (end range)	4	0
Straight leg, raising (bilateral)	59	58

Data from E. Andersson et al., 1995, "The role of the psoas and iliacus muscles for stability and movement of the lumbar spine, pelvis and hip," *Scandinavian Journal of Medicine and Science in Sports* 5: 10-16.

A stability function for the posterior fibers of the psoas has been proposed (Gibbons 2001). These smaller fibers attach from the transverse processes of the lumbar vertebrae and are located closer to the axis of spinal rotation than are the anterior fibers. They attach directly to the deep layer of the TLF and fill the intertransverse interval (Jemmett et al. 2004). Within the "drum" of the intra-abdominal pressure (IAP) mechanism (p. 55), the lid of the drum is the diaphragm and the base the pelvic floor. The posterior fibers of the psoas may form a link between the IAP lid and floor through the medial arcuate ligament to the diaphragm and the psoas fascia to the pelvic floor (Gibbons 1999). Mathematical modeling has shown the psoas to have potential stabilizing effects in upright stance (Penning 2000). We have seen that the multifidus muscle reduces in CSA as a result of back pain, and Barker and colleagues (2004) showed similar CSA changes in the psoas. Their study revealed positive correlations between the percentage decrease in CSA of the psoas on the affected side of the lumbar spine and (a) pain rating, (b) reported nerve root compression, and (c) duration of symptoms.

Abdominal Muscles

The abdominal muscle group consists of four muscles, divided into two groups. The deep (anterolateral) abdominals are transversus abdominis (TrA) and internal oblique; the superficial (front) abdominals are the rectus abdominis and external oblique.

Anatomy of the Superficial Abdominals

The rectus abdominis (figure 3.9) is positioned vertically at the front of the abdomen. It attaches from the symphysis pubis and pubic crest and runs to the xiphoid process and fifth, sixth, and seventh ribs, being broader superiorly. The lateral border (semilunaris) can be seen in lean subjects, as can the central separation between the two

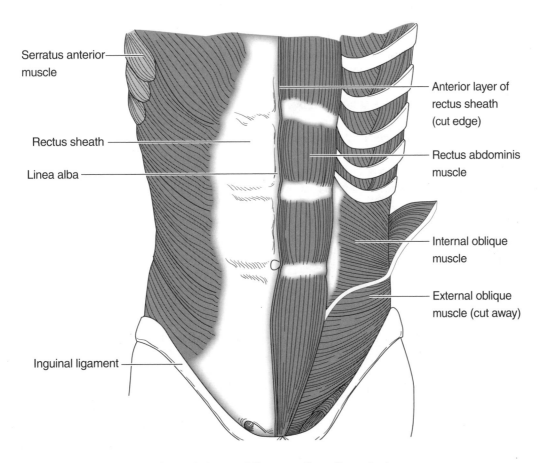

Figure 3.9   Muscles of the abdomen I (intermediate dissection).

muscles, the linea alba. Of the three noticeable tendinous intersections of this muscle, one is level with the umbilicus, one is level with the xiphoid, and one is midway between the two. Each rectus muscle is enclosed within a fibrous sheath (the rectus sheath) formed from the aponeuroses of the internal and external oblique muscles and of the transversus abdominis. These aponeuroses join centrally to form the linea alba. The rectus sheath changes at a level midway between the pubic symphysis and the umbilicus. In the upper area of the muscle, above this point, the aponeurosis of internal oblique splits into two, one part passing behind the rectus and the other in front. The aponeurosis of transversus abdominis fuses with the posterior portion of the sheath, whereas the aponeurosis of external oblique fuses with the anterior sheath. In the lower portion of the muscle (below the midpoint between the pubis and umbilicus), the oblique abdominal and transversus abdominis aponeuroses pass in front of the rectus, and as a result the rectus is less visible in this region (Palastanga et al. 1994).

The external oblique (figure 3.9) is positioned on the anterolateral aspect of the abdomen, with its fibers running downward and medially. It attaches from the outer borders of the lower eight ribs (and their costal cartilages) and then passes toward the midline. The muscle interdigitates with the serratus anterior (above) and latissimus dorsi (below). The lateral fibers are almost vertical and attach to the iliac crest, whereas the medial fibers attach into the rectus sheath. The lower border of the muscle aponeurosis passes between the pubic tubercle and the anterior superior iliac spine to form the inguinal ligament.

Key point: The outermost (lateral) fibers of the external oblique run vertically and work in flexion actions with the rectus abdominis.

Anatomy of the Deep Abdominals

The internal oblique (figure 3.9) is deep to the external oblique and attaches from the lateral two thirds of the inguinal ligament and the anterior two thirds of the iliac crest. It also takes attachment from the thoracolumbar fascia. The fibers fan outward and upward (the posterior fibers being almost vertical) to attach to the inferior borders of the lower four ribs. The anterior fibers pass medially to help form the rectus sheath (figure 3.10). The portion of the muscle that attaches to the inguinal ligament joins its neighboring fibers from transversus abdominis to form the conjoint tendon.

The TrA (figure 3.10) is the deepest of the sheet-like abdominal muscles and attaches from the lateral third of the inguinal ligament and the anterior two thirds of the inner lip of the iliac crest (Palastanga et al. 1994). In addition, it has an attachment from the thoracolumbar fascia (where it merges with the internal oblique to form the lateral raphe) and from the lower six ribs, where it interdigitates with the diaphragm. Its fibers pass horizontally to merge into the rectus sheath (figure 3.11), with the lower fibers attaching to the inguinal ligament and merging with the fibers of the internal oblique to form the conjoint tendon. The lower part of the transversus abdominis forms into the transversalis fascia in which lies the deep inguinal ring.

Functions of the Abdominals

The rectus abdominis and lateral fibers of external oblique are the prime movers of trunk flexion; the internal oblique and transversus abdominis are the major stabilizers. The rectus and external oblique are superficial muscles that often dominate trunk actions. The transversus and internal oblique are more deeply placed, and patients often are unable to contract them voluntarily.

The rectus abdominis flexes the trunk by approximating the pelvis and rib cage to which it attaches (i.e., moving them closer together). EMG investigation has shown that trunk flexion emphasizes the supraumbilical portion, whereas posterior pelvic tilt shows greater activity in the infraumbilical portion (Guimaraes et al. 1991; Lipetz and Gutin 1970).

Abdominal hollowing activates the internal oblique and transversus muscles (Richardson et al. 1992), and the transversus acts at the initiation of movement to stabilize the trunk in overhead and lower-limb actions (Hodges and Richardson 1996). Differentiation has been made between the various regions of the TrA (Urquhart et al. 2005; Urquhart and Hodges 2005). When the TrA is used for postural maintenance during limb motion, the EMG onset of the upper region

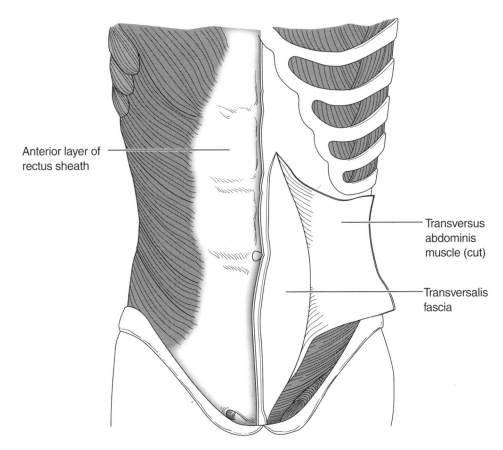

Anterior layer of
rectus sheath

Transversus
abdominis
muscle (cut)

Transversalis
fascia

Figure 3.10 Muscles of the abdomen II (deep dissection).

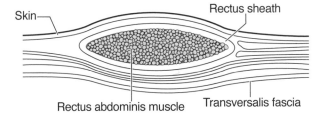

Skin

Rectus sheath

Rectus abdominis muscle

Transversalis fascia

Figure 3.11 Cross section of the rectus sheath.

of TrA is later than that of the middle and lower regions. A similar picture emerges during active trunk rotation, with the recruitment patterns of the upper muscle fascicles being opposite to those of the middle and lower fascicles. During left trunk rotation, the lower and middle TrA regions of the opposite side (contralateral) muscle are more active, but in right trunk rotation the upper region of the same side (ipsilateral) muscle is more active.

Key point: The upper, middle, and lower regions of the transversus abdominis muscle have slightly different functions.

In resisted actions such as sport or lifting, the abdominal muscles stabilize the trunk and provide a firm base of support for the arms and legs to work against. If stability is poor (in relation to total power of the subject), some of the energy of the limb actions can displace the pelvis and trunk instead of provide the desired limb movement. Compare what would happen if a baseball batter wearing sneakers were standing on ice when he connected with the ball, rather than having his feet dug into firm ground: Much of the energy of the swing would be lost, and his body would twist awkwardly. In the same way, if trunk stability is poor, limb power suffers and additional stress is placed on the spinal tissues if they move to full end range.

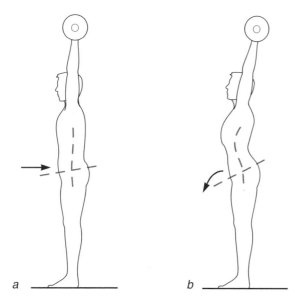

Figure 3.12 Trunk stability in overhead lifting: *(a)* active stability of the trunk through tight abdominals and level pelvis, resulting in reduced stress on lumbar tissues; *(b)* passive stability of the trunk through lax abdominals and tilted pelvis, resulting in increased stress on lumbar tissues.

Reprinted from *Sports injuries: Diagnosis and management,* 2nd ed., C.M. Norris, page 175. Copyright 1998, with permission from Elsevier.

Consider an overhead lifting action performed with an unstable spine (figure 3.12): If the pelvis tilts forward, lumbar lordosis increases and the abdominal muscles overstretch as the lumbar spine moves into full extension. In this case, what trunk stability is present comes from facet joint approximation and elastic recoil of noncontractile tissues (passive stability) rather than from muscle action (active stability) (see p. 40). The key to safe and effective abdominal training in sport is to train for trunk stability before training for trunk muscle performance. Thus, the athlete is performing exercises on a spine made stable by muscle rather than placing excessive stress on spinal joints before muscle stability has been established.

Key point: Stability forms the foundation of all trunk exercise. People should train for trunk stability before training for muscle performance.

Patterns of Coordination Among the Abdominals During Spinal Movement

In terms of spinal stabilization, the contraction speed of the abdominals is more critical than their strength when they react to a force tending to displace the lumbar spine (Saal and Saal 1989). Moreover, the ability of a patient to dissociate deep abdominal function from that of the superficial abdominals is important, and the key to lumbar stabilization appears to be the ratio rather than the intensity of muscle activity. Abdominal hollowing (rather than a sit-up movement) works the transversus abdominis and internal oblique (not the rectus abdominis and the external oblique) (Richardson et al. 1992). O'Sullivan and colleagues (1997) found that patients with chronic low back pain (CLBP) were poorer at using the internal oblique than using the rectus abdominis and external oblique, reflecting a shift in the pattern of motor activity. As CLBP patients attempted an abdominal hollowing action, they tended to substitute the superficial muscles that override the deep abdominals. When expressed as a ratio of internal oblique over rectus abdominis, the value from the control group (non-LBP) was 8.74 whereas the CLBP group had a ratio of only 2.41—indicating a much larger proportional contribution to hollowing by the internal oblique in the control group (figure 3.13). Pain inhibition

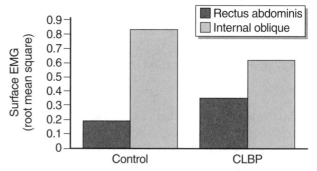

Figure 3.13 Abdominal muscle activation in chronic low back pain (CLBP). EMG = electromyograph.

Data from P.B. O'Sullivan, L.T. Twomey, and G.T. Allison, 1997, "Evaluation of specific stabilizing exercise in the treatment of chronic low back pain with radiologic diagnosis of spondylolysis or spondylolisthesis," *Spine* 22: 2959-2967.

in the subjects with CLBP may have led to altered muscle recruitment and compensatory strategies (O'Sullivan et al. 1997).

EMG measurements of trunk muscles have shown that the muscles do not simply work as prime movers of the spine but show antagonistic activity during various movements. The oblique abdominals are more active than predicted, to help stabilize the trunk. Zetterberg and colleagues (1987) reported that subjects' abdominal muscle activities during maximum trunk extension ranged from 32% to 68% of their longissimus activities. As would be expected, the ipsilateral muscles showed maximum activity in resisted lateral flexion, but the contralateral muscles were also active at about 10% to 20% of the maximum values.

The coordinated patterns among the abdominal muscles are task-specific. But the only muscle that is active in all patterns is the transversus abdominis. During maximum voluntary isometric trunk extension, the transversus abdominis is the only one of the abdominal muscles to show marked activity. It is also the muscle most consistently related to changes in intra-abdominal pressure (IAP) (Cresswell et al. 1992). Not only does the transversus abdominis contract whenever the trunk moves in any direction, but its activity always precedes the contraction of the other trunk muscles in the normal (non-LBP) subject (Cresswell et al. 1994). The ability of the transversus abdominis to contract before other abdominal muscles is a feature of motor control (as described subsequently).

Key point: The transversus abdominis is active in trunk movements in all directions. Its activity always precedes that of the other abdominal muscles in normal subjects.

INTRA-ABDOMINAL PRESSURE MECHANISM

Intra-abdominal pressure (IAP) is sometimes described as intratruncal pressure (Watkins 1999), although this term includes both intra-abdominal and intrathoracic pressure. Intrathoracic pressure is created during inspiration by expanding

the lungs within the rib cage to coincide with a lift or other effort. Although intrathoracic pressure can be useful in competitive sport, I do not emphasize it within this text because the rather complex coordination between it and abdominal hollowing (described later) makes intrathoracic pressure unsuitable for most rehabilitation programs. Timing inspiration with effort, moreover, can lead to use of the Valsalva maneuver, where the breath is held to maintain increased intrathoracic pressure. If done during exercise, the Valsalva can raise blood pressure to dangerous levels (Linsenbardt et al. 1992), an inappropriate situation given the poor health status of many people with back pain.

IAP involves synchronous contraction of the abdominal muscles, the diaphragm, and the muscles of the pelvic floor. The deep abdominals (transversus abdominis and internal oblique) are the most important of the abdominal muscle groups in this respect because they are visceral compressors rather than flexors. Most people experience IAP in everyday life, for example, when the muscles contract reflexively to defend the abdomen from a direct blow. The theoretical basis for the IAP mechanism is that pressure within the abdomen, acting like an inflated balloon against the pelvis and diaphragm, provides additional extensor torque to the spine (figure 3.14); moreover, the "inflated balloon" acts on a

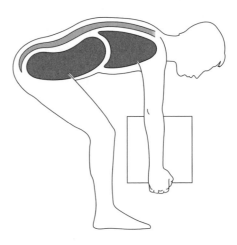

Figure 3.14 Intra-abdominal pressure mechanism. Pressure within the abdomen acting against the pelvis and diaphragm provides additional extensor torque to the spine.

torque arm that is as much as three times greater than that of the erector spinae.

Key point: Intra-abdominal pressure is created by synchronous contraction of the abdominal muscles, the diaphragm, and the muscles of the pelvic floor.

Contraction of the transversus abdominis and the internal oblique increases IAP, providing the glottis is closed. Imagine the trunk as a cylinder. The top of the cylinder is formed by the diaphragm, the bottom the pelvic floor, and the walls the deep abdominals (transversus and internal oblique). As the abdominal wall is pulled in and up, the walls of the cylinder are effectively pulled in. If a deep breath is taken, the diaphragm is lowered, compressing the cylinder from the top. If the pelvic floor (the bottom of the cylinder) is intact, the cylinder is pressurized and made more solid. In this way, it is able to resist any bending stress applied to it.

The IAP is greater if the breath is held following a deep inspiration (Valsalva maneuver) because the diaphragm is lower and the comparative size of the abdominal cavity (the cylinder) is reduced. During lifting, the pelvic floor muscles (the floor of the cylinder) contract to maintain pelvic integrity and prevent urination. The Valsalva maneuver is therefore appropriate for normal subjects during heavy lifting as long as it occurs only briefly. However, because blood pressure changes may not be desirable in subjects with poor cardiopulmonary health, heavy lifting is not recommended for this group.

Making the trunk into a more solid cylinder reduces axial compression and shear loads and transmits loads over a wider area (Twomey and Taylor 1987). IAP may also help to protect the spine from excessive indirect loads (those not acting directly on the spine but through limb loading), with the muscles acting to involuntarily fix the rib cage. IAP is greater when heavy lifts are performed and when the lift is rapid (Davis and Troup 1964).

Abdominal muscle strength affects IAP—strong athletes can produce very large IAP values (Harman et al. 1988). Yet strengthening the abdominal muscles with movements such as sit-ups does not permanently increase IAP (Hemborg et al. 1983) because these exercises usually do not mimic the coordination among abdominal muscles that is inherent in the IAP mechanism (Oliver and Middleditch 1991). Investigating the effect of abdominal muscle training on IAP, Hemborg and colleagues (1985) used isometric trunk curl and twist exercises. Increased recruitment of motor units in the oblique abdominal muscles clearly demonstrated muscle strengthening, yet EMG activity of these muscles decreased during lifting, implying that the subjects did not make functional use of their increased ability to recruit more motor units. The differentiation between strength and functional ability is important: If an exercise is not specific to a task, the physiological adaptation of the musculoskeletal system may be inappropriate. See page 87 for more discussion of training specificity.

Key point: Sit-ups will not permanently raise intra-abdominal pressure.

A number of important criticisms have been made against the IAP mechanism when it has been presented as the only stabilizing process for the spine (Bogduk and Twomey 1987). First, to fully stabilize the spine during the lifting of heavy weights, the IAP would have to exceed the systolic pressure within the aorta, effectively cutting off the blood flow to the viscera and lower limbs. Competitive weightlifters have been known to black out when lifting extremely heavy weight, perhaps because of very high IAP (McGill et al. 1990). At the onset of a lift, there is an initial rapid increase in IAP—known as the snatch pressure—that may last for less than 0.5 s. The pressure declines during the remainder of the lift. Hemborg and colleagues (1985) calculated that a peak IAP of 250 mmHg would be required to lift a 100 kg weight. Second, the muscle force required to create a sufficiently high IAP is greater than the **hoop pressure** possible from the abdominal muscles (Gracovetsky et al. 1985). Third, if the rectus abdominis contracts to increase IAP, it produces a flexion torque that counteracts the antiflexion effect of IAP created as the diaphragm and pelvic floor spread apart. These criticisms of IAP have led to reexamination of its contribution to back stability. Originally, IAP was believed to reduce the compression acting on the lumbar spine by as much as 40% (Eie 1966), but more recent studies have shown this to be only 7% (McGill et al. 1990).

Key point: Intra-abdominal pressure has been estimated to reduce the compression acting on the lumbar spine by only 7%.

To train IAP voluntarily, the subject must contract the pelvic floor muscles and transversus abdominis simultaneously. Ultrasound scanning has shown the thickness of the TrA to be greater (65.8% increase) when contracted with the pelvic floor muscles than without (49.7% increase) (Critchley 2002). Breathing should also be emphasized when retraining IAP, because diaphragm action is important to this mechanism. Using direct stimulation of the phrenic nerve, Hodges and colleagues (2005) showed IAP increases of 31% without TrA contraction—the increase coming from diaphragm action alone.

Key point: Both pelvic floor action and breathing control must be used alongside transversus abdominis action (abdominal hollowing) to train the IAP mechanism.

It may be tempting to see the TrA as the key to the lumbar spine, but just as with the multifidus, isolation of this muscle alone is not enough for full rehabilitation. Many of the studies quoted as targeting the TrA actually used a drawing-in action—abdominal hollowing—described on page 113. Using MRI scanning, Hides and colleagues

(2006) showed that this action significantly increased the CSA of not just the TrA but the internal oblique as well.

Motor Control Strategies

The body's central nervous system (CNS) must continually monitor the forces acting on the spine and the spinal movements themselves. In so doing, the CNS must analyze the present state of stiffness (stability) in the spine and either reduce it to allow unimpeded movement or increase it to reduce unwanted motion. To do this, the CNS receives continuous signals from nerve sensors in the spinal tissues including the joints, discs, ligaments, and muscles.

When people engage in repeated movements, their bodies anticipate the predictable load and the muscles brace themselves accordingly. When back stability is controlled in advance in this way, it is know as *feedforward control*. Using fine-wire electrodes, Hodges and Richardson (1996) assessed abdominal muscle action during 10 repetitions of shoulder flexion, extension, and abduction. They found that the transversus abdominis contracted before the shoulder muscles by as much as 38.9 ms. The reaction time for the deltoid was on average 188 ms, with the abdominal muscles (except transversus) following the deltoid contraction by 9.84 ms. With subjects who had a history of low back pain, however, the contraction of the transversus failed to precede that of the deltoid, indicating that the subjects had lost the anticipatory nature of stability (figure 3.15). This highly significant finding

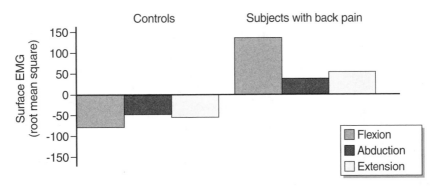

Figure 3.15 Activity of the transversus abdominis muscle during shoulder movements. Note that subjects with back pain had a longer transversus reaction time. Point 0 represents the onset of shoulder movement. EMG = electromyograph.

reveals a uniform dysfunction in the motor control of the transversus abdominis in people with low back pain—the problem is not simply one of muscle strength. It appears that the anticipatory nature of the transversus may be lost in those with low back pain, leaving open the possibility that this mechanism may be redeveloped therapeutically.

Key point: Patients with chronic low back pain exhibit a motor control deficit (alteration in muscle reaction timing and anticipatory bracing) in the transversus abdominis.

A number of authors have highlighted contraction of the abdominal muscles before the initiation of limb movement as an example of a feedforward postural reaction (Aruin and Latash 1995; Friedli et al. 1984). In these cases, as would be expected, the erector spinae and the external oblique contract before arm flexion, whereas the rectus abdominis contracts before arm extension. In each case, the trunk muscles limit the reactive body movement toward the moving limb. Contraction of the transversus before the other abdominal muscle was described by Cresswell and colleagues (1994) in response to trunk movements, but anticipatory contraction of this type during limb movements is a newer finding. The transversus abdominis seems to contract during posture not simply to bring the body back closer to the posture line but to increase the stiffness of the lumbar region and enhance stability (Hodges et al. 1996).

When working in this way, the CNS is predicting the types of stresses that the spine is likely to encounter in an action. How does it know? Throughout life, as we perform actions over and over again, we build up a movement vocabulary, which we are able to use as a reference point against which to compare a new movement. In this process, when the CNS recognizes a familiar movement pattern, it is able to use feedforward motion control to plan ahead and contract the stability muscles by just the right amount to optimally stabilize the spine, without stiffening the spine so much that free movement is compromised. This is a highly skilled action and occurs in many seemingly mundane actions through our daily lives.

Key point: Feedforward motor control anticipates what stability will be required by comparing against an internal reference map of familiar actions.

When more complex actions are performed, especially those that demand a subject's close attention, the contraction latency (waiting time before contraction occurs) of muscles will change. If the brain has to throw its attention into catching a ball, for example, the muscle contraction of a moving limb seems to hesitate and so the limb contraction latency is longer. However, the latency period for the stabilizing muscles of the spine has been shown not to change (Hodges and Richardson 1999), suggesting that stability is an automatic action that does not require a lot of thinking—it is not under higher center control.

When movements are not predictable, the CNS measures stress imposed on the lumbar tissues, and when it determines that this stress is excessive, the CNS invokes a protective response; this is an example of feedback motor control. This is partially attributable to rapid protective reflexes such as the stretch reflex within the muscle spindles of the spinal muscles themselves. This type of reflex is short loop (local to the spinal cord) and has also been shown to occur in spinal muscles through stimulation of the disc annulus (Holm et al. 2002), ligaments, and facet joint capsules (Indahl et al. 1997). Long-loop reflexes occur more slowly, involve the spinal cord and brain, and are thought to have a greater role in postural error correction (Hodges 2004).

Key point: Feedback motor control measures stress imposed on spinal tissues and causes muscle responses after the stress has occurred.

SUMMARY

- The human spine is inherently unstable without its musculature.
- The interspinous and supraspinous ligaments, facet joint capsules, and thoracolumbar fascia (TLF) together provide passive

support for the spine sufficient to balance between 24% and 55% of imposed flexion stress.

- The posterior ligamentous system stabilizes the spine passively and through elastic recoil.

- The TLF stabilizes the spine through three primary mechanisms: (1) passive resistance through its connections with the transversus abdominis muscle; (2) hydraulic amplification, as it restricts expansion of the erector spinae; and (3) form closure and force closure of the sacroiliac joint.

- Of the deep intersegmental muscles, the multifidus is most important for stabilizing the spine by helping to control lordosis and for neutralizing spinal flexion. Following low back injury, exercise therapy is required to restore multifidus function.

- Of the superficial back muscles, the erector spinae is most significant for back stabilization. The endurance rather than strength of this muscle is particularly important.

- Of the abdominal muscles, the internal oblique and transversus abdominis are the major back stabilizers rather than the more superficial external oblique and rectus abdominis. The ratio in which these muscles are used is more important than mere muscle strength.

- The key to effective abdominal training in sport is to train for trunk stability before training for trunk muscle performance.

- People with low back pain tend to favor the more external abdominal muscles. Abdominal hollowing (rather than sit-ups), however, activates the internal oblique and transversus muscles, and because an important aim of rehabilitation is to help patients learn to dissociate use of the deeper muscles from use of the more superficial muscles, learning to practice abdominal hollowing is a vital part of rehabilitation.

- During movements, the deep abdominals are recruited to stabilize the spine through both feedforward and feedback motor control.

Chapter 4
Principles
of Muscle Imbalance

Muscle imbalance occurs when one muscle (the **agonist**) is significantly stronger than the opposing muscle (the **antagonist**) or when one or the other is abnormally shortened or lengthened. The body's attempts to compensate for imbalance cause an impairment in movement, or *movement dysfunction*. This impairment generally exacerbates the problem and can lead to serious disability. This chapter presents the theory of muscle balance and imbalance, and chapter 6 details tests to identify such problems.

BASIC CONCEPTS

We can categorize muscles into two nondistinct groups (Janda and Schmid 1980; Richardson 1992): Muscles that primarily stabilize a joint and approximate the joint surfaces are known as stabilizers or postural muscles, and muscles primarily responsible for movement (those that develop angular rotation more effectively than the stabilizers), are called mobilizers or task muscles.

Key point: Stabilizers (postural muscles) primarily fix a joint and prevent excessive movement. Mobilizers (task muscles) primarily create motion of a body part.

Stability muscles tend to be more deeply placed in the body and are usually monoarticular (one-joint) muscles, whereas mobilizers are superficial and are often biarticular (two-joint) muscles. For example, in the leg, the rectus femoris is classified as a mobilizer, whereas the other quadriceps muscles are stabilizers. Stabilizer function is more

slow-twitch (type I) or tonic in nature, whereas the mobilizers tend toward fast-twitch (type II) action. This physiology suits the functional requirements of the muscles, enabling mobilizers to contract and develop maximal tension rapidly but also to fatigue quickly. The stabilizer muscles build tension slowly and perform well at lower tensions over longer periods, being more fatigue resistant. Take as an example the calf muscles. The gastrocnemius is classified as a mobilizer, powering us away from the blocks in a sprint. The soleus muscle is a stabilizer, being responsible for postural body sway in standing.

Stabilizers can be subdivided into primary and secondary types (Jull 1994) (table 4.1). The primary stabilizers (e.g., multifidus, transversus abdominis, and vastus medialis oblique) have very deep attachments, lying close to the axis of rotation of the joint. In this position, they are unable to contribute any significant torque but will approximate the joint. In addition, many of these smaller muscles have important proprioceptive functions (Bastide et al. 1989). For example, the intertransversarii muscles of the lumbar spine, which attach between the transverse processes, and the interspinales muscles lying between the spinous processes both have a dense concentration of muscle spindles indicating a significant proprioceptive function (Adams et al. 2002). The secondary stabilizers (e.g., gluteals and oblique abdominals) are the main torque producers, being large monoarticular muscles attaching via extensive aponeuroses. Their multipennate fiber arrangement makes them powerful and able to absorb large amounts of force through eccentric action. The mobilizers (e.g., rectus femoris and hamstrings) act as stabilizers only in conditions of extreme need. When they do, the precision of movement is often lost, creating an observable

Table 4.1 Muscle Types

The following characteristics are not absolute but are only tendencies within these sometimes inexact categories of muscles.

Stablilizers		Mobilizers
Primarily responsible for stabilizing and approximating joints		Primarily responsible for movement, including angular rotation
Examples: multifidus, transversus abdominis, vastus medialis oblique		Examples: rectus femoris, hamstrings
PRIMARY STABILIZERS	SECONDARY STABILIZERS	
Deep, close to joint	Intermediate depth	Superficial
Slow twitch	Slow twitch	Fast twitch
Usually monoarticular (1 joint)	Usually monoarticular	Often biarticular (2 joints)
No significant torque	Primary source of torque	Secondary source of torque
Short fibers	Attachments are multipennate	
Build tension slowly, more fatigue resistant		Build tension rapidly, fatigue quickly
Better activated at low levels of resistance		Better activated at high levels of resistance
More effective in closed chain movement		More effective in open chain movements
In muscle imbalance, tend to weaken and lengthen		In muscle imbalance, tend to tighten and shorten

movement dysfunction. They are fusiform in shape—a less powerful fiber arrangement but one able to produce large ranges of motion.

Key point: If stabilizer muscles fail to function, stability may be temporarily provided by mobilizer muscles instead. The precision of movement is lost, leading to an observable movement dysfunction.

Stabilizer muscles are better activated at low resistance levels—about 30% to 40% of the maximum voluntary contraction—whereas mobilizer muscles are generally better activated above this level. Reeducating the muscles of back stability, therefore, calls for low-level contractions, not the extreme workouts that well-meaning trainers sometimes prescribe for low back pain. In addition, stabilizer muscles respond better to closed kinetic chain actions, where movement occurs proximally on a stabilized distal segment; in standing, this would be with the foot on the ground for the lower limb or the hand on a wall for the upper limb. Mobilizer function is more effective in an open chain situation, where free movement occurs without distal fixation. In the lower limb, the swing phase of gait is open chain; in the upper limb, throwing is a prime example. The structure and functional characteristics of the two muscle categories make the stabilizers better equipped for postural holding and antigravity function. The mobilizers are better designed for the rapid ballistic movements seen in competitive

Table 4.2   Stabilizer and Mobilizer Muscles That Affect the Low Back

Stabilizers	Mobilizers
Primary stabilizers	Iliopsoas*
Multifidus	Hamstrings
Transversus abdominis	Rectus femoris
Internal oblique	Tensor fasciae lata
Gluteus medius	Hip adductors
Vastus medialis	Piriformis
Serratus anterior	Rectus abdominis
Lower trapezius	External oblique
Deep neck flexors	Quadratus lumborum*
	Erector spinae
Secondary stabilizers	Sternomastoid
Gluteus maximus	Upper trapezius*
Quadriceps	Levator scapulae
Iliopsoas*	Rhomboids
Subscapularis	Pectoralis minor
Infraspinatus	Pectoralis major
Upper trapezius*	Scalenes
Quadratus lumborum*	

*Can act as both stabilizers and mobilizers in different situations.

sport. Stabilizer and mobilizer muscles affecting the low back are listed in table 4.2.

Three fundamental changes appear when there is muscle imbalance: The first is tightening of mobilizer (two-joint) muscles, and the second is loss of endurance (holding) within the inner range of motion of the single-joint stabilizer muscles, which arises from their being abnormally stretched. These two changes are used as tests for the degree of muscle imbalance present. Because changes in length and tension alter muscle pull around a joint, they may alter either static or dynamic alignment, giving rise to the third fundamental change: movement impairment or dysfunction.

Key point: Muscle imbalance is identified through tight muscles, lax muscles, and movement impairment.

Changes in body segment alignment and the degree of segmental control (the ability to move one body segment without moving any others) form the basis of the movement impairment tests used to assess muscle imbalance. The mixture of tightness and weakness in muscle imbalance alters body segment alignment and changes the equilibrium point of a joint. Normally, the equal resting tone of agonist and antagonist muscles allows the joint to assume a balanced resting position, with the joint surfaces evenly loaded and the joint's inert tissues not excessively stressed. However, if the muscles on one side of a joint are tight and the opposing muscles are lax, the joint will be pulled out of alignment toward the tight muscle (figure 4.1). This alteration in alignment throws weight-bearing stress onto a smaller region of the joint surface, increasing pressure per unit area. Furthermore, the inert tissues on the shortened (closed) side of the joint will contract over time.

The combination of stiffness (hypoflexibility) in one body segment and laxity (hyperflexibility) in an adjacent segment leads to the development of relative flexibility (White and Sahrmann 1994). In a chain of movement, the body seems to take the path of least resistance, with the more flexible segment always contributing more to the total movement range. Consider two pieces of rubber tubing of unequal strengths that are attached to one another (figure 4.2). If the movement begins at C and A is fixed, the more flexible area B–C

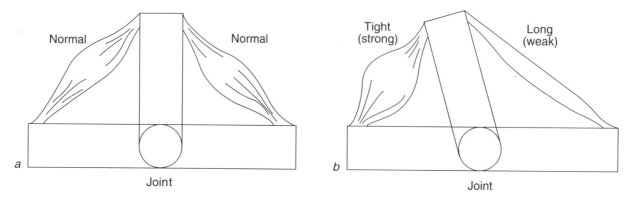

Figure 4.1   Posture and muscle imbalance. *(a)* Equal muscle tone gives correct joint alignment. *(b)* Unequal muscle tone pulls joint out of alignment, resulting in faulty posture.

Reprinted, by permission, from J.C. Griffin, 1998, *Client-centered exercise prescription* (Champaign, IL: Human Kinetics), 176.

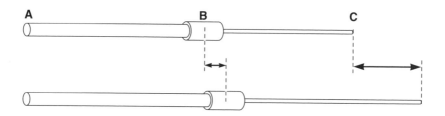

Figure 4.2   Relative flexibility. When the attached cords are stretched, the tighter cord (A–B) moves less than the looser cord (B–C).

Reprinted from *Sports injuries: Diagnosis and management*, 2nd ed., C.M. Norris, page. Copyright 1998, with permission from Elsevier.

moves more. This will still be the case if C is held immobile and A moves.

To relate the example in figure 4.2 to the human body, figure 4.3 shows a toe-touching exercise. The two areas of interest for relative flexibility are the hamstrings and lumbar spine tissues. As we flex forward, movement should occur through a combination of anterior pelvic tilt and lumbar spinal flexion. Many people have tight hamstrings and excessively lax lumbar tissues attributable to excessive bending (lumbar flexion) during everyday activities. During this flexing action, greater movement (and therefore greater tissue strain) always occurs at the lumbar spine. Relative stiffness in this case makes the toe-touching exercise ineffective as a hamstring stretch unless the trunk muscles are tightened to stabilize the lumbar spine.

Key point: Muscle imbalance can lead to changes in both function and structure of the body tissues.

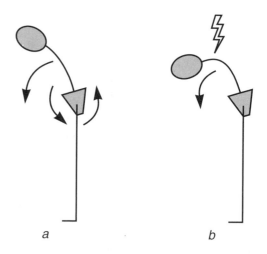

Figure 4.3   Relative stiffness in the body. *(a)* Forward flexion should combine equal pelvic tilt and spinal flexion. *(b)* Tight hamstrings limit pelvic tilt, stressing the more lax spinal tissues.

Reprinted from *Sports injuries: Diagnosis and management*, 2nd ed., C.M. Norris, page 145. Copyright 1998, with permission from Elsevier.

MUSCLE ADAPTATION TO INCREASED AND DECREASED USAGE

Different kinds of muscles react differently to injury and immobilization. *Injury* is normally accompanied by pain and swelling, both stimuli for muscle inhibition. *Immobilization* involves an enforced reduction in activity and is often studied in patients undergoing bed rest. This must be differentiated from *deload,* in which there is a reduction in weight bearing even though some activity may continue. Deload is normally studied using weightlessness and microgravity studies.

Immobilization and Deload

By studying immobilized limbs, Appell (1990) found that the greatest tissue changes occur within the first few days of disuse. Strength loss can be as much as 6% per day for the first 8 days, with minimal loss after this period.

Type I and Type II muscle fibers differ considerably in response to disuse, with Type I fibers showing greater reduction in size and greater loss of total fiber numbers than Type II. In fact, the number of Type II fibers actually increases—demonstrating a process of selective atrophy of the Type I fibers (Templeton et al. 1984). However, not all muscles show an equal amount of Type I fiber atrophy. Atrophy is largely related to change in use relative to normal function, with the initial percentage of Type I fibers that a muscle contains being a good indicator of likely atrophy pattern. Those muscles with a predominantly antigravity function, which cross one joint and have a large proportion of Type I fibers (e.g., the soleus and vastus medialis muscles), show greatest selective atrophy. Predominantly slow-twitch antigravity muscles that cross multiple joints are next in order of atrophy (e.g., erector spinae). Finally, the phasic, predominantly fast Type II muscles (e.g., biceps) can be immobilized with less loss of strength than the other two groups (Lieber 1992).

The loss of Type I fiber density is very noticeable. Haggmark and colleagues (1986) demonstrated a decrease in Type I fiber area in a cross-country skier from 81% to 58% in just 6 weeks of inactivity. Selective atrophy is equally dramatic; a rat model was used to demonstrate Type I area decrease of 60% for the soleus (stabilizer muscle, single joint) but only 17% for the plantaris (mobilizer muscle, two joint) in the calf (Thomason et al. 1987).

The muscle fiber changes that occur are attributable to two mechanisms (Thompson 2002). For the first 3 days of immobilization and deload, there is a significant decrease in myofibril synthesis; following this period synthesis stabilizes and protein loss is attributed to an increase in degradation rate.

Key point: Loss of Type I fibers through immobilization and deload occurs through two distinct mechanisms: decreased myofibril synthesis and increased fiber degradation rate.

Pain and Swelling

We discussed in chapter 3 that the multifidus muscle shows a rapid reduction in cross-sectional area (CSA) in patients with low back pain (Hides et al. 1994) that is accompanied later by a reduction in Type I (slow twitch) muscle fibers attributable to cessation of normal physical activity. This initial CSA change is thought to occur through inhibition attributable to pain and swelling, described as *arthrogenous inhibition.* Similar changes have been shown in the knee, where the oblique fibers of vastus medialis are affected (Stokes and Young 1984), and in the hip, where the gluteus medius changes. This CSA reduction is not simply attributable to the presence of pain, however, but occurs more through stimuli from the joint. Investigating the effects of pain on quadriceps inhibition following knee surgery, Shakespeare and colleagues (1985) gave subjects an interarticular injection of local anesthesia and found muscle inhibition to still be at 35% 10 days postoperatively even though pain had gone.

Muscle inhibition and atrophy of this type are highly selective, with significant quadriceps wastage but little change to the hamstrings. This change is thought to occur through stimulation of joint receptors that have flexor excitatory and extensor inhibitory actions (Young et al. 1987). Clearly, joint arthrogenous inhibition of this type is one cause of muscle imbalance.

Key point: Arthrogenous inhibition occurs following swelling in a joint. Atrophy is selective, creating muscle imbalance.

Training

Training also causes selective changes in muscle. In the knee, rapid flexion–extension actions can selectively increase activity in the rectus femoris and hamstrings (biarticular mobilizers) but not in the vasti (monoarticular stabilizers). In a study by Richardson and Bullock (1986) comparing speeds of 75°/s and 195°/s, mean muscle activity for the rectus femoris increased from 23.0 mV to 69.9 mV. In contrast, muscle activity for the vastus medialis increased from 35.5 mV to only 42.3 mV (figure 4.4). The pattern of muscle activity was also noticeably different after training. The rectus femoris and hamstrings displayed phasic (on-and-off) activity at the fastest speeds, whereas the vastus medialis showed a tonic (continuous) pattern. The graphs in figure 4.5 show an electromyographic trace of the electrical activity produced when a muscle contracts. The general trend of the graph shape is important, rather than each individual line. Note that there are clear groups of electrical spikes for the rectus femoris and the hamstrings, indicating that activity occurred in these muscles at specific points in the total movement. For the vastus medialis there are no clear groups, indicating that the activity occurred continually throughout the movement.

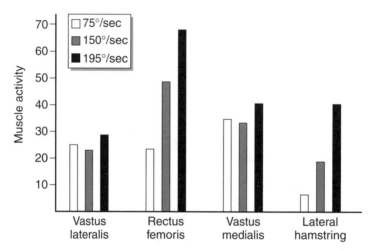

Figure 4.4　**Muscle activity changes with increases in speed.**

Reprinted, by permission, from C.A. Richardson and M.I Bullock, 1986, "Changes in muscle activity during fast, alternating flexion-extension movements of the knee," *Scandinavian Journal of Rehabilitation Medicine* 18: 51-58.

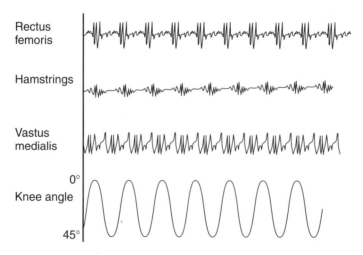

Figure 4.5　**Muscle activity patterns during rapid alternating knee flexion–extension. Note that biarticular muscles are phasic, whereas monoarticular muscles are tonic.**

Reprinted, by permission, from C.A. Richardson and M.I Bullock, 1986, "Changes in muscle activity during fast, alternating flexion-extension movements of the knee," *Scandinavian Journal of Rehabilitation Medicine* 18: 51-58.

Ng and Richardson (1990) found similar changes even in the more functional closed kinetic chain position. A 4-week training period of rapid plantar flexion (in standing position) gave significant increases in jump height (gastrocnemius, biarticular) but also significant losses of static function of the soleus (monoarticular).

Recruitment patterns of low back muscles also change depending on the type of training used (O'Sullivan et al. 1998). Subjects followed a 10-week training program involving either abdominal hollowing (15 min daily, progressed with limb loading) or gym exercise that included trunk curls. Electromyographic activity of the internal oblique (more important for back stability) increased in the hollowing group, whereas that of the rectus abdominis remained relatively unchanged. Trunk curls (but not hollowing) led to an increase in rectus abdominis activity and a reduction in activity of the internal oblique (figure 4.6).

Key point: Selective muscle changes occur following training. This feature can cause muscle imbalance or can be used to rebalance the muscle system.

TRAINING SPECIFICITY

The differences in responses of stabilizer and mobilizer muscles illustrate the importance of training specificity. Responses to training closely correspond to the type of exercise used. For example, if runners want to reduce their marathon running time, sprint training will not be effective. This is because sprinting is primarily an anaerobic activity (energy supplied from stores within the body), whereas marathon training is predominantly aerobic (energy supplied by using oxygen and food as fuel). We can say in this case that although the sprint training caused an increase in fitness, the aspect of fitness that improved was not strictly relevant to the event that the training was designed for. The training was not specific to the event.

In the same way, we have seen that high-speed muscle training leads to recruitment of mobilizer muscles. In the example from Richardson and Bullock (1986) described previously, the rectus femoris increased its activity markedly at high-speed (195°/s) movements. If we used this high-speed training to try to improve the vastus medialis, it would not be very effective. To retrain this muscle we would do better to choose slower exercise at lighter resistances, emphasizing precision of movement.

Specificity can be remembered by a simple mnemonic, SAID, which stands for specific adaptation to imposed demand. The change occurring in the body (the adaptation) is specific to (exactly matches) the training used (the imposed demand). You can adequately address your clients' muscle imbalances only by using quite specific exercises—and this in turn requires accurate muscle assessment. The tests described in chapter 6 will help you target the right muscles.

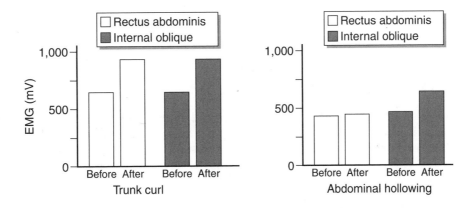

Figure 4.6 Altered abdominal muscle recruitment pattern with training. EMG = electromyograph.

Data from P.B. O'Sullivan, L. Twomey, and G.T. Allison, 1998, "Altered abdominal muscle recruitment in patients with chronic back pain following a specific exercise intervention," *Journal of Orthopedic and Sports Physical Therapy* 27: 114-124.

Key point: Training specificity dictates that when designing an exercise program for a client, you must consider factors such as functional requirement, muscle contraction type, and movement range and speed.

CHANGES IN MUSCLE LENGTH

Changes in muscle length do not occur in a uniform manner throughout the body. An overly simplistic but useful description is that stabilizer muscles tend to weaken (sag), whereas mobilizers tend to shorten (tighten). Exercise therapy aimed at muscle must therefore be selective rather than general, seeking to lengthen (stretch) tight mobilizer muscles and shorten and build endurance of inactive stabilizer muscles.

Chronic Muscle Lengthening

The weakening of stabilizer muscles has been termed *stretch weakness* (Kendall et al. 1993): The muscle remains in an elongated position, beyond its normal resting position but within its normal range. This is different from overstretch, in which the muscle is elongated beyond its normal range.

The length–tension relationship of a muscle (p. 34) dictates that a stretched muscle, where the actin and myosin filaments are pulled apart, can exert less force than a muscle at normal resting length. Where the stretch is maintained, however, this short-term response (reduced force output) becomes a long-term adaptation: The muscle adds more sarcomeres to its ends in an attempt to move its actin and myosin filaments closer together (figure 4.7). This adaptation, known as an increase in serial sarcomere number (SSN), can lengthen a muscle by up to 20% (Gossman et al. 1982).

Key point: Stretched muscle exerts less contractile form because its fibers are drawn apart. When the stretch is maintained, structural changes occur in the fibers.

The length–tension curve of an adaptively lengthened muscle moves to the right (figure 4.8). The peak tension that such a muscle can produce in the laboratory is up to 35% greater than that of a normal-length muscle (Williams and Goldspink 1978). However, this peak tension occurs at approximately the position where the muscle has been immobilized (point *a*, figure 4.8). If the strength of the lengthened muscle is tested with the joint in midrange or inner range (point

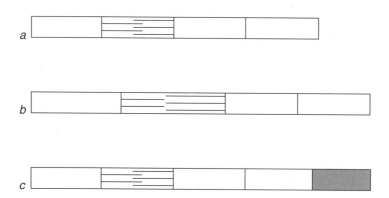

Figure 4.7 Muscle length adaptation. *(a)* Normal muscle length. *(b)* In stretched muscle, the filaments move apart, resulting in loss of muscle tension. *(c)* Normal filament alignment is restored by increases in serial sarcomere number, resulting in chronic abnormal muscle length.

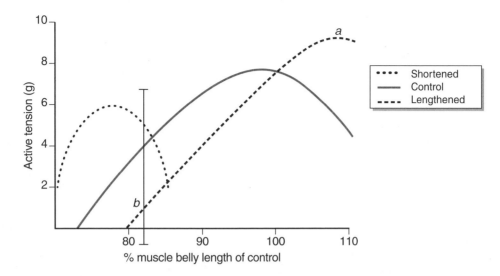

Figure 4.8 Effects of immobilizing a muscle in shortened and lengthened positions (see text for explanation).
Reprinted from *Sports injuries: Diagnosis and management,* 2nd ed, C.M. Norris, page 148. Copyright 1998, with permission from Elsevier.

b, figure 4.8), as is common in clinical practice, the muscle cannot produce its peak tension and appears weak. For this reason, manual muscle tests appear to be more accurate indicators of positional strength than are measures of total strength (Sahrmann 1987).

In the laboratory, a lengthened muscle returns to its optimal length within approximately 1 week if placed in a shortened position (Goldspink 1992). Clinically, restoration of optimal length may be achieved by immobilizing the muscle in its physiological rest position (Kendall et al. 1993) or by exercising it in its shortened (inner-range) position (Sahrmann 1990). Enhancement of strength is not the priority in this situation—indeed, the load on the muscle may need to be reduced to ensure correct alignment of the various body segments and correct performance of the relevant movement pattern.

SSN may be partly responsible for changes in muscle strength without parallel changes in hypertrophy (Koh 1995). A number of factors influence SSN, which exhibits marked plasticity. For example, immobilization of rabbit plantar flexors in a lengthened position showed an 8% increase in SSN in only 4 days; applying electrical stimulation to increase muscle force led to an even greater increase (Williams et al. 1986). Stretching

a muscle appears to affect SSN significantly more than does immobilization in a shortened position. Following immobilization in a shortened position for 2 weeks, the mouse soleus decreased SSN by almost 20% (Williams 1990). However, stretching for just 1 hr per day in this study not only eliminated the SSN reduction but actually increased SSN by nearly 10%.

Key point: Reduction of serial sarcomere number (SSN) caused by inactivity or immobilization is reversed by stretching.

Eccentric stimuli appear to cause a greater adaptation of SSN than do concentric stimuli. Morgan and Lynn (1994) subjected rats to uphill or downhill running and found SSN in the vastus intermedius to be 12% greater in the eccentric-trained rats after 1 week. Koh (1995) suggested that if SSN adaptation occurs in humans, strength training may produce such a change if it is performed at a joint angle different from that at which the maximal force is produced during normal activity.

The lengthened muscle is not weak—it merely lacks the ability to maintain full contraction within the inner range. This shows up clinically as a difference between the active and passive inner ranges. If the joint is passively placed in full anatomical inner range, the subject is unable to hold the position. Sometimes the position cannot be held at all, but more usually the contraction cannot be sustained, indicating a lack in slow-twitch endurance capacity.

Clinically, reduction of muscle length is seen as the enhanced ability to hold an inner-range contraction. This may or may not represent a reduction in SSN but is a required functional improvement in postural control for muscles that are abnormally lengthened. Muscle shortening appears in the dorsiflexors of equestrians, who clearly do not hold the shortened position permanently, as with splinting, but rather show a training response. Following pregnancy, SSN increases in the rectus abdominis in combination with diastasis. Again, length of the muscle gradually reduces in the months following birth. Inner-range training, then, is likely to shorten a lengthened muscle (Goldspink 1992).

SUMMARY

- Muscles can be divided into stabilizer or mobilizer types.
- Stabilizer muscles tend to be deep, to contain mainly slow-twitch fibers, to control only one joint, and primarily to prevent movement while stabilizing a joint. They are the primary postural muscles.
- Mobilizer muscles tend to be more superficial, to contain mainly fast-twitch fibers, to act over two joints, and primarily to create movement.
- Disuse, long-term bed rest, and injury can cause muscle systems to become imbalanced—one muscle is shortened and another lax.
- To train specific muscles, you must carefully target these in your exercise prescriptions.
- You can treat muscle imbalance by prescribing exercises that strengthen or shorten the lax muscle and stretch the shortened muscle.

Part II
Establishing Stability

In part I of this book we established the theory behind back stability, which provides the evidence base for our clinical work with clients. In part II we put this theory into practice. We begin by assessing posture and using our findings to develop an exercise therapy program to optimize posture in chapter 5. As part of this postural optimization, we take a muscle balance approach and use tests to identify specific imbalance faults that we then target in chapter 6. Chapter 7 moves us from this point to the development of core stability. Although these three chapters have been written separately for clarity, when you are working with your client there will be much overlap. This is because you will have to adapt your exercise therapy prescription to the clinical needs of your client and further adapt depending on the how your client reacts to a particular exercise. Some exercises will be more suitable for some clients than others. The old adage, "adopt, adapt, and modify," is very relevant here. Be prepared to modify and fine-tune each exercise to the needs of your client.

Key point: Be flexible with your exercise therapy prescription. Be prepared to modify individual exercises, and alternate between exercises, according to the developing needs of your client.

Chapter 5
Posture

Because postural alignment reflects changes in muscle length, it is usually the first form of assessment you will use to determine muscle imbalance. Before you can diagnose changes in alignment, however, you need a standard of optimal posture. The body moves continually around the optimal position in a process called *body sway,* and back stability is an essential component of this mechanism. In this chapter, I describe four principal types of posture.

OPTIMAL POSTURAL ALIGNMENT

Posture is the arrangement of body parts in a state of balance that protects the supporting structures of the body against injury or progressive deformity—a definition given in 1947 by the Posture Committee of the American Academy of Orthopaedic Surgeons (Cailliet 1983). A good posture is therefore effortless, nonfatiguing, and painless when the person remains erect for reasonable periods (Cailliet 1981). Muscles function most efficiently in such an alignment, and the joints are optimally positioned (Bullock-Saxton 1988).

Optimal posture combines both minimal muscle work and minimal joint loading. The combination of these two factors is important—where optimal posture is lost (e.g., in slouched standing), the muscle activity is clearly reduced, but there is a significant increase in joint loading.

Joint loading should be minimized over time—articular cartilage gains its nutrition through intermittent loading (Norris 1998), and an even distribution of force is preferable to point pressure. Contact pressure is directly proportional to the transmitted force but inversely proportional to area (McConnell 1993). Distributing force over a larger area by optimizing segmental alignment, therefore, reduces joint surface compression and lessens the risk of degenerative changes to a joint. The aim of any posture should be to reduce total energy expenditure and lessen stress on the supporting body structures.

Key point: Good posture reduces total energy expenditure and lessens the stress on the supporting body structures.

Any change in the alignment of one body segment automatically causes neighboring segments to move in an attempt to maintain stability. If one body segment moves forward, for example, another must move backward to keep the body's line of gravity (LOG) within the base of support (figure 5.1). Over time, changes in force per unit area cause tissue adaptation (Norkin and Levangie 1992). Changes in serial sarcomere number within muscles, for example, are adaptations to postural changes over time. Shortening ligaments lead to reduced range of motion, whereas lengthening ligaments reduce a joint's passive stability.

Static posture—when the body is stationary—reflects the alignment of body segments and is affected by both changes in load distribution across joints and resting muscle length. Such postures include standing, sitting, and lying. Dynamic posture—body position during movement—can give information about body segment alignment, muscle actions, and motor skill.

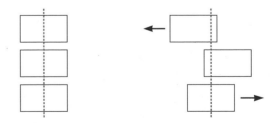

Figure 5.1 When one body segment moves out of alignment, a neighboring segment moves in the opposite direction to maintain the line of gravity within the base of support.

Typical dynamic postures are walking, running, jumping, and lifting. You can use descriptions of both position (kinematic) and force (kinetic) to assess posture.

Excessive changes in posture from the optimal position can give rise to asymmetrical tissue tension. Ultimately, tissue failure can result from repeated passive tissue strain. Avoidance of end-range postures that load the soft tissues excessively may reduce short-term pain as well as long-term pain caused by overuse. Scannell and McGill (2003) studied subjects who had either increased lordosis (hyperlordosis) or reduced lordosis (hypolordosis). The investigators modified subjects' posture using a 12-week exercise program and demonstrated a change in posture toward a midrange (neutral) lordosis.

Key point: Static posture reflects body segment alignment at one moment in time only. Dynamic posture involves alignment during movement.

POSTURAL STABILITY AND BODY SWAY

When standing erect, the human body has a small base of support attributable to its bipedal stance and comparatively high center of gravity (approximately at the second sacral segment). Humans are thus relatively unstable compared with quadrupeds (four-legged animals), which have a larger base of support and lower center of gravity. Maintaining an erect posture takes surprisingly little energy, however, as a result of constant motion brought about by postural control. This motion (postural sway) depends on kinesthesis, or motion sense, which enables us to detect the position of our body parts through organs of proprioception, vision, the vestibular apparatus in the inner ear, and skin receptors. Normal postural sway consists of a small continuous motion in the sagittal plane. This oscillation of the center of gravity results from alternating muscle activity—possibly a relief mechanism to reduce lower-limb fatigue and to aid blood flow (Bullock-Saxton et al. 1991).

Excessive postural sway generally reveals poor balance and stability, a situation commonly seen in elderly and inactive people. Heavy people

also may exhibit greater body sway (Sugano and Takeya 1970), as may tall people (Murray et al. 1975). Training usually can reduce postural sway. In elderly people, strength training may improve stability and limit postural sway (Hughes et al. 1996). Following ankle injury, postural sway increases, but balance and coordination training can return body sway to normal values (Bernier and Perrin 1998). Levels of postural sway can predict risk of recurrent falls among frail nursing home residents (Thapa et al. 1996). Lord and colleagues (1996) reduced fracture risk in women (ages 60-85) using a general aerobic exercise program whose effect was to improve postural sway rather than to change bone density.

Key point: Postural body sway is greater when balance and stability are poor. Exercise that includes balance and coordination training can restore body sway to normal values.

BASIC POSTURAL ASSESSMENT

Basic postural assessment gives you an overview of your client's alignment. It enables you to focus more closely on areas of poor alignment with more specific tests.

Line of Gravity

You can assess static posture through comparisons to a standard reference line (Kendall et al. 1993) that represents the line of gravity (LOG). This method has been shown to be as effective as projected shadow measures and electromagnetic evaluation to assess suboptimal posture (McLean et al. 1996).

The laws of physics dictate that the LOG must pass within the body's base of support to maintain stability. The closer the body segments are to the LOG, the less torque there is around a joint. Where the LOG passes through the joint axis, no torque is created around that joint at all. If the LOG passes some distance from the joint axis, gravitational torque would tend to move the body segment toward the line of gravity were the segment not counterbalanced by elastic recoil of soft tissue and

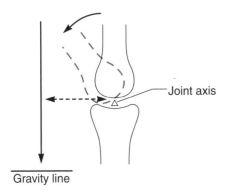

Joint axis

Gravity line

Figure 5.2 When the gravity line falls outside a joint, the proximal body segment tends to move toward the gravity line.

muscle action (Norkin and Levangie 1992). With the LOG anterior to the joint axis, the proximal segment of the body connected to the joint tends to move anteriorly (figure 5.2); posterior motion tends to occur when the LOG is posterior to the joint axis.

In the standard posture viewed from the side, the subject is positioned with a plumb line representing the LOG, passing just in front of the **lateral malleolus** (the bulge on the outside of the ankle). In an ideal posture, this line should pass just anterior to the midline of the knee and then through the greater trochanter, bodies of the lumbar vertebrae, shoulder joint, bodies of the cervical vertebrae, and lobe of the ear (figure 5.3). Because the LOG is anterior to the ankle joint, gravity is continuously pulling the tibia anteriorly. This would result in enough dorsiflexion to unbalance the body were it not for constant opposing resistance provided by muscle action from the soleus (Norkin and Levangie 1992). The LOG passes in front of the knee joint axis (but behind the patella), forcing the femur anteriorly and creating an extension torque resisted by the posterior knee structures. Table 5.1 shows the gravitational torques created by the position of the LOG and the opposing structures resisting these torques.

When viewed from the front, with the feet 3 to 4 in. (7-10 cm) apart, the LOG should bisect the body into two equal halves. The anterior superior iliac spines (ASIS) should be approximately in the same horizontal plane, and the pubis and ASIS should be in the same vertical plane (Kendall et al. 1993). This alignment defines the neutral lumbar–pelvic alignment, which typically is about

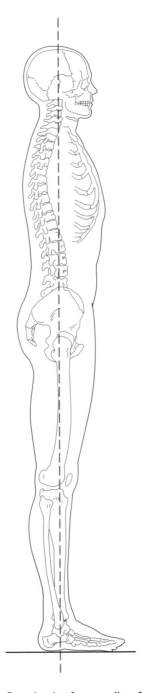

Figure 5.3 Standard reference line for posture.
Reprinted, by permission, from J.C. Griffin, 1998, *Client-centered exercise prescription* (Champaign, IL: Human Kinetics), 66.

5° to the horizontal. The joint axes of the hips, knees, and ankles should be equidistant from the LOG, and the LOG should transect the vertebral bodies (Norkin and Levangie 1992). The gravitational torque imposed on one side of the body should equal that of the other side.

Table 5.1 Normal Alignment in the Sagittal Plane

Joints	Line of gravity	Gravitational torque	OPPOSING FORCES Passive opposing forces	Active opposing forces
Atlanto-occipital	Anterior to transverse axis for flexion and extension	Flexion	Ligamentum nuchae; tectorial membrane	Posterior neck muscles
Cervical	Posterior	Extension	Anterior longitudinal ligament	
Thoracic	Anterior	Flexion	Posterior longitudinal ligament; ligamentum flavum; supraspinous ligament	Extensors
Lumbar	Posterior	Extension	Anterior longitudinal ligament	
Sacroiliac joint	Anterior	Flexion type motion	Sacrotuberous ligament; sacrospinous ligament; sacroiliac ligament	
Hip joint	Posterior	Extension	Iliofemoral ligament	Iliopsoas
Knee joint	Anterior	Extension	Posterior joint capsule	
Ankle joint	Anterior	Dorsiflexion		Soleus

From Norkin, CC and Levangie, PK: Joint structure and function: A comprehensive analysis, 2nd ed. FA Davis, Philadelphia, 1992, p. 433, with permission.

Anatomical landmarks that provide comparisons for horizontal level on the right and left sides of the body include the knee creases, buttock creases, pelvic rim, inferior angle of the scapulae, acromion processes, ears, and external occipital protuberances. You also can observe alignment of the spinous processes and rib angles; minor scoliosis becomes more evident when assessed in Adam's position (forward flexion in standing). Unequal distances between arms and trunk (referred to as the *keyhole*), various skin creases, or unequal muscle bulk should prompt closer examination. You should also assess foot and ankle alignment.

Using the Posture Charts

Tables 5.2 and 5.3 provide simple checklists for postural assessment in the clinic. For each, view the subject from behind (table 5.2) and then the side (table 5.3). When viewing from behind, assess the symmetry of each body part shown in the first column of table 5.2 by comparing the right and left sides of the body. Record your observations in the

Table 5.2   Assessing Standing Posture From Behind

	Position of body part	Notes
	Head position	
	Shoulder level	
	Position of shoulder blade alignment	
	Skin creases at waist and spinal alignment	
	Level of buttock creases	
	Level of knee creases	
	Calf muscle bulk and Achilles alignment	
	Flat foot or high arch	

Reprinted from *Sports injuries: Diagnosis and management,* 2nd ed., C.M. Norris, copyright 1998, with permission from Elsevier.

Table 5.3 Posture Assessment From the Side

	Position of body part	Notes
	Head position	
	Shoulder position	
	Upper spine	
	Ribcage	
	Lower spine	
	Pelvis	
	Knee	
	Calf	

section headed Notes (e.g., head tilted to right, left shoulder higher than right, left scapula lower). These notes will highlight the region of the body that requires local testing of muscle length and joint movement by yourself or another therapist. When viewing from the side, stand the subject behind a plumb line positioned just in front of the lateral malleolus of the ankle. Note the position of each body part in relation to the plumb line and compare with the standard reference line shown in figure 5.3. Record (on table 5.3) any deviations from this ideal (e.g., in front of plumb line) and note any shape changes (e.g., rib cage flatter, thoracic spine rounded). These score sheets give you your **baseline** assessment to compare against as you progress your client through a posture-based exercise program.

Key point: Posture assessment provides a baseline with which to plan a posture-based exercise program.

Posture Grid and Digital Images

Another way to assess static posture is to use a posture grid. The posture grid again uses a plumb line as a reference, but the subject stands behind a screen divided into 10 cm squares to aid inspection of body part alignment. As an alternative, digitally photograph your client standing, and use your computer to overlay a grid onto the digital image. The advantages of a digital photograph are that it can be added to the client's notes and can be used for client education. Ensure that clients give written consent for you to photograph them and store their image on a computer or in paper form. Do not share this image with another person (therapist or instructor at another establishment) without first obtaining your client's consent.

For each digital image that you take of a client, stand the same distance from the client and at the same angle to him to ensure test–retest reliability. If you stand closer when taking one photograph, his body will appear larger, which will make comparison difficult. If you are at a different angle to the subject when you take a second image, any rotation of a body segment that was noted (e.g., rib cage rotation) cannot be compared accurately.

To ensure reliability of the plumb line assessment for a given client, perform it at the same time of day to help remove diurnal variability (Tyrrell et al. 1985). Have subjects stand with their feet 10 cm apart. They should walk on the spot (10 paces) and then come to rest, to aid general body relaxation. Instruct your clients to maintain their normal posture rather than modify or attempt to improve it.

Key point: Digital pictures provide a useful record of posture and can be used to show changes over the months of an exercise program.

Body Segment Measures

You can refine whole-body posture analysis by measuring alignment of individual body segments. You can assess pelvic tilt with a pelvic **inclinometer,** which measures the angle of pelvic tilt relative to the horizontal. The inclinometer consists of a protractor mounted on a base plate and attached to a pair of bone calipers. The inclinometer reads $0°$ when the caliper arms are horizontal. The ends of the arms are positioned over the posterior superior iliac spine and the anterior superior iliac spine of one side of the body. The inclinometer dial shows the angle of pelvic tilt in the sagittal plane. This method of assessing pelvic tilt appears to be accurate to within $±1/4°$ (Toppenberg and Bullock 1986).

Inclinometers are highly reliable and quite valid compared with lateral radiographs (Crowell et al. 1994). Pelvic tilt and lumbar lordosis are intimately linked, with changes in pelvic tilt significantly altering the depth of the lordosis (Day et al. 1984). Bullock-Saxton (1993) demonstrated that inclinometer measurement is repeatable in both normal and symptomatic females: Subjects were measured three times on a single day with 3 min intervals between consecutive tests and then over three separate days with a 4-day rest period between each test.

You can use a **flexible ruler** to measure the depth of lordosis. Locate the spinous process of the second sacral segment (S2), which lies between the posterior superior iliac spines. Palpate each spinous process from S2, counting back to the first lumbar vertebra (L1) (figure 5.4). Record the

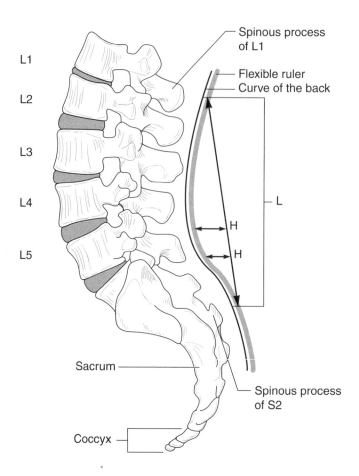

Figure 5.4 S2 lies between the posterior superior iliac spines. Palpate each spinous process cephalically from S2 up to L1. Use a flexible ruler to assess the depth of lumbar lordosis.

length (radius) of the traced curvature (L) of the lordosis from L1 to S2 and the depth of the lordosis (H) from the line joining L1-S2 to the deepest part of the lordotic curve, as shown in figure 5.4. Calculate the lordotic index (U) using the arctan formula, $U = 4 \arctan(2H/L)$.

Arctan is a trigonometric term that can be calculated on most scientific calculators or computer spreadsheet programs. The flexible ruler method of assessing lordosis is highly reliable, as verified by lateral radiographs (Hart and Rose 1986; Lovell et al. 1989). Lordosis measured in this manner showed average (mean) values of 50.9° in normal people and 40.4° in subjects who demonstrated lower abdominal weakness, confirmed as an inability to maintain alignment on supine leg-lowering tasks (Levine et al. 1997).

Detect head position relative to trunk position with a stadiometer, an apparatus used to measure horizontal displacement of body segments relative to each other. The stadiometer consists of two or more sliding arms mounted on a vertical frame. The arms may be raised or lowered to the level of the body segments being measured and then adjusted forward and backward (horizontally). A scale on the side of the horizontal arm shows the distance of each body segment from the vertical arm. Record the craniovertebral (CV) angle by measuring the degree of forward shift of the head that pulls the suboccipital region into hyperextension (Watson 1994). The CV angle is that formed between a horizontal line through the C7 spinous process and the tragus (the prominence on the inner side of the ear) (figure 5.5).

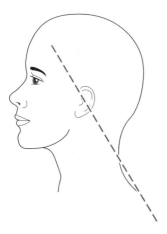

Figure 5.5 Using a stadiometer to measure the craniovertebral angle.

The average CV angle in asymptomatic subjects is 50° (range 48.6-52.0°); people who complain of cervical headaches have reduced angles (44.3°) (Watson 1994), indicating a head-held-forward posture as described by McKenzie (1990).

Key point: Local low-tech measures of posture can be valid, reliable, and reproducible.

PRINCIPLES OF POSTURAL CORRECTION

Correcting posture requires a combination of several factors, embracing the approach to muscle imbalance described in chapter 4. Shortened muscles must be stretched and lengthened muscles shortened. Static stretching and proprioceptive neuromuscular facilitation can stretch muscles, whereas inner-range holding techniques can shorten lengthened muscles and build postural holding time. You must use principles of motor skill training (Norris 1998).

Use the three stages of motor skill training to help your clients regain segmental control (table 5.4). In the cognitive stage, your client must learn objectively the requirements of a skill. In terms of postural reeducation, this often involves passive positioning of optimal posture—you place your clients passively into the optimal postural alignment by correcting pelvic tilt, for example, and instruct them to hold this position. This is a hands-on approach, and you must attain your clients' consent to touch them. Some clients may not be comfortable with this, so respect their wishes. If you are a personal trainer or therapist working alone, consider having a chaperone during

Table 5.4 Stages of Motor Skill Learning

Cognitive	Motor	Automatic
The stage of understanding.	Movement is effective.	Movement "runs by itself."
Environmental cues are important.	Movement is more consistent.	Movement is independent of attention demands.
Person uses information from past experiences.	Person is able to identify his own mistakes.	Action is very fast.
Person is poorly coordinated.	Proprioception is more important than visual cues.	
Person is unable to identify his own mistakes.		
Visual and verbal cues are more important than proprioceptive cues.		
Much coaching is needed.		

this process. Invite your client to have a friend or member of their family accompany her during the early stages of postural education.

Key point: The first stages of postural correction require a hands-on technique. Respect your clients' wishes when it comes to touching their body, and invite them to bring a friend or family member to their sessions.

During this passive positioning stage of posture correction, give your clients as much information as possible to enable them to appreciate body position. Provide cues to body position through touch, or have the client lean against a wall for tactile cueing. You can use vision, for example, using a mirror or digital camera to give feedback (visual cueing), or use instructions and the tone of your voice (auditory cueing). The more methods you use (multisensory cueing), the greater the chance that your client will get it right.

Repeat passive positioning several times until your clients are able to recreate the optimal position themselves. This signifies that they have progressed to the second stage of skill training (motor). During the second stage, the key factor is that people can now identify their own mistakes. In the case of posture, this means that they can consciously move into the optimal posture. To do this they self-monitor by comparing their posture to the optimal. Once they have achieved this ability, they are ready to perform a home exercise program designed to build endurance of the postural muscles.

Key point: Only give home exercises when your client is able to identify her own movement errors and self-monitor.

Only after many thousands of repetitions of a movement will a person move into the third and final stage of motor training (automatic). Now, he is able to maintain an optimal postural alignment without conscious control because the action has become automatic.

The process of learning to drive a car illustrates the three stages of motor learning. When we first learn to drive, the actions are difficult and we must concentrate on many separate activities. The

actions become easier with repetition, as we begin to integrate the independent actions into a whole. Eventually, driving becomes largely automatic. Similarly, the separate components of postural control must be corrected individually and then pieced together to form a more complex single movement. By dividing the total movement into a number of component sequences, you can help your client learn the action more easily.

Correcting a posture so that the correction becomes automatic is extremely difficult. If poor posture is held by shortened tissue, stretching can sufficiently lengthen tissue so that posture can change permanently—assuming that the tissue is not allowed to shorten again through poor postural alignment. If poor posture is the result of muscle weakness brought on through injury (wasting or pain inhibition), muscle strengthening after the pain has eased may optimize posture.

For many cases of poor stability, progressive exercises and proprioceptive training can enhance stability and produce positive postural changes. When posture has been suboptimal for many years, however, full correction probably is not possible. Certainly improvements can be made, and these may be clinically significant (especially in relieving pain), but they will be limited.

Postural Correction Example

As an example of postural reeducation, consider how you might treat a client with a common lordotic posture. This posture typically combines the following imbalance features:

- Lengthening of the rectus abdominis, with poor tone of the gluteus maximus
- Shortening of hamstrings, hip flexors, and spinal extensors
- Poor lumbar stability and poor coordination of lumbar–pelvic rhythm in bending activities

All three of these features need to be addressed, and the order in which they are addressed is usually dictated by pain. Often the tight erector spinae is a source of pain, so reeducation of posture begins in this instance with posterior pelvic tilting to stretch the spinal extensors and shorten the abdominals. To stretch the hamstrings and hip flexors, adequate stability is required to control the pelvis as the muscles are placed on stretch. So stability training is addressed second and stretching third.

Once stability and stretching have been used, your client could then combine the two separate activities, using a hamstring stretch in sitting position while maintaining spinal alignment. Hip flexor stretching is used as described on page 119. Following work to improve recruitment of the gluteals, she should begin whole-body postural reeducation using standing, walking, sitting, and bending movements depending on her functional requirements. Finally, she would begin proprioceptive training as described on page 191.

Especially in the early stages of learning, you could use taping to give your client feedback. The taping performs two functions: Structural taping or bracing can support a hypermobile segment of the body, and functional taping can provide tactile feedback. In the latter case, skin drag will remind your client that her posture has moved away from the optimal alignment (place breathable undertaping under zinc oxide tape to protect the skin) (Norris 1994a).

POSTURE TYPES AND HOW TO CORRECT THEM

There are four classic abnormal posture types (figure 5.6). In the lordotic posture, the main feature is excessive anterior pelvic tilt (figure 5.6*a*). Anterior displacement of the pelvis characterizes the swayback (figure 5.6*b*), whereas the flat-back posture has slight posterior pelvic tilting and loss of lumbar lordosis (figure 5.6*c*). In the kyphotic posture, the thoracic curve is excessive (figure 5.6*d*).

Lordotic Posture

See pages 88-89

In the classic lordotic or hollow-back posture, the greater trochanter remains on the LOG, but the pelvis tilts anteriorly, moving the anterior superior iliac spine (ASIS) forward and downward in relation to the pubic bone. The abdominal muscles and gluteals are typically lengthened and have poor tone. Over time, the hip flexors may shorten, and pelvic tilt is limited by tightness in the overactive and tight hamstrings (Jull and Janda 1987). In an extreme lordotic posture seen in chronic obesity, the lumbar spine rests in extension with the lumbar facet joints impacted; the elastic recoil of the hamstrings allows the pelvis to hang. Janda and Schmid (1980) called this posture the *pelvic crossed syndrome:* High contact pressures occur in the facet joints, with the inferior articular processes impinging on the lamina below. Increased weight bearing of the facet joints in turn reduces the compression force on the lumbar discs (Adams et al. 1994).

Key point: In the lordotic posture, the facet joints are placed under excessive pressure.

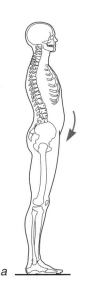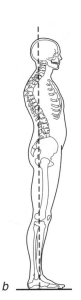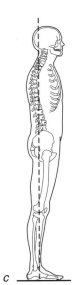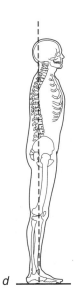

Figure 5.6   Classic abnormal posture types: *(a)* lordotic, *(b)* swayback, *(c)* flat-back, and *(d)* kyphotic.

Lordotic posture is common in dancers and in young gymnasts, for whom this posture is a requirement of the activity. It is the posture most noticeable in women after childbirth, especially multiple births. In the case of childbirth, however, lengthening of the rectus abdominis through serial sarcomere adaptation is accompanied by diastasis, which may or may not resolve spontaneously.

Correction of lordotic posture requires shortening the abdominal muscles and lengthening the hip flexors. The rectus abdominis must be shortened by combining a posterior pelvic tilt with spinal flexion—but only after developing effective deep abdominal muscles to prevent bowstringing, where the abdominal muscles contract and bulge outward instead of pulling flat. This is different from the diastasis that occurs during pregnancy. With bowstringing there is no long-term structural change in the muscle, nor does the linea alba (the tendinous line between the two rectus abdominis muscles) split.

Swayback

In the swayback or slouched posture, the pelvis remains level but the hip joint is pushed forward, the greater trochanter lying anterior to the LOG. Whereas in normal posture the sternum is the most anterior structure, now the pelvis has shifted and become the more anterior body segment, with the LOG moving from the ankle to the midfoot and toes (see figure 5.3). The hip is effectively extended, lengthening the hip flexors, and the body "hangs" on the hip ligaments and anterior hip structures. The lordosis now changes shape from an even curve to a deeper, shorter curve with a prominent crease normally at L3 level. The kyphosis is now longer and may extend into the lumbar spine. The lower lumbar region is flatter than normal, and the pelvis may be minimally posteriorly tilted.

Key point: In the swayback posture, the pelvis is placed forward of the chest.

A person with this posture will often be able to point to the exact point of pain, which normally occurs after prolonged standing. Swayback is common in youth and is the most common posture in athletes 18 to 28 years old (Norris and Berry 1998).

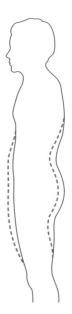

Figure 5.7 Changing length of the oblique abdominals in swayback posture.

The rectus abdominis remains relatively unchanged in the swayback posture because the pubic bone and lower ribs in general retain their anatomical relationship. However, because of the direction of the fibers of the oblique abdominals, the external oblique is lengthened and the internal oblique unchanged or shortened (figure 5.7); in the latter case, the upper fibers are affected (Kendall et al. 1993).

See pages 93-94
The swayback posture may be combined with dominance of one leg in standing (hanging on the hip), especially in adolescents. In this case, weakness in the gluteus medius allows the pelvis to tip laterally, a situation partially compensated by increased tone in the tensor fasciae latae. Shortening is seen in the iliotibial band (ITB), with a prominent groove apparent on the lateral aspect of the thigh, as the tight fascial band pulls on the skin. You can assess tightness in the ITB using the Ober test (see p. 115), which you may also use to stretch the tight muscle. Assess the ability of the gluteus medius to maintain pelvic stability in single-leg standing by using the Trendelenburg sign test (see p. 141). Page 112 shows the inner-range holding test position of this muscle in side lying. Correction of swayback relies on two essential points of the posture type: (a) The pelvis

is the most anteriorly placed structure instead of the sternum, and (b) the posture results in height loss. To correct the posture, you must help your client change the relative alignment of chest and pelvis.

If you have observed single-leg dominance with the swayback posture, help your client correct it by stretching the adductor muscle group on the tight side and enhancing the endurance of the abductors (gluteus medius especially) on the lax side. Symmetry between the two legs is essential. Use the Ober test (p. 115) on both legs to determine the length of the hip abductors. Determine hip adductor length by passively stretching your client's straightened leg into an abducted position; a total of 90° hip abduction (45° on each leg) is desirable.

Use these two exercises to assess the range of hip abduction and to develop it. The first assesses tightness in only the short adductors inserting above the knee (adductor longus, adductor brevis, adductor magnus) because the knee is allowed to bend. The second targets the long adductor inserting below the knee (gracilis) by keeping the knee straight throughout the stretch.

Because swayback posture is common in youth but is not associated with marked muscle tightening or weakening, it can be difficult to correct. The emphasis is on reeducation, with postural awareness playing an important part in the process. You can increase postural awareness by using proprioception during the spinal lengthening exercise at the end of the chapter.

Flat-Back Posture

The main problem with the flat-back posture is lack of mobility in the lumbar spine and a flattening of the lordosis (lumbar flexion). This posture reflects the extension dysfunction described by McKenzie (1981) and is common in chronic low back pain after extended periods of inactivity. The pelvis may be posteriorly tilted compared with the reference line, and the lumbar tissues are often thickened and immobile. The flat-back posture is also seen in subjects who practice a high number of sit-up type exercises (repeated lumbar flexion). In this case, the lumbar spine may be mobile, but

the rectus abdominis is strong and tight and is by far the dominant member of the abdominal muscle group.

Flat-back posture is corrected by regaining appropriate mobility in the lumbar spine through passive and active extension movements.

Kyphotic Back

In the kyphotic posture, the shoulder joint moves anteriorly to the posture line, increasing the thoracic kyphosis. In optimal upper-body alignment (table 5.5), the scapulae should be approximately the width of three fingers from the spine, and the medial borders of the scapulae should be vertical. The scapulae should be held lightly but firmly onto the rib cage through action of the scapular stabilizing muscles, mainly the serratus anterior assisted by the lower fibers of the trapezius muscle. When the scapula is held in position against the rib cage, it is actually quite difficult to see. This gives us a clue for postural assessment—if you can see the medial border of the scapular standing out like a knife edge (figure 5.9a), the scapula has been allowed to move because of poor recruitment of the scapular stabilizing muscles.

Key point: The scapula should be fixed to the rib cage through muscle action. If you see its edge jutting out, scapular alignment is suboptimal and stability is likely to be poor.

Assess optimal positioning of the shoulder by comparing the head of the humerus in relation to the acromion process. In optimal positioning, no more than one third of the humeral head should be anterior to the point of the acromion. The humerus should be held with the cubital fossa (elbow crease) at 45° to the sagittal plane in relaxed standing. A smaller angle indicates excessive medial rotation, indicating tightness in the medial rotators (especially the pectoralis major) and lengthening of the lateral rotators. Visualizing how this would appear from above may be helpful. When the arm is held in medial rotation, the crease of the elbow is oriented more forward and inward; when lateral rotation is greater than normal, the elbow crease faces farther outward.

Table 5.5 Correct Alignment of the Shoulder Girdle

From behind	From the side
Medial border of scapula vertical	Line from ear canal to center of shoulder joint perpendicular to floor
Medial border of scapula no more than three finger breadths from the spinous processes	No more than one third of head of humerus anterior to acromion
Spine of scapular T3-T4 level, inferior angle at T7	Humerus held with elbow crease 45° to sagittal plane
Scapula flat against thoracic wall	

Deviation from the ideal is often described as a *round-shouldered posture,* a term that covers a number of scenarios. Tightness in the anterior structures pulls the shoulder forward, away from the posture line. The weight of the arm moves farther from the upper body's center of gravity, dramatically increasing the leverage forces transmitted to the thorax. Eventually, thoracic kyphosis increases. Tightness in the pectoralis minor pulls on the coracoid process, tilting the scapula forward (figure 5.8a). Tightness in the pectoralis major causes both excessive medial rotation at the glenohumeral joint and anterior displacement of the humeral head (figure 5.8b). Lengthening of the lower trapezius and serratus anterior may cause excessive abduction (figure 5.8c) and downward rotation (figure 5.8d) of the scapula. Excessive elevation (figure 5.8e) and upward rotation may result from tightness in the upper fibers of the trapezius.

Correction of kyphotic posture depends on flexibility of the thoracic spine. Where the kyphosis appears fixed and thoracic motion is grossly reduced, thoracic joint mobilization by a PT is required as a first step. Once some mobility has been gained passively by manual therapy, you can use exercise therapy to maintain the newly gained motion. The sternal lift action (p. 103) is the exercise of choice. If the subject is younger and the thoracic spine is mobile, only scapular repositioning is required.

Figures 5.9 and 5.10 give examples of suboptimal scapular positions. Figure 5.9a shows the appearance of scapular tipping combined with abduction at rest. At initiation of arm abduction (figure 5.9b), the scapula is not held stable against the rib cage but rotates downward instead. When stress is placed on the arm, scapular instability becomes even more noticeable. Figure 5.10a shows the appearance of scapular instability in four-point kneeling (hands-and-knees position). As the arms are bent during the eccentric (lowering) phase of a press-up exercise from this position, the shoulder muscles pull on the scapula, which should remain fixed to the rib cage. As stability fails, the scapulae fall together, showing marked adduction, and actually move farther

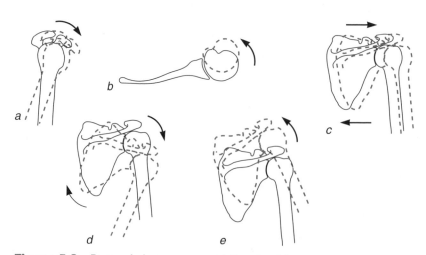

Figure 5.8 Postural changes around the shoulder.

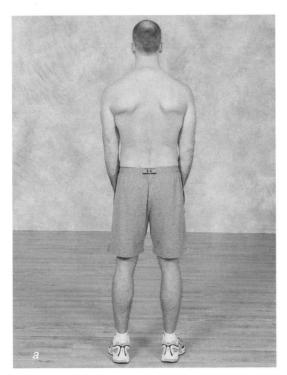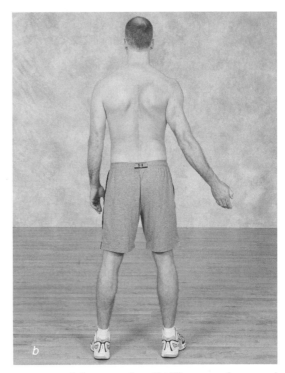

Figure 5.9 *(a)* Poor scapular alignment at rest. Note the contours of the scapulae. *(b)* The scapular muscles work hard to fix the scapula to the ribcage.

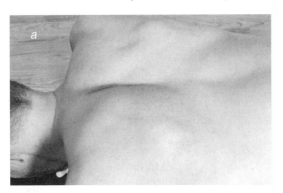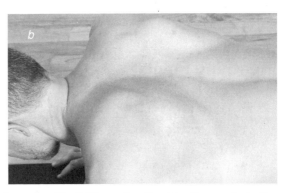

Figure 5.10 *(a)* Scapulae move inward when stabilizers do not work. *(b)* Scapulae fixed to ribcage but alignment is still poor. Note the flaring of medial borders.

away from the rib cage rather than being drawn in toward it (figure 5.10*b*).

SUMMARY

- Posture is the arrangement of body parts in a state of balance that protects the supporting structures of the body against injury or progressive deformity.

- Postural sway consists of a small continuous motion in the sagittal plane—an oscillation of the center of gravity that may reduce lower-limb fatigue and aid blood flow.

- You can assess clients' postures by use of a plumb line or a posture grid.

- There are four basic types of abnormal posture:

  1. Lordotic posture is characterized by excessive anterior pelvic tilt.

  2. Swayback is characterized by anterior displacement of the pelvis.

  3. Flat-back posture is characterized by slight posterior pelvic tilting and loss of lumbar lordosis.

  4. Kyphosis is characterized by excessive thoracic curve.

Modified Trunk Curl

Goal: Shorten and strengthen the rectus abdominis muscle.

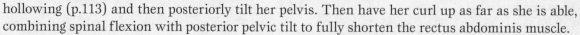

The modified trunk curl action can help correct lordotic posture. Where full inner-range motion is lacking because of muscle lengthening, your client can perform the modified trunk curl in progressive stages.

Stage 1: Your client lies supine with her knees bent. Have her perform abdominal hollowing (p.113) and then posteriorly tilt her pelvis. Then have her curl up as far as she is able, combining spinal flexion with posterior pelvic tilt to fully shorten the rectus abdominis muscle.

Stage 2: Provide assistance for inner-range work. You can gently pull your client into a slightly higher position, or she can pull herself higher by gripping her thighs. The extra lift should be no more than 2 in. (5 cm) and must be performed slowly and with care to avoid jolting the spine.

Stage 3: After your client has lifted herself into the upper position and released, she should slow her descent back to the floor as much as possible. Initially she may fall back to the floor in less than 1 s. With practice, she should be able to lower herself more slowly, taking 1 to 2 s and then 4 to 5 s and finally a full 10 s. When the client has achieved this level of strength, she can progress to holding the full upper position in stage 4.

Stage 4: Have your client hold the upper position with an isometric contraction, gradually building up the holding time from 1 to 2 s to 4 to 5 s and finally 10 s, at all times breathing normally.

Teaching Points

▶ This exercise is a progression in four stages; make sure your client masters each stage before going to the next.

▶ The muscle activity in this exercise is intense, and people tend to hold their breath. This dramatically raises blood pressure, however, and must not be allowed.

▶ Instruct the client to avoid bowstringing at all times by drawing the abdominal wall inward (stage 1) and keeping this alignment.

▶ Do not force the inner-range position (maximum trunk flexion). Allow your client to pull into the position with her own muscle strength.

▶ Do not allow high-momentum movement by permitting bouncing or bobbing movement at the end of the motion range.

How will you know if the abdominal muscles are lengthened and require shortening by this full inner-range holding method? In chapter 4, we saw that the length–tension curve moves to the right for lengthened muscles (see figure 4.8), indicating that they are unable to hold a joint at full inner range (i.e., to close the joint fully). When your clients perform the trunk curl, they are attempting full spinal flexion. If, in an attempt to pull the spine into full flexion, they fall back away from the inner-range position while performing the extra lift (with your help or by pulling on their thighs), you can safely conclude that the muscle is lengthened and requires this type of training to shorten it.

Normally, full-range flexion of the spine is not recommended for general back care. People with lordotic posture, however, have been maintaining the lumbar spine in extension. Full flexion is therefore a treatment of choice for such people and is widely used within physical therapy practice (McKenzie 1981).

Gluteus Maximus Inner-Range Exercise

Goal: Contract and fully shorten the gluteus maximus.

The gluteus maximus muscles must be tightened and shortened by working them in inner range. Have your client lie prone and flex one knee to 90°. She should then extend her hip, trying to emphasize the action of the gluteal muscles. If she is unable to lift the leg into full inner range, lift the leg for her. Then she should try either to hold this position (isometric) or to control the leg as it descends (eccentric). She even-

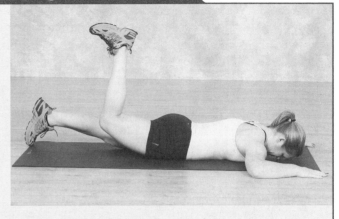

tually should attain full inner-range holding ability, with holding times built up from 3 to 5 s to 30 to 60 s.

Take a gradual, progressive approach for those who are unable to lift the leg, always remembering to adapt the program to your client's individual level of progress. Begin with muscle reeducation, encouraging your client simply to contract the gluteus in prone lying. Use of electromyographic feedback and manual muscle stimulation is helpful at this stage if the person is completely unable to perform a static contraction. Tapping or brushing the gluteus with the fingers adds to multisensory cueing, making the task easier by increasing the amount of information that accompanies the movement. By making the contractions forceful, your client can increase the holding time until she can contract and hold the muscle for 10 s. Once she can do that, the next step is to lift the femur into 10° to 15° of extension and place the knee on a block or cushion to maintain the extended hip position. She then contracts and holds the muscle as before, but in this new starting position. Eventually, she will develop sufficient strength so that you can remove the cushion and ask her to hold the extended position by herself.

If your client is unable to hold this nonsupported position, have her use eccentric lowering. After you have raised her hip into 15° extension, instruct her to hold it there as you release the leg. Encourage her to use the same intensity of muscle contraction as for the first two movements. If she is unable to hold the leg into extension (i.e., off the examination table), she should try to lower it in a controlled way rather than allowing it to drop. Have her gradually increase the time required to lower the leg to at least 10 s.

The next stage is for your client to forcibly contract the gluteal muscles and simultaneously try to lift her leg off the table into extension. Suggest that she bend her knee to reduce the hamstrings' contribution to extension. She should begin with 2 to 5 repetitions, lifting her leg as high as possible without allowing the pelvis to tilt. Try placing your hand just above your client's heel on the lifting leg and then encouraging her to lift the leg until her heel touches your hand.

The final progression is first to lift the leg to full extension and hold this inner-range position for a full 10 s and then to perform 10 repetitions of this movement.

If clients have both poor tone in the gluteals and poor control of hip extension in the prone position, have them begin a progression of exercises leading toward the goal of performing 10 repetitions, with each contraction held 10 s, at each exercise session. For the first week, they should perform the exercises only every other day to reduce the likelihood of muscle soreness. They should perform 2 sets of 10 repetitions, one in the morning and one in the evening, for the first two exercise days, then 3 sets (morning, late afternoon, and evening) on the next two exercise days. Instruct clients

(continued)

to work gradually on increasing reps and holding time—perhaps starting with 3 repetitions, held as long as possible, and then alternating between adding to the number of reps and increasing the holding time. Once they can hold a full contraction in both prone position and in extension, they should do the exercises 10 times twice per day for 2 days followed by 10 reps three times per day for 2 days. They should take a full day's rest after each 4-day cycle. They should follow the sequence of 2 sets per day for 2 days, then 3 sets per day for 2 days, and then 1 day of rest for each progression until they can consistently perform 10 reps at each session, holding each rep for 10 s.

Teaching Points

▶ In extreme cases, no contraction of the gluteus maximus may be detected, and the leg may be lifted with the hamstrings instead. Observe your client closely to detect this.

▶ This is an open-chain exercise, and some clients may find this difficult to initiate. If this is the case, have your client press her foot upward against resistance provided by your hand.

▶ If the exercise is poorly performed, turn your client over into crook lying (hook lying) to perform a bridge action instead.

Although inner-range exercises may shorten the previously lengthened rectus abdominis and gluteus maximus, excessive pelvic tilt will be corrected only if the tight hip flexors are stretched to release the pull on the pelvis through the iliacus muscle. Tightness of the hip flexors (if attributable to increased muscle tone rather than to adaptive shortening of connective tissue) inhibits the activity of the hip extensors through a process called pseudoparesis (Janda 1986). When this is the case, a person must reduce muscle tone in the hip flexors before engaging in exercises to strengthen the hip extensors. The Thomas test can show whether the hip flexors are tight and whether the rectus femoris or iliopsoas is the tighter muscle. You also can prescribe the Thomas test for initial stretching of the hip flexors, later using the half lunge to combine lumbar stability with hip flexor stretching.

Half Lunge Without Chair

Goal: Stretch the hip flexors while maintaining back stability.

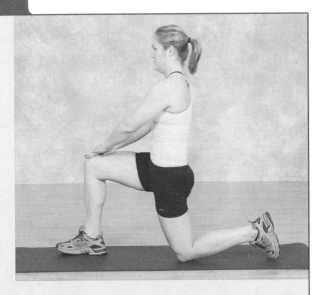

Instruct your client to assume a half-kneeling position and to tighten her abdominal muscles (using a hollowing action) to stabilize the pelvis. From this position, she should press her pelvis or midsection forward to force the trailing hip into extension. Providing the pelvis is not allowed to anteriorly tilt, the hip flexors will be stretched. Prescribe twice-daily exercise for 4 days, 10 repetitions per session, holding the position 20 to 30 s for each repetition. Instruct your client to rest for a day and then repeat the 4-day cycle until she has gained the desired range of motion or until range improvement has stopped. The long-term maintenance exercise schedule should be 10 repetitions, three times per week. A chair may be useful for the client to hold (p. 119) if she finds the balance of this exercise difficult.

Teaching Points

▶ If the hip is very tight, your client may not be able to contract her abdominals powerfully enough to fix the pelvis. If this is the case, use an alternative hip stretch such as the Thomas test (p. 114).

▶ Both the rectus femoris and iliopsoas are stretched using this action. To increase the emphasis on the rectus, put the foot of the trailing leg onto a block to increase knee flexion.

▶ Clients with patellar pain should kneel on a thick, soft cushion to reduce patellofemoral compression.

Back Flattening

Goal: Stretch hip flexors and build endurance in the abdominal muscles while learning posture control.

Once a client has corrected the muscle imbalance of the lordotic posture, he should practice assuming optimal posture. A back-flattening exercise can help. Have your client stand with his back flat against a wall and his feet 6 in. (15 cm) from the wall. He should then tighten the abdominal muscles and gluteals in order to posteriorly tilt the pelvis while his legs remain fully extended. The posterior pelvic tilting will effectively stretch the hip flexors. The client can gradually increase the holding time, starting at 3 to 5 s and building to 30 to 60 s, breathing normally throughout the exercise. Prescribe exercises twice daily for 10 repetitions, with each repetition held 5 s and a rest day taken after every four exercise days.

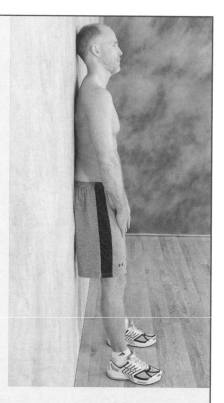

Strengthening the abdominal muscles is not sufficient to correct a lordotic posture. Unless a person modifies hip flexor tightness and corrects abnormal lengthening of abdominal muscles, abdominal strength changes will have little effect on pelvic tilt or lumbar lordosis. Walker and colleagues (1987) and Levine and colleagues (1997) both examined the effects of abdominal strengthening alone and found no changes in postural variables.

Teaching Points

▶ Use your hands to guide your client's pelvis into posterior tilt.

▶ Place your flat hand behind your client's back to give him something to press against.

▶ Ensure that your client does not hold his breath when pressing his back into the wall.

▶ Use a mirror in front of your client to enforce muscle contraction or to the side of your client to guide back flattening.

Chest–Pelvis Stacking

Goal: Reeducate body segment positioning.

Have your client stand with his pelvis against the top of a table; it is useful to have the feet back slightly, so that the body weight presses the thighs against the table. From this position he presses his chest forward, shifting it as a single segment and avoiding any spinal flexion. The aim is to align the chest and pelvis as though stacking two bricks. At the same time, he performs abdominal hollowing to reeducate the flat abdomen alignment. Remember that a key feature of the swayback is loss of height attributable to the curvature of the body line. A useful cue is to tell your client to grow taller by lengthening his spine.

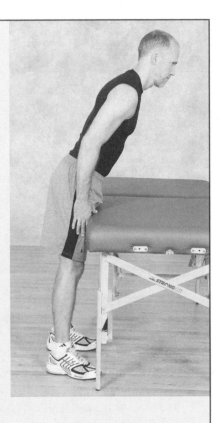

Teaching Points

▶ Hold the hair on the top of your client's head and gently pull upward to give a tactile cue for spinal lengthening.

▶ Place your hand just in front of your client's sternum to encourage him to press the sternum forward.

▶ Note that this model is performing the exercise poorly. He has angled the trunk on the hip rather than stacked it. The movement should be from swayack (pelvis thrust forward) to optimal alignment.

Sitting Bilateral Hip Adductor Stretch

Goal: Stretch the hip adductors, excluding the gracilis.

Have your client sit on the floor on a folded towel that is 2 in. (5 cm) thick, her back supported against a wall. She should place the soles of her feet together, grip her feet, and press down on her knees using her elbows, holding the full stretch for 5 to 10 s while maintaining back alignment. A desirable range of motion is for the knees to fall to within 3 to 4 in. (7-10 cm) of the floor. Prescribe 10 repetitions daily.

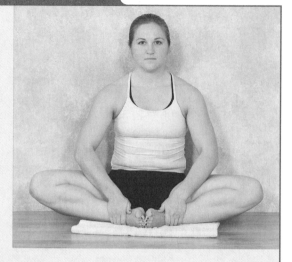

Teaching Points

▶ If your client's lumbar spine is very rounded, have her sit on a wedge with the wider edge to the rear to anteriorly tilt her pelvis.

▶ Clients with very long bodies find it difficult to grip their feet and press their elbows against their knees while keeping their spine straight. These clients should release their feet and press directly on their knees with their hands.

▶ Ensure that your client avoids bouncing or bobbing actions at the end of the hip motion.

▶ The pull of the adductors onto the pubis will stress the pubic symphysis, making this exercise contraindicated within 3 months of childbirth and in those with symphysis pubis dysfunction.

Sitting Wide Splits

Goal: Stretch all the hip adductor muscles.

Have your client sit on the floor in an upright posture with her arms behind her, hands on the floor to stop her from leaning back too far, legs straight. The body should be as vertical as possible. Instruct her to abduct her legs as far as possible, allowing the pelvis to posteriorly tilt. This posterior tilt will take the stretch off the adductors slightly, enabling the subject to get into the position comfortably. Then, she can increase the stretch by maintaining the position of the feet and pressing her hands

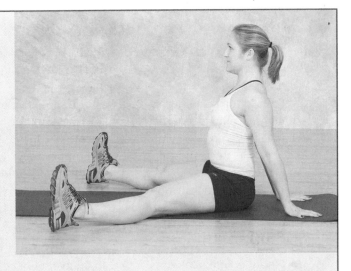

against the floor to lengthen the trunk (tell her to grow taller or to reach her head up to the ceiling). As this occurs, the subject attempts to anteriorly tilt her pelvis, which will move the pubic bone (the upper insertion of the adductor muscles) backward and so increase the stretch. A desirable range of motion is a total of 90° hip abduction between both legs. She should hold the full stretch for 5 to 10 s. Prescribe 10 repetitions daily.

Teaching Points

▶ It is common for a client to flex at the top of her spine rather than tilt her pelvis. To prevent this, place a stick along the length of your client's spine to encourage her to move her spine as a single unit rather than flex.

▶ If your client finds it difficult to anteriorly tilt her pelvis, have her sit on a wedge with the wider edge to the rear to anteriorly tilt her pelvis.

▶ The pull of the adductors onto the pubis will stress the pubic symphysis, making this exercise contraindicated within 3 months of childbirth and in those with symphysis pubis dysfunction.

Spinal Lengthening

Goal: Improve awareness of body position.

Your client needs a partner for this exercise. As your client stands in her normal resting posture, her partner places a hand 1 to 2 in. (2.5-5.0 cm) above the crown of the client's head. Instruct your client to lengthen her spine (tell her to grow taller) as she attempts to touch her partner's hand with the top of her head. The client must not look up (cervical extension) in an attempt to lengthen her neck and must not stand on her toes!

Once the client has mastered this action, she should attempt the same lengthening action without the help of a partner. The instruction is again to grow taller.

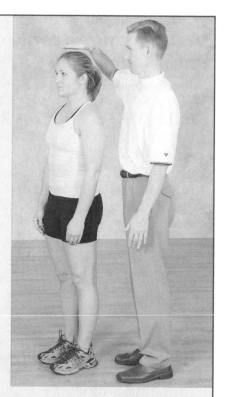

Teaching Points

► Placing a light book or beanbag on the client's head provides sensory feedback and can help her focus her attention on moving the top of her head upward.

► Initially she practices simple lengthening at whatever speed is comfortable, with the beanbag on her head. Eventually she should slow the lengthening action, attempting to hold the lengthened position for 5 to 10 s while breathing normally (do not allow her to take a deep breath and hold it—this can lead to lightheadedness).

► The lengthened position should be relatively relaxed and not stiff—comparisons with a puppet rather than a wooden stick can illustrate the difference between stability (spine lengthened and aligned) and rigidity (spine fixed).

► When your client is able to perform the movement and hold the corrected body position, she can progress to walking while holding the lengthened position and then to simple activities such as sitting down or standing up from a chair to increase the variety of movements.

To provide sensory feedback when the swayback posture is incorrectly stretching the muscle, try applying nonelastic tape on the skin over the external oblique, taking up any skin slack. Attach the tape to the lower lateral aspect of the abdomen, out toward the anterior rim of the pelvis. Pull the tape tight from this point up to the posterolateral aspect of the lower ribs. Although the tape is not strong enough to prevent the pelvis from moving forward in relation to the rib cage, it will remind your client when this is happening and encourage her to correct the posture. The more times she makes the correction, the more likely it is that optimal postural alignment will become automatic. Either a physical therapist or athletic trainer should apply the tape, and it should be done immediately following the spinal lengthening exercise to encourage the client to maintain correct alignment between exercise bouts.

Another way to reinforce automatic alignment is to build correction into daily activities. Encourage your client to perform the pelvis–chest realignment exercise regularly throughout the day. Office workers, for example, can perform the exercise whenever the telephone rings, and students can perform it each time a bell rings to end class.

If the iliopsoas is lengthened by the extended position of the hip (the Thomas test will reveal this; see chapter 6), its inner-range holding must be redeveloped.

Key point: Build postural awareness and correction into everyday activities.

Sitting Hip Flexor Shortening

Goal: Shorten the iliopsoas and rectus femoris muscles and build their endurance.

While your client is sitting, passively flex her hip to the maximum degree possible without pain (approximately 110°) or to the point where the pelvis just begins to posteriorly rotate. Tell her to hold this position for 10 s while maintaining a neutral lordosis. Inability to hold at full inner range for 10 repetitions (10 s each) is a sign of postural lengthening. If the iliopsoas is lengthened, the leg may drop or the pelvis may drop back into posterior tilt, moving the iliopsoas into its lengthened position. Your client can redevelop inner-range holding of the iliopsoas by using first eccentric and then isometric inner-range hip flexor exercises while maintaining a neutral lordosis.

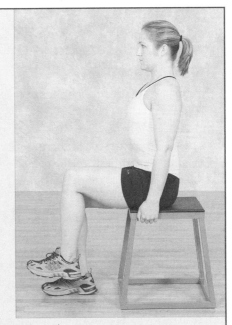

While your client is in the sitting position, ask her to lift her leg to full flexion. You try to lift her leg farther (increasing hip flexion) without altering the position of the spine or pelvis. Remember that a lengthened muscle cannot contract powerfully to pull a limb into its fully closed (inner-range) position. If your client's hip flexors are lengthened, further passive movement will be possible because she will not have been able to pull her own leg into full inner range. Have her attempt to hold this new (passive) inner-range position. If she is able to do so, instruct her to start with a holding time of 1 to 2 s and increase to 10 s while performing the exercise daily for 2 weeks—her target is 10 repetitions of the 10-s hold.

Teaching Points

▶ If your client is not able to hold the passive inner-range position, she should use controlled lowering (eccentric). From the passive inner-range position, she attempts to slow the descent of the leg after you release it from its fully flexed position. She should continue the controlled lowering until she can slow the descent sufficiently to hold the leg still.

▶ Progress to holding at reducing joint angles. For example, assume that the active inner-range position (with your client using her own muscles) is 90° hip flexion, and the passive inner-range position (as you lift the leg farther into flexion) is 120°. The target for active flexion and holding is about 110°. You lift her leg to 120° hip flexion and release the leg. She then controls the lowering back to the 90° starting position.

▶ Once she can do this consistently, you lift your client's leg to 90° to 100° and she attempts to hold it. Once she can hold this position, you repeat the exercise, beginning again with 110° to 120° of passive flexion.

Your client should perform each holding or lowering exercise only five times before taking a rest period, because the muscle fatigues quickly with this exercise and alignment will be lost. Prescribe 3 sets of 5 repetitions twice daily for 4 days (a family member can provide the passive flexion), followed by a single day of rest, then another 5-day cycle, and so on. The goal is for her to actively flex her leg to 110° and hold it for 10 s for each exercise set.

Lying Passive Back Extension

Goal: Improve the passive range of extension in the lumbar spine.

Performed in the lying position, extension exercises first mobilize the upper lumbar levels, with proportionally less caudal movement (McKenzie 1981). Instruct your client to lie prone on the lab table (or floor), with her hands by her shoulders in a push-up position *(a)*. She should extend her arms while keeping her pelvis on the table, thereby forcing extension of the spine *(b)*.

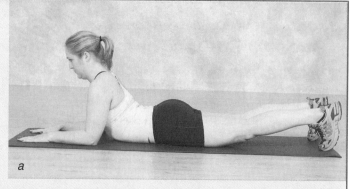

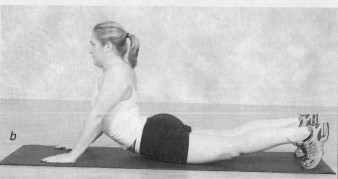

Teaching Points

▶ Initially, some people may need to push up only with their forearms on the floor, gradually building up to full arm extension.

▶ If your client finds that pressing on flat hands makes her wrists sore, have her press on her open fist (fingers flexed at the knuckles but not tightly curled) instead.

▶ To emphasize the motion of the spine rather than the pelvis, try fixing the client's pelvis to the table with a webbing belt.

If your client experiences any pain in the lumbar region during this exercise, refer her to a physical therapist (PT). Often, instead of the whole lumbar spine being stiff to extension, one or two vertebrae may be stiffer than others. These stiff units require a specific manual therapy technique called *joint mobilization* either before or during the exercise program. When a specific stiff area has started to move (the PT will assess this), you can move the webbing belt up or down within the lumbar region to form a fulcrum around which the movement occurs. In this way, the extension action is focused more exactly on a single lumbar joint.

See that your clients practice the passive extension movement often, but for only a short time each session, to allow the movement to develop without causing too much reactionary pain. Suggest 10 repetitions every 2 hr throughout the waking day, with a full day's rest after every 4 days. The exercise should continue until the person has achieved the desired movement range.

Sitting Pelvic Tilt Reeducation

Goal: Regain both range and quality of movement in the lumbar spine.

If the lower lumbar spine has reduced extension, the pelvic tilting action may be effective in correcting it. Instruct your client to sit on a low stool with his feet on the ground. Keeping his shoulders still, he should try to tilt his pelvis forward and down.

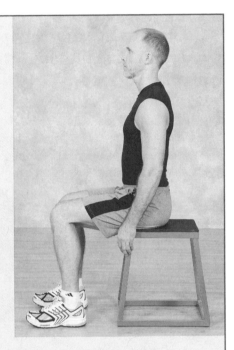

Teaching Points

▶ Tell your client to think of his pelvis as a bowl full of water, and that by tilting the bowl he can pour the water onto the ground between his feet. He should try to bring the back of the bowl up as he pushes the front of it down, always keeping his shoulders still and his sternum up.

▶ When the motion is especially poor, provide passive assistance. Wrap a webbing belt around your client's waist and, fixing the sternum, pull the lumbar spine into extension as he attempts to tilt his pelvis (sitting assisted pelvic tilt, p. 144).

Refer to chapter 4 for a fuller discussion of pelvic tilt.

Thoracic Joint Mobilization

Goal: Increase mobility of thoracic joints, using manual therapy, in preparation for exercise therapy.

With your client in the prone lying position, work with a PT to use posterior–anterior vertebral pressures or gross extension pressures to isolate the thoracic spine. With your client sitting, you can combine mobilization with overpressure. Have her sit facing a treatment table, with her arms folded and placed on the table. As you press the thoracic spine into extension, instruct her to try to follow the action. If thoracic mobility is quite limited, at first you will simply press the spine passively into extension. As your client gains mobility, encourage her to follow your motion with her own active movement while you gradually reduce the pressure you apply.

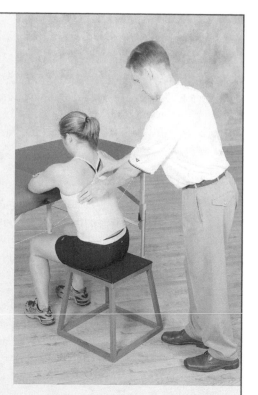

Teaching Points

▶ The first step in this active process is for the subject to feel the movement. Many people with a kyphotic posture have a poor ability to control the quality of motion in the thoracic spine, and this type of guided exercise can help them improve their control.

▶ If your client is still unable to perform active thoracic extension even after regaining passive extension, suggest a visualization technique: Encourage her to imagine herself performing the action. Either you or a model should demonstrate the correct action to your client.

▶ You can also use video to enable your client to see the action from behind, while a mirror provides a view from the front. Then have her repeat her attempt at active thoracic extension.

Key point: Use visualization to improve your client's exercise control.

Your client may need to cycle through a series of visualization sessions, passive extension, and attempts at active extension before she can finally sense what active extension feels like. Once that happens, she can proceed to daily exercises. She should perform the exercise daily for 10 to 15 repetitions. In the early stages, because mobility is very poor, some soreness can be expected following the exercise, so a greater number of repetitions should not be performed.

Many clients have a rounded thoracic spine, and most will respond to exercise therapy. However, older clients may have spinal pathology that requires management by a PT. Arthritis may affect the spinal joints, stiffening them and limiting range of available motion, and an X ray will reveal the extent of bone degeneration. Osteoporosis can also affect clients, mainly women, and although exercise is a key treatment for this condition, your client's physician should measure bone mineral density to determine the degree of osteoporosis and recommend treatment.

Scapula Repositioning

Goal: **Improve control of scapular retraction and depression.**

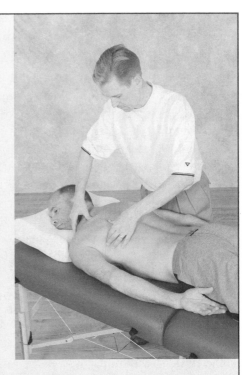

If the thoracic spine is mobile, you can correct kyphotic posture by repositioning the scapulae—shortening the shoulder retractors and enhancing the scapular stabilizers (especially lower trapezius and serratus anterior). The aim here is to improve control of movement rather than simply increase strength. By combining strength, muscle endurance, and movement quality (coordination and timing), these exercises differ from many traditional weight-training programs, whose primary aims are gains in strength and muscle size.

With your client lying prone, passively place his scapula into optimal alignment—the medial borders vertical, three finger widths from the spine. The scapula should be firmly anchored to the thorax (by action of the serratus anterior and lower trapezius muscles) rather than being separated from the rib cage. Frequently this involves passively depressing and adducting the scapula, but the amount of passive movement of the scapula that is required depends on the postural alignment of the subject. More movement is needed in subjects who have grossly abducted scapulae (medial border of scapula 5-6 in. [13-15 cm] from the spine) than for those with minimal abduction (medial border 3-4 in. [8-10 cm] from the spine).

Teaching Points

▶ Subjects often tend to brace their shoulders back. Discourage this reaction, because it requires maximal muscle activity. Encourage your client to "let go" until the scapula just begins to move away from the corrected position and then to hold the muscles slightly tight.

▶ Progressively increase the amount of time that this position is held with minimal muscle work: 1 to 2 s, then 3 to 4 s, and eventually 10 s.

▶ The aim is to build up to 10 reps, holding each for 10 s, with the minimal amount of scapular muscle work that is required to maintain good scapular alignment.

▶ To prevent your client's neck being rotated to extreme range, place a folded towel beneath his forehead and have him look forward into the couch.

Tight anterior structures must be stretched to allow the shoulders to retract fully. Check for tightness in the pectoralis major and pectoralis minor, and if necessary prescribe stretching exercises as detailed in the following sections.

Door Frame Stretch

Goal: Stretch the pectoralis major muscles.

Instruct your client to lean forward onto a door frame, her upper arms horizontal and her forearms vertical against the frame. She then pushes her arms back into extension by leaning into the doorway opening, holding the position for 20 s. Have your client do this exercise three times a day, with 2 repetitions each time.

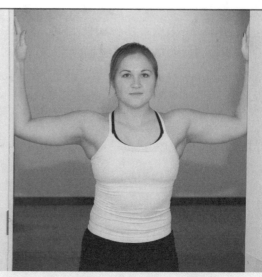

Teaching Points

▶ Make sure that your client lowers herself gradually into this movement. Falling forward into the stretch can cause severe injury.

▶ It is common for clients to be asymmetrical, that is, one shoulder less flexible than the other. Spend more time stretching the less flexible shoulder, and then when both are equal perform the same number of reps on each.

This action presses the upper arm bone (humerus) backward and in so doing anteriorly displaces the head of the humerus. It is therefore contraindicated for anyone with a history of shoulder dislocation.

Weight Bag Passive Stretch

Goal: Stretch the pectoralis minor muscles.

A tight pectoralis minor can pull the scapula down and forward. Have your client lie in a supine position. Place a 3 to 5 lb (1.3-2.3 kg) weight bag over the anterior aspect of her shoulder. She should relax and allow the bag to press her shoulder back into position for 30 s. The weight bag will help press the shoulder back into retraction, passively stretching the anterior structures. To use a contract–relax technique, the client presses the shoulder into protraction for 2 s, trying to lift the weight bag, and then relaxes for 5 to 10 s, allowing the weight bag to press the shoulder farther back. A static stretch may also be used, where the client simply lies relaxed, allowing the weight bag to press her shoulders back.

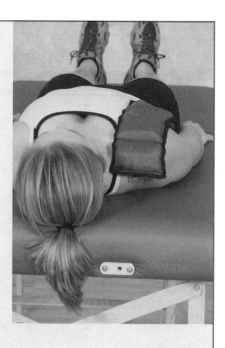

Teaching Points

▶ It may take some time for your client to learn to relax into this position. Tell her not to expect significant progress for three to five stretching sessions.

▶ Because the pectoralis minor is a small muscle, your client may experience some pain. If the pain is unpleasant, use a smaller weight bag and only increase the weight when the pain has subsided.

Sternal Lift

Goal: Combine thoracic extension and scapular repositioning.

While sitting, your client should lift his sternum using thoracic extension (rather than simply taking a deep breath) *(a)*. At the same time, he should draw the scapulae down and in toward their optimal alignment. He may prefer to perform the action against a wall, where he rolls the thoracic spine up the wall while keeping the lumbar spine stable and avoiding any increase in the depth of the lumbar lordosis *(b)*.

Teaching Points

▶ If the client's lumbar spine stability is particularly poor and he is unable to avoid hyperflexion, modify the starting position by having him sit on a bench, with his feet on a chair to bring the femur above the horizontal. This position posteriorly tilts the pelvis and flattens or reverses the lumbar lordosis.

▶ Older clients or those with chest pathologies may have stiff rib cages. It is still important for them to practice this action, but expect progress to be slower.

▶ Note that this client's head is thrust forward. Ensure that your client maintains good cervical alignment and "sits tall."

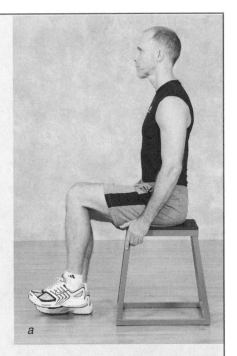

a

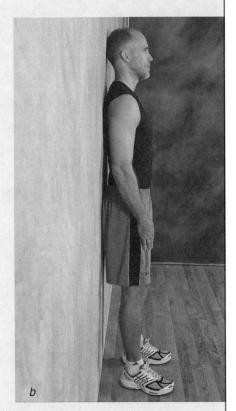

b

Chapter 6
Muscle Balance Tests

In chapter 4 we saw that muscle imbalance can give rise to three changes: stretched or lax muscles, tight or short muscles, and altered static alignment and movement quality. Chapter 5 looked at the gross effects of these changes in general posture. In chapter 6 we use a series of specific tests to identify muscle imbalance. These measures form a baseline for us to develop an exercise program to correct muscle imbalance and enhance back stability.

ASSESSING STRETCHED MUSCLES—TESTING INNER-RANGE HOLDING ABILITY

Figure 4.8 demonstrated that the length–tension curve of a lengthened muscle moves to the right, indicating that the muscle is unable to produce significant power within the full inner range. This fact forms the basis for assessing stabilizer muscle length by inner-range holding tests. Tests for the most important stabilizing muscles are described here.

Key point: Lengthened muscle cannot shorten sufficiently to open or close a joint fully.

Low Back and Hip Muscles—Inner-Range Holding Tests

The ability of a stabilizer to maintain a low-load isometric contraction over a period of time is vital to its antigravity function and may be assessed using the standard muscle test position (Richardson 1992; Richardson and Sims 1991). In all the assessments, ask your clients to maintain a contraction in full inner range,

the key factor being the length of time they can maintain the static hold before developing jerky (phasic) movements. In each case, you will place the limb passively into the full inner range. If the limb drops on release, the passive range of motion differs from the active range—an important indicator of poor stabilizer function. Full stabilizing function is present only when a subject can maintain the inner-range position for a prolonged period, which represents muscle endurance. Typically, values of 10 repetitions of 10 s duration are quoted (Jull 1994). In all the tests, your subjects should attempt all 10 repetitions; often they will perform the first two or three normally, with the deficit becoming apparent only in later repetitions.

Deep Abdominal Muscles—Inner-Range Holding Tests

Rather than deal with specific abdominal muscles as I did with the hip muscles, in this section I focus on the entire system of deep abdominal muscles that affect lumbar stability and that often are abnormally stretched (and therefore weak in their inner ranges). You can test a client's ability to hold the inner range of the deep abdominals by assessing her ability to hollow the abdomen and by monitoring her lumbar lordosis and pelvic tilt while overloading the stability system. You can assess both actions by accurate palpation and motion recording, but I also recommend using pressure biofeedback, which will make the assessment considerably easier. The pressure biofeedback unit can also be used by the client for continuing exercises to provide useful tactile and visual feedback.

To assess limb function relative to lumbar-pelvic stability, you can use a number of starting positions—two of which I describe in detail on pages 110-111.

ASSESSING SHORTENED MUSCLES

Mobilizer muscles have a tendency to tighten. Tightness in the hamstrings (mobilizers), for example, is common, whereas tightness in the gluteals (stabilizers) is rare. In addition to reducing range of motion, muscle tightening may lead to development of trigger points (Travell and Simmons 1983)—small hypersensitive regions within a muscle that stimulate afferent nerve fibers, causing pain. The sensation created is a deep tenderness with an overlying increase in tone, creating a palpably tender band of muscle. These muscles demonstrate spontaneous electrical activity, often being activated for no reason during daily activities. When palpated deeply, the trigger point creates a local muscle spasm, called the jump sign (Janda 1993). Because tight muscles have a lowered irritability threshold, they are activated earlier than normal in a movement sequence, and they have less slack to take up before contraction begins. In addition, tight muscles have increased afferent input via the stretch receptors (Sahrmann 1990).

You should assess the tightness of your client's mobilizer muscles for several reasons. First, because limited range of motion may not allow sufficient movement for correct body segment alignment, limbs may be pulled into positions that stress joint surfaces and collateral ligaments. Second, tightness in a muscle may, through reciprocal innervation, inhibit the opposing muscle through the process of pseudoparesis (Janda 1986). Third, stability must be relative to flexibility. Consider the straight-leg raise (see p. 117): Poor stability can lead the pelvis to tilt very early in the range of motion. Normally, the pelvis only tilts when the hamstring muscles reach the end of their stretch—they are fully wound up—and this may not occur until 80° to 90° of hip flexion. If pelvic tilt is seen before this (in a flexible individual), an imbalance exists. The individual's level of stability is not sufficient for her level of flexibility; she has lost active muscular control over a portion of her total range of motion, a fundamental feature in the difference between hypermobility and instability.

If you find muscle tightness, you can use the test movements as starting positions for stretch-

ing. But before prescribing stretching exercises, be sure that they will not place excessive strain on adjacent body parts because of relative stiffness. Your clients often will require some stability work before beginning the stretches. The need for stability work is indicated if the subject's alignment is degraded (partially lost) as a stretch is applied.

Key point: Do not stretch muscles if impaired core stability causes poor body alignment. Doing so may place excessive stress on joint structures.

To assess tightness in those muscles that are most likely to exacerbate low back problems, there are six principal tests—each of which will help you to assess restriction of pelvic motion: the modified Thomas test, the Ober test, the hip abduction test, the straight-leg raise test, the side flexion test, and the tripod test. The first five of these are described next. The tripod test position is described on page 125. Carefully note whether any of the movements in these tests reproduces the pain for which the patient has sought treatment; note also if the range is significantly less than the optimal position.

PRINCIPLES OF MUSCLE STRETCHING

Five methods of stretching are generally recognized: ballistic, static, active, and two proprioceptive neuromuscular facilitation (PNF) techniques (table 6.1). PNF stretching has been adopted by the sporting world from neurological physiotherapy treatments. These techniques, which involve alternately contracting and relaxing muscles, capitalize on various muscle reflexes to achieve a greater level of relaxation during the stretch. The back stability program uses two PNF techniques: contract–relax (CR), and contract–relax–agonist–contract (CRAC). PNF stretching was believed at one time to be the most effective type of stretching (Etnyre and Abraham 1986; Holt and Smith 1983), with CRAC methods generally being better than CR. The data are not consistent, however. Moore and Kukulka (1991) found CRAC to cause more pain than either CR or static stretching; moreover, they found that static stretching appeared to be

Table 6.1 Principal Stretching Techniques

Method	Action
Ballistic	Rapidly jerking at end of range to force the tissues to stretch.
Static	Slowly and passively stretching the muscle to full range and maintaining this stretched position for a set period—usually from 15 to 30 s.
Active	Contracting the agonist muscle to full inner range to impart a stretch on the antagonist.
Contract–relax (CR)	Isometrically contracting the stretched muscle and then relaxing and passively stretching the muscle still farther. This action is usually performed by a partner.
Contract–relax–agonist–contract (CRAC)	The same as CR, except that during the final stages of the stretching phase, the muscle opposite the one being stretched is contracted.

the most effective of all the techniques, leading to less pain and more range of motion. I recommend that you select stretching techniques on a client-by-client basis. See what works best for each person. The advantage of static stretching, of course, is that it does not require your presence or that of anyone else.

Here are the basic five stretching methods:

1. Ballistic stretching involves taking the limb to the end of its movement range and adding repetitive bouncing movements. This method is increasingly out of favor because it appears that it may cause injury and muscle soreness (Etnyre and Lee 1987). Although not recommended for regular training, ballistic stretching may have a place in the final stages of rehabilitation for athletes whose sport requires ballistic actions (e.g., high kicks in martial arts practice) (Norris 1998).

2. During static stretching, a muscle is stretched to the point of slight discomfort and held there for an extended period. A holding time of 30 s has been shown to be optimal, with 15 s being less effective and 60 s being not more effective (Bandy and Irion 1994). Repeating the stretch is important, with the greatest stretching effects occurring within the first four repetitions (Taylor et al. 1990). Easily remembered, basic guidelines for static stretching are 5 repetitions,

holding each for 30 s, with 30 s rest between each movement.

3. Active stretching involves pulling a limb into full inner range so that the antagonist muscle is stretched passively while the agonist is strengthened. This type of stretch can be important when correcting muscle imbalance. The inner-range contraction helps shorten a lengthened (lax) muscle, while the shortened muscle is stretched using a functionally relevant movement. Webright and colleagues (1997) found static and active stretching equally effective when used daily for 6 weeks. Static stretching involves less coordination and fewer repetitions than active stretching, so it is more appropriate during early treatment stages. Active stretching involves more complex coordination and requires greater segmental control, making it more useful in later stages of rehabilitation.

4. The CR PNF technique involves lengthening a muscle until a comfortable stretch is felt. From this position, the muscle is isometrically contracted and held for a set period. The muscle is relaxed again and then taken to a new lengthened position until the subject again feels the full stretch. The rationale behind the CR method is that the contracted muscle will relax as a result of autogenic inhibition, as the Golgi tendon organ (GTO) fires to inhibit tension. Some authors argue

that a maximal isometric contraction is needed to initiate relaxation through the GTO mechanism (Janda 1992). Others recommend the use of minimal isometric contractions (Lewit 1991), which seem more appropriate in situations where pain is present. A window of opportunity exists after isometric muscle contraction—because the stretch reflex is suppressed for about 10 s following isometric contraction (Moore and Kukulka 1991), the stretch must be imposed during this time.

5. With the CRAC PNF technique, the muscle is stretched as just described, but in the final stages of the stretch, the opposing muscle groups are isometrically contracted to use reciprocal inhibition of the agonist and to reduce its tension.

To illustrate each of these procedures, consider stretching the hamstrings.

1. A ballistic stretch could involve keeping the leg straight while standing and vigorously reaching for the toes with a bouncing action. Although the rapid action may actually tighten the muscle by increasing its tone, it may stretch other soft tissues, including the noncontractile muscle elements, muscle tendons, and ligaments surrounding the hip, knee, and spine. In this particular exercise, moreover, repeated spinal flexion may increase intradiscal pressure within the lumbar discs, potentially leading to discal migration (McKenzie 1981) or discal herniation. For this reason, ballistic stretching should only be performed in the presence of good lumbar stability and optimal segmental alignment.

2. An easy static stretch for the hamstrings involves lying supine on the floor in a doorway, with the hips just inside the door frame. With the leg farthest from the door frame flat on the ground and the back in neutral position, raise the other leg, keeping it straight, until it rests on the door frame. To increase or decrease the stretch, move the body closer to or farther away from the door frame. The stretch is held for 30 s.

3. An active stretch could be performed by standing, holding onto a wall bar for support, and lifting the straight leg upward using the force of the hip flexors.

4. A person could perform the CR technique for the hamstrings while lying on his back. A training partner lifts his leg, keeping the knee straight. After holding the stretch for 10 s, the subject contracts his hamstrings by pulling the straight leg down toward the floor against his partner's resistance. He holds the tension for 10 to 20 s—sufficient time to allow the GTO to override the stretch reflex. He then releases the tension, and the training partner reapplies the stretch.

5. The CRAC technique takes this stretch even further: As the stretch is applied, the subject tries to increase the stretch himself by pulling the straight leg up toward his head, tensing his hip flexors. In this situation, the hamstrings are relaxed still further through reciprocal inhibition, and the stretch becomes even more effective.

STRETCHING TARGET MUSCLES

Several mobilizer muscles within the lumbar–pelvic region are commonly tight and may require stretching. It is generally best to begin with passive static stretching, followed by CR techniques. Finally, the opposing muscles are shortened to full inner range to stretch the antagonist actively.

ASSESSING SEGMENTAL CONTROL

The combination of tight muscles and lax muscles will alter body alignment. Static alignment is reflected in postural changes identified in chapter 5. Dynamic alignment changes are seen when one body segment moves relative to another, a process termed *segmental control* or *movement dysfunction*. In each of these tests, instruct your client to repeat the action three or four times while you observe him closely. Movement analysis of this type is easier if you focus your attention on one part of the body with each repetition. For example, if you are interested in pelvic and lumbar movement, focus on the pelvis on the first repetition and the lumbar spine on the second.

We will use some basic screening tests that are covered in greater detail in chapter 7, where they are used to redevelop segmental control. It is often helpful to use the test movement as the first exercise during rehabilitation, because the client is already familiar with the movement and so learning is facilitated.

Key point: Use the test movement as the first exercise during rehabilitation. Because the client is already familiar with this movement, learning will be easier.

SUMMARY

- Inner range holding is used to test muscle laxity.
- The gluteals (maximus and medius), iliopsoas, and deep abdominals are the main lax muscles of concern for back stability.
- Pressure biofeedback may be used to monitor an increase or decrease in the depth of the lumbar lordosis.
- Muscle length tests are used to assess short muscles.
- Tests used to assess muscle imbalance may be used as the initial exercises to retrain muscles.
- Five methods of muscle stretching are described in this chapter.
- Segmental control measures your client's ability to move one body segment in isolation to another.

Assessing Muscle Balance in the Iliopsoas

Goal: Determine if the iliopsoas muscle is capable of holding the hip at full inner range flexion.

While sitting, your client flexes her hip maximally while maintaining 90° knee flexion so that the foot is lifted clear of the ground. Have her hold this position as long as she can, while you record the time at which phasic movements begin. Note also the position of the pelvis and lumbar spine. Where the iliopsoas is lengthened, one of two things may happen. (1) If lumbar stability is poor, the pelvis will drop back into posterior tilt, flattening or even reversing the lumbar lordosis. (2) If lumbar stability is good, your client will be able to maintain the neutral position of the lumbar spine and pelvis, but the knee will simply drop, indicating that the hip flexor muscles have lengthened (but not necessarily weakened) and are unable to hold the full inner-range position.

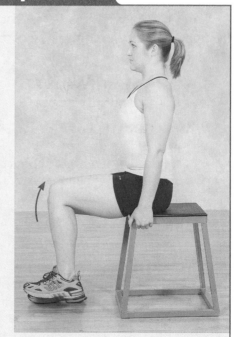

Hip pain during this action should be assessed by a physical therapist (PT). Pressure on the psoas bursa will be painful if the bursa is inflamed. Also, the joint may glide anteriorly because of imbalance of the hip lateral rotators. Normally, these muscles (especially quadratus femoris) hold the head of the femur back against the anteriorly directed force of the hip flexors. In a swayback posture, the hip lies in extension, and the posterior muscles may be lax or wasted. As flexion progresses, the head of the femur may glide anteriorly, stressing the hip structures and causing pain (Sahrmann 2002).

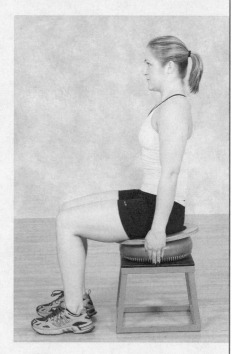

Assessing Muscle Balance in the Gluteus Maximus

Goal: Determine if the gluteus maximus muscle is capable of holding the hip in full inner-range extension.

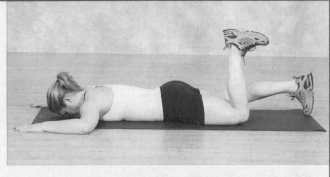

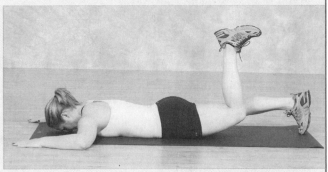

Have your client lie in a prone position with her knee flexed to 90°. Then she should lift her hip to the inner range of extension and hold it steady. Using palpation, note the order of muscle contraction during the hip extension. Normally, the hamstrings should contract first, followed by the gluteus maximus, then the contralateral erector spinae, and finally the ipsilateral erector spinae (Lewit 1991). In many cases of imbalance, the gluteus is poorly recruited or even inhibited (**pseudoparesis**) by tightness in the opposing hip flexors (Janda 1986). Where this is the case, the order of muscle contraction changes. If the gluteals do not function adequately, the hamstrings dominate the movement—little gluteal activity is apparent, and the muscle mass remains flaccid. Note how long your client can hold the position steady before phasic movement begins.

Performing the test with the knee bent reduces the contribution that the hamstrings make to the movement by shortening them. The contribution of the gluteus is therefore more apparent. Your ability to see and feel the subtle changes that indicate the order of muscle contraction, however, takes time to develop. Until you have gained experience in this area of examination, you can use dual-channel electromyography to show the intensity and timing of muscle contraction. Watch carefully to see if your client performs a false hip extension movement; in this action, the pelvis anteriorly tilts because of the powerful action of the erector spinae, and the relationship between the hip and pelvis remains the same.

Explain to your client which muscles she should use to perform this activity and in which order. If she tends to make a false hip extension, hold her pelvis down while she raises her leg using only her gluteals, so that she learns what the correct movement feels like.

When the gluteus maximus is poorly recruited, hip hyperextension power will be lost. You can see this if you ask your client to walk backward. If the gluteus is poorly recruited, clients will often anteriorly tilt their pelvis and hyperextend their lumbar spine in an attempt to make up for the loss of extension power at the hip.

Key point: Backward walking can make gluteus maximus weakness readily apparent.

Assessing Muscle Balance in the Gluteus Medius

Goal: Determine if the gluteus medius muscle is capable of holding the hip in full inner-range combined abduction and external rotation.

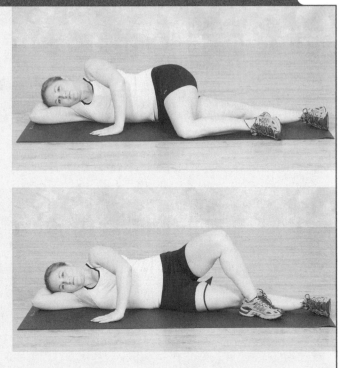

The action in this test is combined hip abduction, with slight lateral rotation to emphasize the posterior fibers of the muscle (Jull 1994). Have your client lie on her side with her knees flexed and feet together. Place a small cushion or folded towel between her feet for comfort. Instruct her to abduct and externally rotate her upper leg as high as possible.

This position will identify where muscle tone is poor. Athletes should rotate their trunk forward until the chest is on the couch and allow the knee to drop over the couch side. From this position they lift the leg as before. Although this is basically the same action, the difference is one of leverage. In the first movement (the nonathlete), as the movement progresses the femur approaches the vertical and so leverage decreases and the muscle work gets easier toward the inner range. In the second movement, because the body has turned through 90°, the femur (moving from below couch level) approaches the horizontal as the movement progresses, and so leverage and muscle work increase toward inner range—a much more difficult action altogether.

Prone Abdominal Hollowing Test Using Pressure Biofeedback

Goal: Assess client's ability to hold the inner range of the deep abdominals.

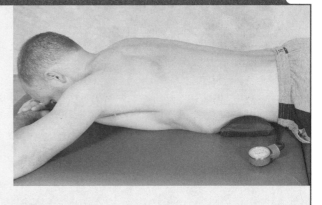

With your subject lying prone, place the pressure biofeedback unit beneath his abdomen with the upper edge of the device's bladder below his navel. Inflate the unit to 70 mmHg, and instruct your client to perform abdominal hollowing (see chapter 4). The aim is to reduce the pressure reading on the biofeedback unit by 6 to 10 mmHg and to maintain this contraction for 10 repetitions of 10 s each while breathing normally (Richardson and Hodges 1996).

This test relies on your client's being relatively lean. For an obese subject, the test is not suitable, because abdominal soft tissue contact will be maintained throughout the abdominal hollowing action, nullifying the test.

Heel Slide Maneuver Using Pressure Biofeedback

Goal: Assess the ability of the deep abdominals to maintain spinal stability.

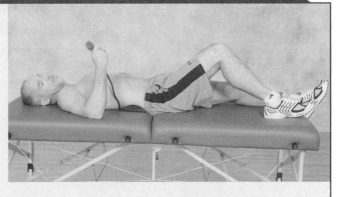

The subject begins in a crook-lying position with the spine in a neutral position and the pressure biofeedback unit positioned beneath his lower spine. While you palpate the anterior superior iliac spine, instruct him to gradually straighten one leg, sliding the heel along the ground to take the weight off the limb. During this action, the hip flexors work eccentrically and pull on the pelvis and lumbar spine. If the strong pull of these muscles is sufficient to displace the pelvis, you will be able to feel the pelvis tilt; moreover, the pressure shown on the dial of the biofeedback unit will change. If your client cannot complete the action without altering pelvic tilt or depth of lordosis, palpate the abdominal muscle action. Often subjects will substitute their rectus abdominis or external oblique in an attempt to fix the pelvis rather than using transversus abdominis and internal oblique. Where this is the case, these deeper abdominal muscles will need to be reeducated.

Restoration of abdominal muscle function is covered in chapter 7.

Thomas Test

Goal: Assess the length of the hip flexors.

The patient begins in crook-lying position at the end of the examination table. Instruct her to lift both knees up to her chest, keeping her back flattened to a point where the sacrum just begins to lift away from the examination table surface, but not farther. You can monitor the movement of the pelvis and lumbar spine using a pressure biofeedback unit. As she holds one leg close to her chest to maintain the pelvic position, have her lower the other leg over the end of the table, maintaining a 90° angle at the knee (a). Optimal alignment occurs with the femur horizontal and aligned with the sagittal plane (no abduction) and with the subject's shoulder, hip, and knee more or less in line. The tibia should hang vertically (90° knee flexion) and be aligned with the sagittal plane (no hip rotation—see c). If the femur rests above the horizontal and the knee is flexed less than 90°, tightness may be present in either the iliopsoas or rectus femoris. If the rectus is tight, straightening the knee will take the stretch off the muscle and the leg will drop down (b). If the knee is straightened and the leg stays in place, this indicates tightness in the iliopsoas. Use palpation to distinguish between the psoas and iliacus. Psoas can be palpated deep in the abdomen at the side of the lumbar spine. Iliacus is found on the inner side of the pelvis. Both muscles take experience to palpate, because they lie beneath the abdominal contents (see figure 3.12b).

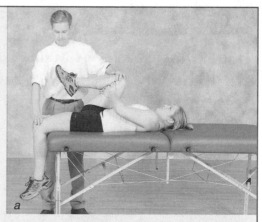

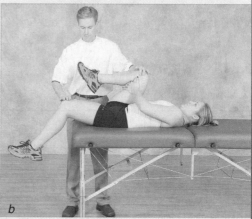

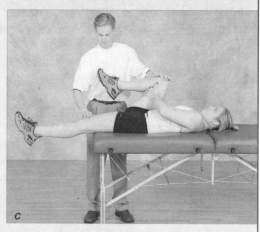

Ober Test

Goal: Assess both the length of tensor fasciae lata muscle and the tightness of the iliotibial band (ITB).

The modified Ober test begins in side-lying position with the pelvis in a neutral position *(a)*. Have your client bend her lower leg to improve overall body stability while you stabilize the pelvis to avoid lateral pelvic dipping. The examination table should be low enough to allow you to place pressure through the subject's iliac crest in the direction of the lower shoulder. You may monitor the position of the spine and pelvis using pressure biofeedback. While she maintains the neutral pelvic position, have your client abduct her upper leg to 15° above the horizontal and then extend her hip about 15°. She should then adduct her leg while maintaining extension. For an athlete, optimal muscle length would be confirmed if she is able to lower her upper leg to the level of the table; the nonathlete should be able to lower her leg to the horizontal *(b)*. A false

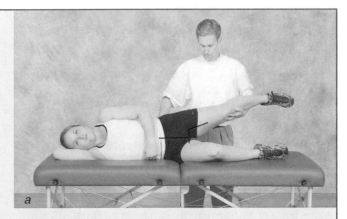

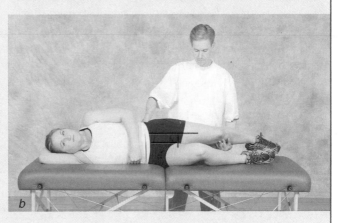

reading is obtained if the pelvis is allowed to tip and the lumbar spine to laterally flex. You can still proceed with the test when hip extension is limited, but you should further assess the hip tightness to determine whether it results from muscular, capsular, or osteological factors—an examination for which you should refer the subject to an orthopedic physical therapist.

Bending the knee during the Ober test will wind up the ITB more and place a greater emphasis on the portion closer to the knee, a useful procedure if testing for ITB friction syndrome at the knee (see Norris 2004b, page 222, and Norris 2004a. This latter paper is available online at www.norrisassociates.co.uk/library/6-11MITB.pdf).

Hip Abduction Test

Goal: Assess tightness in the hip abductor muscles.

Have your client lie on his back on a couch, closer to the far edge of the couch. Hook his far heel lightly over the couch edge to stop the leg from sliding. Grasp the near leg using a hook grip or your forearm and use your other hand to monitor the pelvis. Take up a broad walk stance, and abduct your client's hip while monitoring pelvic position. For a normal value, you should be able to abduct the hip to 45° to the midline. Bear in mind that the hamstrings, if tight, may also limit the abduction range. If you suspect this to be the case, flex your client's knee slightly (unlock it) and repeat the test. If abduction range has increased, the hamstrings are contributing to abduction range loss.

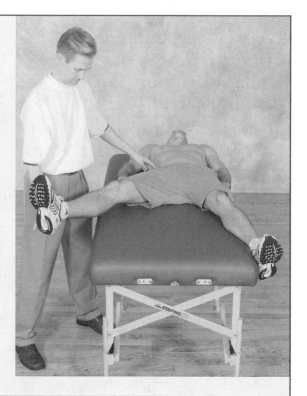

Straight-Leg Raise Test

Goal: Assess tightness in hamstrings.

Have your client lie supine on the examination table, one leg slightly bent. Have him raise the other leg, keeping it completely straight. Palpate the anterior rim of the pelvis to note the point at which the pelvis begins to posteriorly tilt because of hamstring tightness—this is the point at which a stable base is no longer being provided for the hamstrings to stretch against. Two body segments are moving here; this is a prime example of relative flexibility, as mentioned on page 64. As the maximal range of hamstring flexibility is reached, the pelvis will begin to tilt posteriorly, bringing the ischial tuberosity of the pelvis forward in an attempt to reduce tension in the hamstrings. Look for pelvic tilt, which will occur before the hamstrings are fully stretched to their end range. For example, if your client can stretch his hamstrings to 90° hip flexion, does the pelvis move at 80° to 90° as it should because the tension in the hamstrings is maximal? Or does the pelvis begin to tilt at perhaps 40° to 50°, when the tension in the hamstrings is only moderate? The latter case indicates a lack of muscular control over the pelvis—the individual is unable to create a stable pelvic base (using the trunk stabilizers) for the stretched hamstrings to pull against.

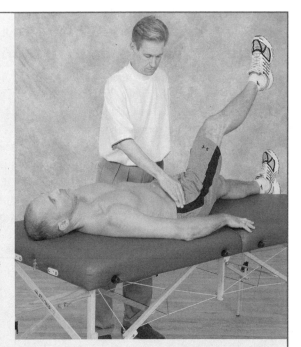

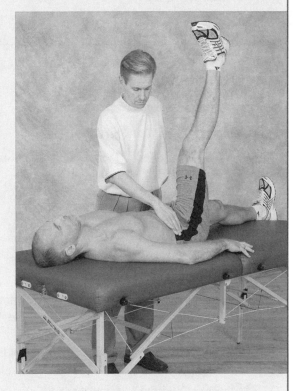

Side Flexion Test

Goal: Assess tightness in the trunk side flexors, especially quadratus lumborum.

Have your client stand with her back to a wall, feet shoulder-width apart. Have her place her hands either behind her head or, if her shoulder flexibility is poor, on her forehead. Ask her to side bend, attempting to put her lower elbow onto her hip area (greater trochanter). Observe (a) the gap between her lower ribs and pelvic rim on the concave side of the body movement, (b) the sternum, and (c) the level of the lower elbow. For normal movement, the rib–pelvic gap should open (get wider) and the client's elbow should lower to within 6 to 8 in. (15-20 cm) of his hip. As she moves, her sternum should remain central and should not deviate to one side, indicating that side flexion has become a trunk shift.

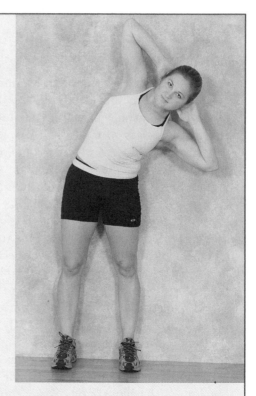

Thomas Test Stretch

Goal: Stretch the hip flexors.

This stretch is performed from the Thomas test position (see p. 114). Any firm surface may be used at home, such as a sturdy coffee table. Your client should hold one knee tightly to her chest and allow the other leg to rest in a stretched position near the horizontal.

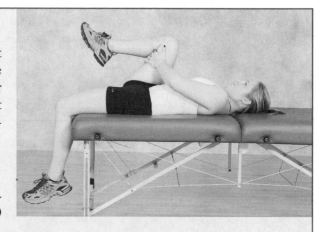

Teaching Points

▶ To increase the emphasis on the rectus femoris muscle, the knee of the lower (horizontal) leg may be bent.

▶ Throughout the movement, the back must remain flat on the table and the pelvis must not be allowed to move.

▶ Raising into the stretch position and recovering from it should be performed with control, taking 5 s in each direction.

Your client should hold the stretched position for 10 to 20 s and then lower her leg slowly. Reverse the legs and repeat the cycle two more times. Have her perform this stretch daily until she can perform the Thomas test satisfactorily.

Half Lunge

Goal: Stretch the hip flexors.

Have your client take up the half-kneeling position, with one hand on a chair to aid balance and the other hand pressing into his lumbar spine on the side of the dependent leg (the one with the knee on the floor). Instruct him to keep his abdomen hollowed throughout the exercise to keep the lumbar spine in neutral position. Tell him to lunge his body forward, forcing the dependent hip into extension while avoiding increasing the lordosis. He should hold this stretched position for 10 s.

Instruct your client to perform this exercise three times a day, each session consisting of 10 lunges on each side.

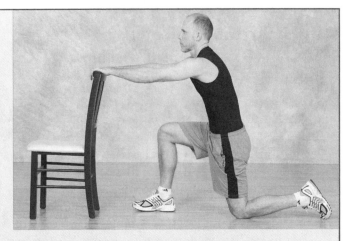

Teaching Points

▶ If his hip is very tight, your client may not be able to contract his abdominals powerfully enough to fix the pelvis. If this is the case, use an alternative hip stretch such as the Thomas test (p. 114).

▶ Both the rectus femoris and iliopsoas are stretched using this action. To increase the emphasis on the rectus, put the foot of the trailing leg onto a block to increase knee flexion.

▶ Clients with patellar pain should kneel on a thick, soft cushion to reduce patellofemoral compression.

▶ This client is too far from the chair, causing him to flex his spine. Make sure your client maintains spinal alignment throughout the exercise.

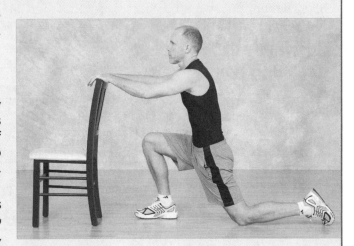

Ober Test Stretch

Goal: Stretch the iliotibial band (ITB) and tensor fasciae lata (TFL).

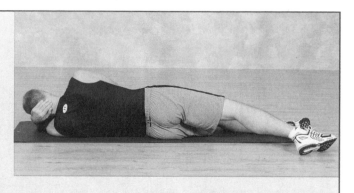

The ITB and TFL can become overactive and tight to compensate for a weak or inactive gluteus medius muscle. When this occurs, tightness in the ITB–TFL can cause friction of this structure over the greater trochanter of the femur or the lateral epicondyle of the femur. Both of these areas are common sites for ITB friction syndrome—a common overuse condition, particularly among distance runners, that results from muscle imbalance.

Beginning in a side-lying position, your client first performs the hip hitch described on page 184. Then he continues with the Ober test actions (see p. 115): He abducts the upper leg to 15° above the horizontal, extends it to 15°, and then lowers it into adduction (toward the floor or couch) while maintaining an immobile pelvis.

Teaching Points

▶ The exercise is complex because it requires the control of two body parts simultaneously. Supervise your client closely, watching the pelvic rim to note any unwanted pelvic movement and noting whether the hip extension is maintained.

▶ When the hip extension is lost, the leg falls forward into flexion and the stretch is lost from the TFL.

▶ If your client is unable to maintain stability of his pelvis, assist him by holding the pelvis in place with your hands.

Active Knee Extension, Holding Thigh

Goal: Stretch the hamstrings.

Have your client lie supine and then raise one leg to 90° hip flexion, comfortably bent at the knee, and hold it with his hands beneath the thigh. Then instruct him to straighten the leg as much as possible. The sensation should be one of deep stretching rather than acute pain. The discomfort should reduce as the stretch is held. He should hold the stretch for 30 s. Instruct him to perform this stretch at home three times a day, with two repetitions for each leg at each session.

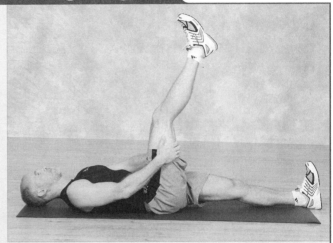

Teaching Points

▶ When extending the leg to lock the knee, people tend to allow the knee to move distally, reducing the stretch. Monitor the vertical position of the thigh throughout the action.

▶ This exercise also stretches the sciatic nerve and may be classified as a neural stretch. To reduce the neural effect, allow your client to plantar flex his foot. To increase the neural effect and target the sciatic nerve, have him dorsiflex the ankle and flex the toes.

Active Knee Extension, Pushing Against Thigh

Goal: Strengthen hip flexors, hip extensors, and hamstrings.

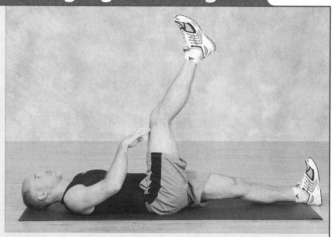

This action stretches the hamstrings while activating the quadriceps against a resistance. Increasing the quadriceps activity should reduce the hamstring tone through reciprocal innervation.

Have your client lie supine and, with one knee comfortably bent, raise that leg until it is at a 60° angle to the floor. Instruct him then to straighten the leg and then slowly raise the straightened leg until it is vertical (90° hip flexion). He should keep the leg completely straight and use only his hip flexor muscles to raise the leg (no use of the hands this time!), without allowing the knee to bend. Once the leg is vertical (or as near vertical as your client can raise it), have him place his hand on the leg just above the knee and use it as a fulcrum to straighten the leg just a little bit more. This is especially helpful in stretching the hamstrings. He should hold this position for 30 s.

Tell your client to do this exercise three times a day, using 3 repetitions for each leg per session.

Teaching Points

▶ The coordination of this movement is actually quite difficult. Encourage your client to take his time until he gets the technique right.

▶ The action is one of knee extension, but clients often also flex their hips. In those with short hip flexors, this can cause painful muscle cramping and so should be discouraged.

Trunk Side Flexor Stretch

Goal: Stretch the quadratus lumborum and lateral portion of the oblique abdominals.

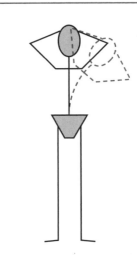

These muscles are commonly tight after prolonged periods of sitting or bed rest. Have your client stand with his back against a wall, his feet shoulder-width apart, and his hands clasped behind his head or placed on his forehead. He should keep his abdomen hollowed throughout the exercise. Instruct him to slowly bend his spine (and only his spine) to one side, being very careful to keep his pelvis level and his knees straight. Until he learns what the proper movement feels like, you should place your hands on his pelvis and let him know when it's bending. Tell him to reach his upper elbow as far toward the ceiling as he can, in an attempt to lengthen his spine, and to hold this position for 30 s. Then he should repeat the exercise to the other side. The height of the upper elbow indicates the range of motion obtained, and the comparative range of each side will reveal your client's degree of symmetry.

Instruct your client to do this stretch three times a day on each side.

Teaching Points

▶ Monitor the position of your client's sternum. It should remain central and not deviate to one side. Sideways motion of the sternum indicates a side shift rather than side flexion action.

▶ It is common for people to have more motion on one side than the other. However, this asymmetry may be attributable to stiffness within individual spinal segments. Intersegmental spinal motion should be checked by a PT.

Cat Stretch

Goal: Stretch the erector spinae.

The erector spinae muscles can tighten during long periods of sitting or bed rest. Have your client assume a four-point kneeling position. Emphasize that throughout this exercise, she must move only her spine, with her shoulders remaining over her hands and her hips remaining over her knees at all times. Have her tilt her pelvis posteriorly and continue flexing her spine until her face points toward her groin. She should hold this position for 30 s and then slowly relax back toward the starting position.

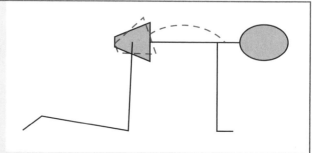

Instruct your client to perform this exercise three times a day, with 6 repetitions per session.

Teaching Points

▶ Although useful, this exercise relies on the ability of the abdominal muscles to shorten sufficiently to pull against the tight spinal extensors. In some clients, abdominal strength may not be good enough to achieve this aim.

▶ Where this is the case, have your client perform sitting trunk flexion with overpressure instead.

Sitting Trunk Flexion With Overpressure

Goal: Stretch the erector spinae using overpressure.

Have your client sit on a gym bench. She should flex her lower lumbar spine by placing her feet on a low stool to posteriorly tilt the pelvis and flatten or reverse the lordosis. The therapist should guide her to flex her spine by drawing the head downward and placing her interlocked hand behind her neck. Encourage her to gently pull on her neck to increase flexion of the spine. Have the client hold the end position for 30 to 40 s and perform 3 repetitions daily.

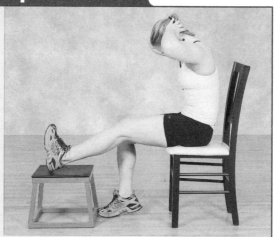

Teaching Points

▶ The action should be one of trunk flexion rather than hip motion. Encourage your client to draw her nose toward her umbilicus rather than pull her face between her knees.

▶ The overpressure affects the delicate neck region, so pressure must be very light indeed, with no bouncing action.

▶ Your client should feel a comfortable lengthening of the spine. If she feels pain, she must stop the movement immediately.

Tripod Position

Goal: Monitor lumbar–pelvic motion as the hamstring muscles are placed on stretch.

Have your client sit upright on the edge of a table, her lumbar spine in its neutral position and her feet hanging over the edge of the table. Have her straighten one leg and visually monitor pelvic tilt and lumbar alignment. At the initiation of hamstring stretch, the lumbar–pelvic region should not move. As the leg is straightened and the hamstring stretch increases, only minimal posterior tilt and lumbar flattening should occur. Poor segment control, shown as pelvic tilt and lumbar flexion, are seen as soon as the leg straightens or if lumbar flexion is exaggerated.

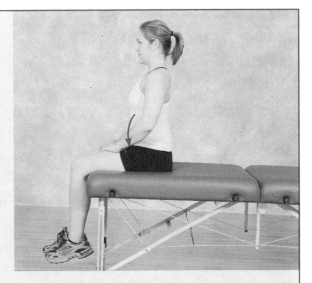

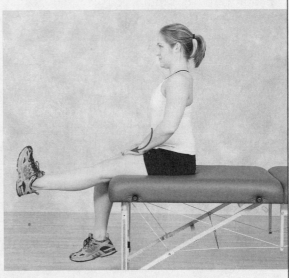

Kneeling Rock-Back

Goal: Determine control of the hip relative to the lumbar–pelvic region while kneeling.

Have your client kneel on a mat on all fours, with her hand directly beneath her shoulder and her knee beneath her hip. The client should begin with the lumbar spine in a neutral position and then rock backward, pulling the hip behind the knees. Monitor the pelvic tilt angle and lumbar lordosis. For optimal segmental control, motion should begin at the hip. Once hip flexion passes about 120° (depending on your client's body proportions), her pelvis should posteriorly tilt and her lumbar spine flatten. Ensure that she moves slowly, and determine whether the sequence is motion at the hip–pelvis–lumbar spine. Poor segmental control is present if at the beginning of the rock-back, the pelvis tilts and the lumbar spine flattens.

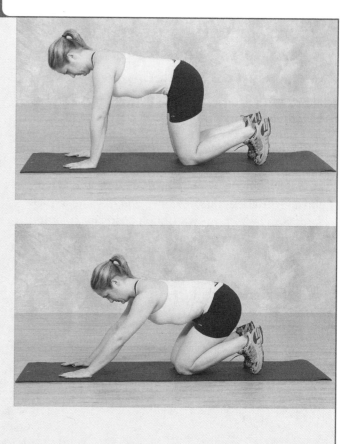

One-Leg Lift

Goal: Assess lumbar–pelvic control during one-leg lifting.

Ask your client to stand side-on to a wall with one hand on the wall for balance if needed. Instruct him to slowly lift one leg, bending at the knee. He should take the leg to a comfortable position (usually above hip height) and then lower. Monitor the lumbar–pelvic region from the front and the side. In optimal alignment, the pelvis should remain level horizontally as the client lifts his leg, and the sequence should be hip motion (flexion) followed by pelvic motion (posterior tilt) followed by lumbar motion (lordosis flattens and then reverses). Poor control exists when the pelvis drops as the leg is lifted, and the lumbar spine flexes during the early stages of the movement.

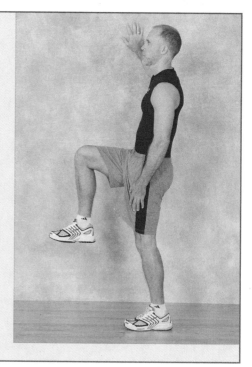

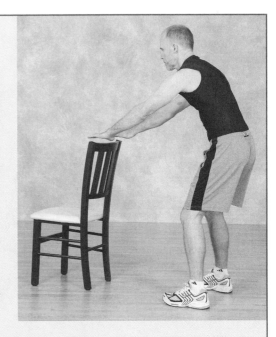

Forward Bending

Goal: Determine lumbar–pelvic control in bending.

Have your client stand with his feet shoulder-width apart, facing the seat of a chair. Instruct him to bend forward to touch the chair seat and then stand back up again. Optimal control has occurred when your client unlocks his knees and anteriorly tilts his pelvis, flexing only slightly at the lumbar spine. Poor control is present when he locks out and hyperextends the knees; he should not tilt his pelvis but instead should flex markedly at the lumbar and thoracic spine.

Exercises to correct segmental control are covered in chapter 7.

Note the increased thoracic kyphosis on this client. When you see this, have your client practice the sternal lift action first.

Chapter 7
Foundation Movements

Your clients must have certain fundamental abilities before they can follow the programs and practices discussed later in this book. This chapter shows you how to teach your clients these skills.

Muscle action can stabilize the trunk by turning it into a solid cylinder. Clients should stabilize in a neutral lumbar position, and they must have sufficient postural awareness to identify this position. The foundation movements, therefore, address two principle aims:

1. To enable your client to contract her stability muscles and maintain that contraction
2. To enable your client to identify her neutral lumbar position and move into this position at will

Once your clients have learned to contract their stability muscles, they must increase the contraction intensity to 30% to 40% of their maximum and sustain this. Your clients must learn to build stability muscle endurance, aiming to perform 10 repetitions and hold each movement for 10 s. Your client must also learn to recognize the neutral position of the lumbar spine, to detect when the lumbar spine has moved away from this neutral position, and to correct the position of the spine using a pelvic tilting action to move back into neutral.

Some of the movements used in this section are the same as those used in chapter 6 as tests of segmental control. This is intentional, because your client is already familiar with the movement, and this makes learning a new action easier. One of the recurring themes that I introduced in chapter 4 is that muscle imbalance consists of three components: **tight muscle,** which limits movement; **lax muscle,** which fails to support the body; and **segmental control** or movement dysfunction, which is lack of control of one body segment relative to another. To establish back stability using a muscle balance approach, we identify imbalance and then correct it using these three components.

Key point: Muscle imbalance consists of changes in muscle (tight or lax) and movement (segmental control).

We saw in chapter 6 how the tests of muscle tightness become stretching exercises and those of muscle laxity can introduce inner range shortening movements. Similarly, the segmental control tests now become exercises. Optimal movement only occurs if muscle balance is present, so why do we not simply focus on that? We could, and if we practice optimal movement over and over again, we will stretch the tight muscles and shorten the lax. However, this is very hard for clients to do: They will have to pull against tight, painful muscles and work very hard to get lax muscles to engage. The effort and coordination that this involves can easily defeat clients, and compliance rates are very low indeed. Instead, we split the movements into their component tasks and practice these individually. This so-called part task training allows your clients to focus closely on one part of the action. When they have mastered this single movement, they can do another and then put the two actions together. In this way they gradually progress to practicing the whole task and correcting their movement dysfunction.

Key point: Part task practice splits a complex action into several simpler components.

TEACHING YOUR CLIENTS TO CONTROL PELVIC TILT

You will need to teach your client how to tilt and hold his pelvis to correct misalignment, so he can confidently move into a neutral lumbar position. As you begin treatment, remember that for some clients, touching may be a sensitive issue. Be alert for words or body language that indicates your client is uncomfortable. Before you touch the client, explain clearly what you are going to do and be sure that he is comfortable with the proposed action and gives consent. If he is not comfortable, try a different approach. With sensitive clients, if you proceed gradually you can usually establish the trust necessary to pursue the most helpful therapeutic course. Therapist–client trust is an essential ingredient for successful treatment, so do everything you can to establish and maintain that trust.

Key point: Get your clients' consent before touching them. Check the policy of your facility, school, or club. For some institutions, verbal (spoken) consent is sufficient. For others, written consent may be required.

Segmental Control

The ability to dissociate the movement of one body segment from that of a neighboring segment depends on stabilization ability and adequate muscle length. The central requirement of segmental control as it applies to back stability is that the pelvis be able to move independently of the lumbar spine in both frontal and sagittal planes.

The combination of movements of the hip on the pelvis and of the lumbar spine on the pelvis increases the range of motion of this body area. The relationship between lumbar and pelvic movement is called lumbar–pelvic rhythm (see p. 131). During forward flexion in standing, when the legs are straight, movement of the pelvis on the hip is limited to about C0° hip flexion. Any further movement, allowing the subject to touch the ground, must occur at the lumbar spine. For lumbar–pelvic rhythm to function correctly, movement of the pelvis on the hip should be equal to or greater than movement of the lumbar spine on the pelvis. In people with a history of back pain, however, the ability to perform pelvic tilting (pelvis moving on hip) is often lost—almost all the movement during forward bending comes from the lumbar spine, which shows excessive flexion laxity but limited, or often blocked, extension. In

the lower trunk, the ability to dissociate lumbar movement from pelvic movement is therefore important, and correction of faulty lumbar–pelvic rhythm is vital.

Key point: The ability to dissociate movement of the lumbar spine from movement of the pelvis is essential for the healthy functioning of the back.

Assessing and Developing Lumbar–Pelvic Dissociation

 See pages 125-127 We begin by repeating some of the screening tests we looked at briefly in chapter 6. With each test, perform the action first to determine the level of lumbar–pelvic dissociation that your client has. Record this as his baseline value and then repeat the same action to begin the process of movement reeducation. The quality of movement rather than quantity is imperative at this stage. The goal of each exercise is simply to perform the action correctly for 3 sets of 5 repetitions before you allow your client to progress to another movement. I have included several movements with similar aims, because you may need to try different exercises to find one to suit your client. For example, a client requiring back stability may also have a knee condition, so you would not want to choose a kneeling condition. Someone whose back pain is exacerbated by standing would find a sitting or kneeling starting position more comfortable. Use the following guidelines for each action:

- Ask your client to perform the action first to determine his level of lumbar–pelvic dissociation.
- Repeat the action giving multisensory cues. Use touch (tactile cues), voice commands (auditory cues), and mirrors and demonstration (visual cues).
- Stop each movement when the quality degrades. Begin again after a rest period.
- Progress the action only when your client can perform the movement several times by himself without coaching.

Building on Correct Lumbar– Pelvic Rhythm

Restoring accurate lumbar–pelvic rhythm is essential for the correct functioning of this region. Rehabilitation of this mechanism begins with your client recognizing the action of pelvic tilt and being able to maintain the neutral lumbar spine.

 Control of lumbar–pelvic rhythm is used extensively during static loading of the stabilizing system covered in chapters 8 through 11. These exercises will help your client gain the essential control of pelvic tilt that is necessary for back stability. The last two exercises use a gym ball and will prepare your client for the more advanced gym ball exercises described in chapter 10.

Key point: The pelvic tilt mechanism is an important key to movements of the lumbar–pelvic region.

TEACHING YOUR CLIENTS TO IDENTIFY AND ASSUME THE NEUTRAL POSITION

Teach your clients to identify and maintain the neutral position of the lumbar spine at each stage of the back stability program, because the neutral position places minimal stress on body tissues. Lumbar neutral position is midway between full flexion and full extension as brought about by posterior and anterior tilting of the pelvis. The discs and facet joints are minimally loaded in this position, and the soft tissues surrounding the lumbar spine are in elastic equilibrium. Because postural alignment is optimal in this position, it is generally the most effective position from which trunk muscles can work.

Key point: Lumbar neutral position is midway between flexion and extension of the lumbar spine. It is the position of least stress on the spinal tissues.

In the healthy, uninjured person, the neutral position corresponds to lumbar alignment in an optimal posture. Individuals with suboptimal posture may increase or reduce their pelvic tilt, causing corresponding changes in the depth of lumbar lordosis. In either case, the neutral position remains midway between end-range flexion and end-range extension; in cases of postural malalignment, however, part of the treatment aim is to restore optimal posture by rebalancing the length of the surrounding soft tissue elements. Subjects can find neutral position passively (as you move the pelvis) or actively (subject moves her own pelvis through muscle action).

Refer to Optimal Postural Alignment in chapter 5 for a more thorough treatment of the neutral position while standing. In kneeling, your subject attempts similar lumbar alignment by slightly hollowing the lumbar spine. A flat back or excessive lordosis both mean that the subject has moved away from the neutral position and will need to reposition by tilting the pelvis.

With time, your clients will be able to recognize and maintain the neutral position. In the early stages of the program, however, you will need to constantly remind them of their spinal alignment. Proprioceptive exercises will help your clients learn to assume neutral position at will.

Proprioception– Basic Concepts

Because proprioception is vital to back stability during later stages of rehabilitation (Norris 1998), your clients should begin appropriate proprioceptive exercises at the start of their treatment programs. Lephart and Fu (1995) defined **proprioception** as a specialized variation of touch encompassing the sensations of both joint movement and joint position. During acute injury, the reflexes initiated by displacement of mechanoreceptors and muscle spindles occur far more rapidly than those brought about by pain (nociception) (Barrack and Skinner 1990). Effusion (escape of fluid) from joints contributes to a reduction in mechanoreceptor discharge, resulting in inhibition of muscular contraction. This inhibition commonly occurs in the vastus medialis of the knee, for example, where just 60

Table 7.1   Components of Proprioception

Level of neural system	Component of proprioception controlled
Spinal	Muscle stiffness
Brain stem	Static joint positioning
Higher	Kinesthesia (movement sense)

ml of intra-articular effusion may result in 30% to 50% inhibition of quadriceps contraction (Kennedy et al. 1982). Proprioceptive deficits parallel joint degeneration (Barrett et al. 1991), but it is unclear whether this is a cause or a result of degeneration (Lephart and Fu 1995). Proprioceptive exercise is useful from the early stages of rehabilitation to restore normal functioning of the proprioceptive control of the back. And it is nowhere more useful than in helping your clients master neutral position.

From a clinical standpoint, proprioception consists of three interrelating components (Beard et al. 1994) that represent activity at spinal, brain stem, and higher centers (Tyldesley and Grieve 1989) (table 7.1). Individuals beginning back stability training should focus on brain stem activities, characterized especially by static joint positioning, because they must cultivate this ability before proceeding to more advanced training.

Key point: Both joint swelling and joint degeneration reduce proprioception. Seniors and those recovering from joint injury can be expected to have poor proprioception.

Static Joint Positioning

See pages 151–152

Static joint position sense helps us to maintain posture and balance at the brain stem level. Input for these actions is from joint proprioception, from the vestibular centers in the ears, and from the eyes. Balance and postural exercise with the eyes open or closed can enhance static joint posi-

tion sense. Reproduction of passive positioning (RPP) and reproduction of active positioning (RAP) are exercises in which an individual tries to place a joint back in its starting position after either active or passive movement.

Key point: For reproduction of passive positioning (RPP), the client places his joint back into its starting position after it has been moved away by the therapist. It is a *hands-on* approach. For reproduction of active position (RAP), the client repeats an active movement with precision, which is a *hands-off* approach.

TEACHING YOUR CLIENTS TO USE ABDOMINAL HOLLOWING

Individuals with low back pain must reeducate their muscles by learning to isolate the deep (lateral) abdominals from the superficial abdominals. This requires a hollowing action of the abdomen, using the internal oblique and transversus abdominis muscles rather than the traditional lumbar flexion movements (e.g., sit-ups) that emphasize the upper rectus. Before proceeding with the exercises described later in this book, your clients must be able to perform abdominal hollowing well and consistently.

Because the concept of abdominal hollowing is probably less familiar than other major points in this chapter, I devote a disproportionately large portion of the chapter to this discussion.

Abdominal Hollowing— General Considerations

See pages 153-157

Abdominal hollowing is simple in theory and is the same in all positions: The subject pulls his belly in and up at the navel without moving the rib cage, the pelvis, or the spine. Everything else in this section merely elaborates on that basic action and on how you can best help your clients to learn it well.

In comparison with mobilizer muscles, stability muscles are better suited to endurance (postural holding) and are better recruited at low resistance levels. Contraction intensities of 30% to 40% of the maximum voluntary contraction (MVC) work best for the deep (lateral) abdominal muscles. Your clients initially will have little control over the intensity of their contractions. Often they will begin with minimal contractions and then build to high intensities (60-70% MVC). This is acceptable during the early stages of learning and enables your clients to feel their muscles working. Clients eventually must gain accurate control, however, and you should instruct them to master changing the intensity of contraction in all hollowing exercises. An effective way to teach this is to ask for a maximal contraction and then tell your clients to relax by half, and then half again. Once they have achieved minimal contraction, they should then build up the intensity again, in steps, to the maximum. Only when they can control hollowing with minimal muscle intensity over a period of time (10 repetitions each of 30-40% MVC, held for 10 s) should they progress to more advanced exercises.

The position in which the movements are performed is important. Have your clients assume the neutral position of the spine whenever possible—initially, you will need to position your client correctly (you may want to reread the section Optimal Postural Alignment in chapter 5 for the optimal position while standing). If your client is kneeling, have her try to achieve proper alignment by slightly hollowing her lumbar spine—a flat back or excessive lordosis means that the subject has moved away from the neutral position and should appropriately reposition by tilting the pelvis. Even-

tually, your clients will be able to maintain the neutral position throughout their exercises.

Key point: Have your clients maintain the neutral position of the spine throughout all the exercises in this chapter.

Abdominal Hollowing— Starting Positions

Different people require different starting positions, depending on their weight, degree of injury, flexibility, and so on. Next we look at four basic starting positions: four-point kneeling, standing (wall support), prone lying, and sitting.

Four-point kneeling places the fibers of the transversus abdominis muscle vertically. It thereby initiates some stretching in the transversus, making contraction of this muscle easier. The four-point kneeling position is usually more comfortable than the other positions for people with back pain. On the other hand, four-point kneeling requires control of structures in the spine, shoulders, and hips, whereas lying positions require control over only spinal structures. Because controlling a single body segment is considerably easier than controlling three, many people (especially those with poor body control and especially when unsupervised) find exercises in the lying position easier to perform. Moreover, because four-point kneeling places compression on the patellae and the wrists, individuals with pathology in these joints (such as arthritis) may need to modify the kneeling position. Modifications include (a) placing the open fist on the ground rather than the flat of the hand to reduce the wrist extension stress, (b) placing extra padding beneath the shins and leaving the patellae free, (c) taking the body weight on the forearms rather than the wrists, and (d) supporting the upper body with the chest on a chair to reduce the upper-body weight transmitted to the arms and wrists.

Obese subjects often have trouble performing abdominal hollowing in a kneeling position—the sheer weight of their abdominal tissue presents too large an overload for their deep abdominals to work against. For obese individuals, the **standing (wall support)** position is better: Although it is usually a progression from kneeling (standing provides no stretch facilitation of the deep abdominals), obese individuals can control the action more easily. They can use their hands to palpate the abdominal wall, and the action of pulling the abdominals in is often rather familiar in the standing position.

Prone lying is not suitable for obese individuals with poor abdominal muscle tone because of the compression of excess body tissue in this position. Lean people often like the prone position, however, because it provides many sensory cues—the act of hollowing to draw the abdominal wall away from the supporting surface gives useful tactile feedback (especially if a pressure biofeedback unit is used, as described later in this chapter).

Sitting provides the advantage that clients can practice hollowing while at work or in class. The disadvantage for those with back pain is that sitting often exacerbates their pain. If it does so, chose four-point kneeling or lying until subjects are pain free. If you do choose sitting, make sure your client sits up tall and uses a neutral lumbar position. Slouch or slumped sitting places significant stress on the spinal tissues and actually makes abdominal hollowing more difficult to perform.

Table 7.2 gives the pros and cons for each starting position. Use your own judgment to select appropriate starting positions for clients, taking into account body size, body condition, age, and pathology. Be flexible—experiment with different starting positions until your client feels comfortable with the exercise.

Key point: Linking abdominal hollowing with pelvic floor contractions is a useful way to enhance learning in both males and females. For research on this topic, see page 57.

Your clients must be able to differentiate the abdominal hollowing action from pelvic tilting. Ensure that your clients do not flatten their backs completely against the wall, because that would indicate posterior pelvic tilting through action of the rectus abdominis. Once a client has performed wall-standing abdominal hollowing correctly to repetition, have him repeat the action without wall support. There should be no movement of the spine, pelvis, or rib cage.

Tips for Teaching Abdominal Hollowing

Multisensory cues can facilitate learning (Miller and Medeiros 1987). You can provide auditory cues by giving your clients frequent feedback about their performance. To create visual cues, encourage people to look at their muscles as they function and to place a mirror on the floor or couch below the abdomen. For tactile (kinesthetic) cues, encourage subjects to feel the particular action—for example, ask them to feel their stomach being pulled in.

Key point: Multisensory cueing involves increased sensory input through auditory, visual, kinesthetic, and tactile stimuli, in conjunction with visualization of correct exercise technique.

Tactile cues for abdominal hollowing can come from you or from a belt touching your client's abdomen. The first technique involves palpation. Place the heel of your hand over the client's anterior superior iliac spine and point your fingers toward the pubic bone (figure 7.1). Your fingertips will then fall over the retroaponeurotic triangle, which is the most superficial position of transversus abdominis (Walters and Partridge 1957). At this point the external oblique is aponeurotic and, so, not electrically active. This point may be used for placing the electrode of a surface electromyograph (EMG) unit. Because the muscles are sheetlike, they will flatten rather than bulge when they contract. One way to facilitate the contraction is to say, "Stop me from pushing in" as you palpate the abdominal wall. A second way is have clients cough (visceral compression) and hold the muscle contraction they feel beneath your fingers. This cough-and-hold procedure is also useful in conjunction with surface EMG—as the muscle

Table 7.2 Abdominal Hollowing Starting Positions

Starting position	Advantage	Disadvantage
Four-point kneeling	Abdominal wall is stretched to facilitate abdominal hollowing. Different motor pattern to familiar sit-up exercise protocol in sport Position is comfortable for clients with LBP and during pregnancy. Belt or waistband can be used for tactile cueing.	Position places stress on wrists and knees. Position is difficult for obese clients.
Prone lying	Whole body is supported. Position makes it easier to avoid spinal movement. Tactile cue is provided when client pulls abdominal wall away from table. Pressure biofeedback may be used.	Position is inappropriate for obese or pregnant client because of soft tissue contact. Position may be challenging for client with breathing difficulties.
Sitting	Position is useful for daily practice at work. Self-palpation is easily applied. Position rehearses good sitting posture.	Sitting position may exacerbate back pain.
Standing	Tactile cue is provided to pull abdominal wall away from waistband. Position is appropriate for obese clients. Wall support may be used to reduce spinal movement. Position is functional for daily activities.	Weight bearing may not be suitable for client with discal pathology. Clients with extreme postural abnormalities may find position uncomfortable.

LBP = low back pain.

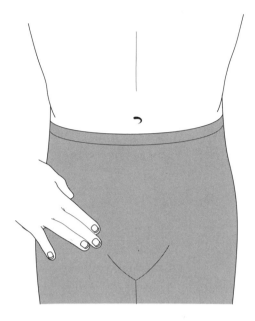

Figure 7.1 Palpation of the deep abdominals—the retroaponeurotic triangle—to teach abdominal hollowing.

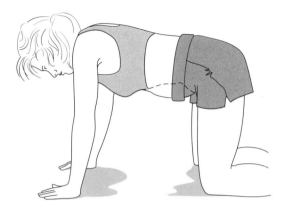

Figure 7.2 Using a belt to teach abdominal hollowing.

contraction shows on the EMG unit, encourage the subject to maintain the contraction while breathing normally. Continue with this exercise until your client can hold the contraction for a single 30 s repetition or for 10 repetitions of 10 s each. Then encourage your client to reduce the contraction intensity of the muscle to the minimum required to maintain the hollow abdomen position.

Here is another tip for tactile cues in the four-point kneeling position: Fasten a webbing belt around your client's abdomen below the navel, with the muscles relaxed and sagging (figure 7.2). The belt should be just tight enough to touch the skin but not to pull in the muscles. Have your client hollow the abdomen, pull the muscles away from the belt, and then relax them completely to fill the belt again. Some people may be unable to draw the muscles away from the belt; others may contract their muscles too strongly, making the abdominal wall rigid and leading to an inability to relax the muscles again to fill the belt. Several days' practice will give your clients full muscle control over both actions. Once they can achieve the appropriate contraction, have them build up the holding time to 10 to 30 s while breathing normally.

A final learning technique is visualization of correct exercise technique following your demonstration. For this mental practice, your clients should relax and imagine themselves performing the exercise. Such visualization has been shown to benefit development of both motor skills (Fansler et al. 1985) and strength (Cornwall et al. 1991). To help your clients visualize the hollowing action, explain the workings of the transversus abdominis and internal oblique muscles—use simple diagrams of the muscles and then demonstrate their location using palpation. Analogies such as "personal muscle corset" or "cylinder of muscles" can be helpful.

Abdominal Hollowing: Common Errors

Be sure that your client's rib cage, shoulders, and pelvis remain still throughout the hollowing action (figure 7.3a). The contour of the abdomen will flatten if a person takes and holds a deep breath, but you will notice the chest expansion (figure 7.3b). If this occurs, instruct your client to exhale and then hold the resulting chest position while performing the exercise. Placing a belt around the lower chest provides helpful feedback about chest movement. If your client is using the external oblique to brace the abdomen, which is also an incorrect technique, the lower ribs will be depressed, and you may observe a horizontal skin crease across the upper abdomen (figure 7.3c). When this occurs, instruct your client to perform pelvic floor contraction at the same time as abdominal hollowing but to avoid contracting the gluteus maximus (use of which leads in this

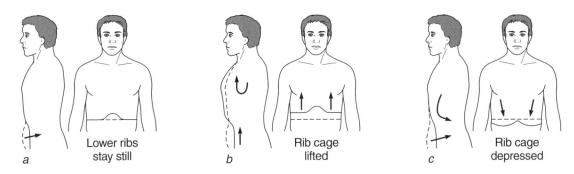

Figure 7.3   Abdominal hollowing in standing: *(a)* is correct, and *(b)* and *(c)* are incorrect.

case to inappropriate motor patterns for trunk stability during dynamic sports activity).

In kneeling, lying, and sitting positions, pressing onto the floor with the feet indicates a failure to isolate the deep abdominal action from that of the hip muscles. Placing your client's feet on a bathroom scale will provide clear feedback about hip extension pressure—ideally, the scales should show no increase in weight during the exercise.

Key point: Your clients should maintain a neutral lumbar position during abdominal hollowing and refrain from significant movement of ribs, pelvis, or hips.

TEACHING YOUR CLIENTS TO CONTRACT THE MULTIFIDUS MUSCLES AT WILL

Multifidus is the key stabilizer muscle within the spinal extensor group. Subjects with low back pain often lose the ability to contract this muscle (probably through pain inhibition), and they do not regain the ability spontaneously (Hides et al. 1996). Two kinds of exercises will help increase your client's basic back stability. The first focuses solely on the multifidus muscles, with an emphasis on helping your client learn

to recognize what it feels like to tense and relax only those particular muscles. The second, using the techniques of proprioception, focuses not only on the multifidus but also on the lateral abdominals, which are also vital for basic stability. Contracting the multifidus together with the other stabilizing muscles rather than in isolation is the ultimate goal.

Basic Exercise for Multifidus Contraction

See pages 158-162

Your help is essential for your client to learn adequate control of this muscle.

SUMMARY

- Safely improving back stability requires your client to learn to contract certain muscles—in particular, the deep abdominal muscles (transversus abdominis and internal oblique) and the multifidus muscles of the back.

- Your client must learn to control pelvic tilt, perform abdominal hollowing, and control neutral position of the lumbar spine.

- Some clients will need to perform isolated multifidus muscle contractions.

Standing Knee Raising

Goal: Differentiate hip, pelvic, and lumbar motion.

The subject stands at a right angle to a wall bar for support and flexes his hip beyond 90° by raising his thigh to his chest and allowing his knee to bend. The movement should ideally occur in three phases. Initially there should be no pelvic or lumbar movement, with phase I consisting of hip flexion alone *(a)*. During phase II, the pelvis should begin to posteriorly tilt as the hip approaches 90°. The lordosis should flatten, but the lumbar spine movement should not be excessive *(b)*. In phase III, no further hip or pelvic movement is available, and the final position is obtained by lumbar flexion alone *(c)*. When control of lumbar–pelvic rhythm is poor, lumbar flexion and pelvic rotation often occur early in phase I, with thoracic movement noticeable as the subject dips his chest downward toward his knee *(d)*.

When lumbar flexion occurs early in the movement, the action of knee raising in standing can be used as a stability exercise in itself. Instruct your client to raise his knee initially by performing 10° to 20° of hip flexion while maintaining stability of the lumbar–pelvic region and avoiding any pelvic tilt. To progress the overload of the exercise, increase the range of hip motion to 30° to 45° and slow the action so that the knee raise takes a total of 10 s.

Teaching Points

▶ As the leg is lifted higher, the lumbar spine will flex, so avoid high lift movements initially.

▶ Begin by asking your client to simply take his foot off the ground. When he can control this, allow him to lift his foot slightly higher with each repetition set.

For the body to remain balanced, the gravity line must pass through the base of support—in the case of the human body, the feet. When a client transfers her weight from two legs to one, she must shift her body weight over her single weight-bearing leg. This is normally accomplished by shifting the pelvis sideways. However, some clients lack the subtlety of control that this requires and move their whole spine instead, markedly laterally flexing. If you see this occurring, stop the exercise and perform the Trendelenburg test (p. 141) and hip hitch (p. 184) first.

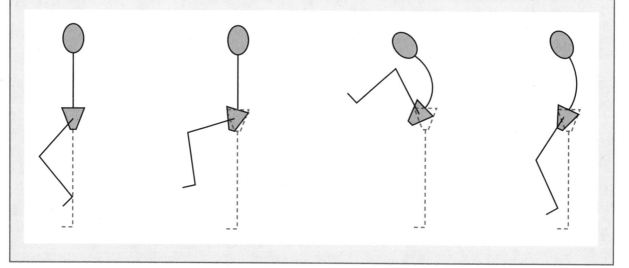

Standing Passive Pelvic Tilt

Goal: Facilitate passive pelvic tilt.

Have your client stand facing a wall. Ask him to stretch out his arms and place his hands flat onto the wall. Grip him below the waist with your forearm placed around the pelvic rim. Place your other hand flat on his sacrum, and use your shoulder to stabilize his thoracic spine. Move your client's pelvis into anterior and then into posterior tilt, assessing how far you can move it in either direction. If your client demonstrates a flat-back posture, the amount of anterior tilt will be reduced; if he demonstrates a lordotic posture, the corresponding amount of posterior tilt will be limited.

Teaching Points

▶ Make sure that your client has his arms locked out when you press against his pelvis; otherwise, you will simply push the whole of his body forward.

▶ If your client has a very stiff lumbar spine attributable to a fixed postural type, his pelvis may not tilt freely.

▶ To further stabilize the thoracic spine, the instructer could bring his right shoulder further forward to press it over the client's right scapula.

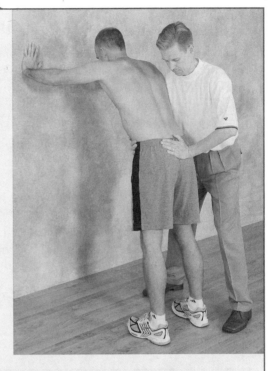

Prone Kneeling Lumbar–Pelvic Rhythm

Goal: Facilitate active pelvic tilt.

Your client kneels on all fours (prone kneeling) with his shoulders directly above his hands and his hip above his knees. Instruct him to begin sitting back toward his ankles. The action should occur in three phases. In phase I, no lumbar or pelvic movement should occur *(a)*; in phase II, posterior pelvic tilt and hip flexion occur *(b)*; and in phase III, lumbar flexion and some thoracic flexion finish the action *(c)*. Faulty lumbar–pelvic rhythm often shows up when lumbar flexion and posterior pelvic tilt occur immediately *(d)*.

Teaching Points

▶ If your client has a flat-back posture, he may not be able to begin this movement from a neutral spine position. Judge the movement quality from wherever his comfortable resting position is.

▶ There will be a specific point at which the spine begins to move. Work around this point, moving your client's body forward and backward encouraging his to keep the spine stable as he moves.

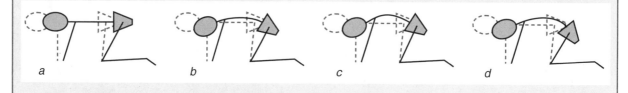

a   *b*   *c*   *d*

Standing Hip Hinge

Goal: Differentiate lumbar flexion from anterior pelvic tilt.

This activity permits you to observe your client's ability to isolate pelvic motion from that of the lumbar spine in the more functional position of standing. Your first aim is to assess the client's forward flexion, because the relative contribution of anterior pelvic tilt to this movement is important. With normal lumbar–pelvic rhythm, unlocked knees

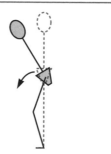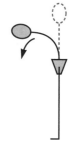

and anterior pelvic tilt reduce the amount of lumbar flexion required to reach downward to below waist height, as when one is standing and working at a low bench *(left)*. Where pelvic tilt is limited, greater lumbar flexion is required. Throughout the day, the number of lumbar flexion movements is greatly increased, leading to accumulated stress on the body tissues in this area *(right)*. Observe the action first, and then reeducate the movement initially asking your client to bend down to place her hands above waist level.

Teaching points:

▶ Begin with your client facing the back of an office chair. Ask her to bend down to touch the top of the chair back.

▶ When this action is perfected, turn the chair around and ask her to bend down to touch the chair seat.

Pelvic Motion Control in the Frontal Plane: The Trendelenburg Sign

Goal: Reeducate the hip abductors muscles to hold the pelvis level.

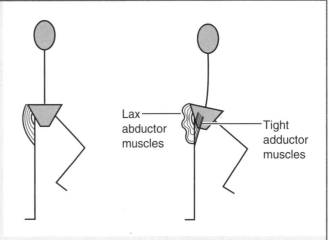

When one leg supports all the body weight, the hip abductors (mainly gluteus medius) of the supporting leg work to prevent the pelvis from dipping *(left)*. When these muscles are unable to hold an inner-range contraction, the pelvis dips downward toward the lifted leg, effectively adducting the weight-bearing limb *(right)*. Persistent use of this action in the swayback posture can lead to an imbalance, combining lengthening of the hip abductors and shortening of the hip adductors.

Have your client (dressed in shorts) stand with his back toward you and his arms outstretched to place his fingertips on a wall for balance. Ask him to slowly walk on the spot, lifting the feet 6 to 12 in. (15-30 cm) from the ground. Focus your attention on the rim of his pelvis (waistband of the shorts) and notice if the pelvis remains level to the horizontal or drops on the side of the bending leg. If the leg drops, have your client focus his attention on his pelvis and try to keep it level initially as he bends one leg, keeping the foot on the ground. When he is able to do this, allow him to lift the foot off the ground.

Teaching Points

▶ Place a stick horizontally across the rim of the client's pelvis in front of him. Have him stand in front of the mirror and note whether the stick dips down as he walks on the spot.

▶ Some clients are unable to perform this action not because of control but because of reduced strength in their hip abductors following injury or surgery (especially hip replacement). For these clients, build the abductor muscles using the hip hitch (p. 184).

Pelvic Motion Control in the Sagittal Plane: Standing Hip Scissor

Goal: Differentiate hip and pelvic motion in standing.

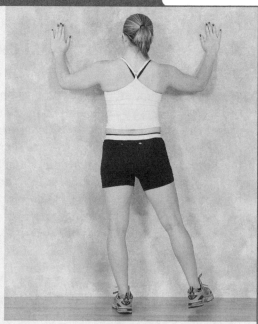

We saw when using the lumbar–pelvic rhythm in prone kneeling (p. 140) that the hip abductors of the supporting leg work to prevent the pelvis from dipping in single leg standing. When these muscles are unable to stabilize the pelvis on the femur, the pelvis dips down toward the lifted leg. With the hip scissor action, this fault is compounded because the dipped pelvis moves with the abducting non-weight-bearing leg.

Have your client (dressed in shorts) stand with her back toward you and her arms outstretched to place her fingertips on a wall for balance. Ask her to slowly lift her right leg out sideways in a scissor action to about 30° of abduction. Focus your attention on the rim of her pelvis (waistband of her shorts), and notice whether the pelvis remains level to the horizontal, while the leg is lifted. You may notice two faults: (a) the pelvis drops on the side of the lifting leg at the initiation of the movement, and (b) as abduction progresses the pelvis and moving leg move as a single unit. The correct sequence is as follows:

1. Pelvis and body shift to the left to unload the right leg.
2. Pelvis remains level as the right leg is lifted into abduction.
3. Pelvis does not move (tip laterally) as leg is lifted; the leg lifts in isolation.
4. Process reverses as leg is lowered.

Teaching Points

▶ Place a stick horizontally across the rim of the client's pelvis in front of her. Have her stand in front of a mirror and note whether the stick dips down as she raises her leg.

▶ The movement is quite subtle, so ensure that your client moves slowly to allow you time to see any movement fault.

▶ Allow only 30° of hip abduction. More movement will force the pelvis to move, not through lack of segmental control but because of lack of motion range at the hip.

Side-Lying Hip Abduction

Goal: Differentiate hip and pelvic motion in lying.

In a non-weight-bearing situation, inactivity of the gluteus medius shows as a false hip abduction movement. Normally when the upper leg is lifted from side-lying position, the pelvis remains level and the hip moves on this stable base *(a)*. When the hip abductors are weak, the subject is unable to abduct his leg correctly *(b)*. Instead, her pelvis tilts laterally on the spine using the trunk side flexors, which gives the false appearance of hip abduction. Although the leg lifts, the relationship between the femur and pelvis remains unchanged, with close inspection showing the movement isolated to the lower spine.

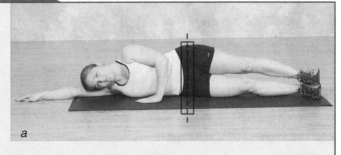

a

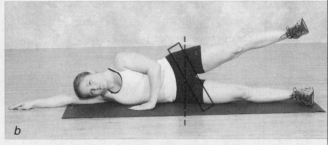

b

Have your client lie on her side, with her top arm forward, hand on the floor to support herself and prevent her from rolling forward. Ask her to lift her top leg in a scissor action so that her feet are 2 ft (61 cm) apart. Repeat this action five times, and notice the degree of pelvic lateral tilt. The client should repeat the movement, attempting to keep the pelvis level vertically.

Teaching Points

▶ Place your hand over your client's upper hip and pelvis to feel if the pelvis is tipping.

▶ Encourage your client to feel this action herself with her own (upper) hand.

▶ Place a stick vertically level with the client's feet. As the leg lifts, encourage your client to reach for the stick with her foot (leg lengthening).

Sitting Assisted Pelvic Tilt

Goal: This exercise is for subjects who are unable to perform a pelvic tilt while sitting. The action is especially useful for individuals whose flat-back posture causes pain after prolonged sitting.

Stand in front of your client and place a webbing belt around his waist. Gripping the belt, place your hand over his sternum to prevent upper-body sway. As you pull the belt, his lumbar lordosis increases and his pelvis tends to tilt anteriorly. This action is made easier if your client sits on a wedge—in this case, the ischial tuberosities are higher than the pubic bone, and the pelvis is forced into anterior tilt.

Initially, most of the power comes from your pulling on the belt, but gradually the belt provides less and less assistance as the subject becomes able to perform the tilting action by himself.

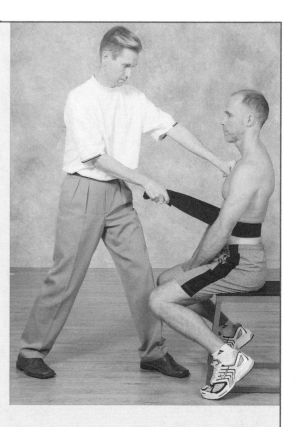

Teaching Points

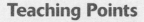 Wrap a towel around the belt if your client complains that it digs into his skin.

▶ Initially pull the belt firmly enough to actually move your client's pelvis. Repeat the action, but gradually reduce the pull on the belt so that your client takes over.

▶ Eventually allow your client to do the action himself, and use the belt only to guide him.

Crook-Lying Assisted Pelvic Tilt

Goal: For subjects who are unable to perform a full active tilt by themselves in any position.

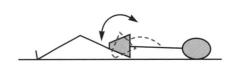

The subject begins in the crook-lying position, as for the heel slide maneuver on page 168. Grip his pelvis over the pelvic rim on each side, and push the pelvis into anterior and then posterior tilt. Encourage your client to visualize the effect of the tilt on the lumbar spine as the lordosis is increased and reduced. Have him attempt first to follow the action using his own musculature (abdominals and gluteals); then gradually reduce your force in tilting the pelvis until he performs the action independently.

Teaching Points

▶ Initially you provide all of the force for this action so it is a true passive movement.

▶ Next, encourage your client to follow your lead, so that you each provide 50% of the force.

▶ Finally, use your hands purely for tactile cueing, providing no force for the movement.

The next exercise begins to load the lumbar spine. If your client is unable to control neutral position in even these basic movements, stop the exercise and take her through abdominal hollowing (p. 154) first.

High (Two-Point) Kneeling (Assisted) Hip Hinge Action

Goal: Use a pelvic tilt action to move the spine forward and backward.

Once your subject can perform pelvic tilting well, he should combine it with classic hip hinge actions—where the trunk moves on the hip in a hinge action and the spine remains straight. With your client in the two-point kneeling position, assist him in performing the pelvic tilt. Encourage him to follow this movement with his shoulders, keeping his spine stable and avoiding any increase or decrease in lumbar lordosis. He should gently draw his abdominal muscles in (abdominal hollowing, see p. 154) and maintain this minimal contraction (feeling tightness only) throughout the movement.

The essence of this action is to angle the spine forward and backward from the hip without flexing or extending the spine.

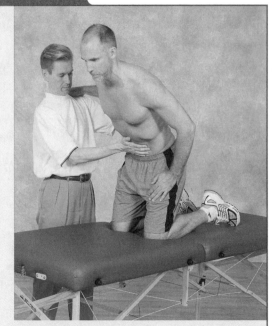

Teaching Points

▶ The movement is made easier if the subject visualizes a rod tipping forward and backward from a single point (the hip) rather than a rope bending.

▶ Provide gentle pressure on the back of your client's shoulders to initiate forward angulation of the spine and pressure over the front of the shoulder to initiate backward angulation.

Hip Hinge With Table Support

Goal: Perform a progression on assisted hip hinge.

The subject stands facing a couch or other object placed just below waist level, with his hands on the couch surface (a). With his knees unlocked to relax the hamstring muscles, he performs the hip hinge action described in the previous exercise, using pelvic tilt and a fully stable spine. As he leans forward, he supports some of his weight with his hands, thus reducing spinal loading. After your client has mastered this supported action, he should move to the free standing position (b).

Teaching Points

▶ Make sure that your client's knees remain unlocked throughout the movement to relax the hamstring muscles. There is a tendency to focus all the attention on the trunk movement and end up with the knees hyperextended.

▶ Your client does not have to bend forward very far for the exercise to be effective. Trunk angles greater than 45° to the vertical are excessive.

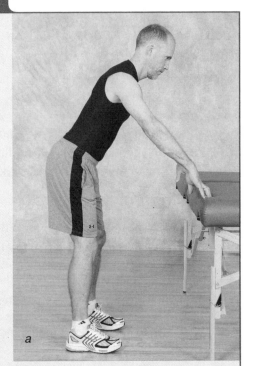

a

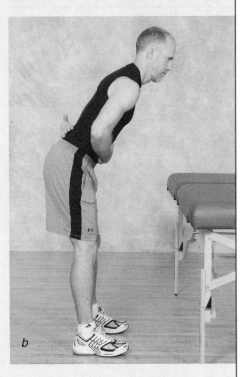

b

Controlled Forward Bending

Goal: Teach segmental control of the lumbar–pelvic region as a precursor to lifting.

Once an individual has mastered the hip hinge actions, permit him a small degree of lumbar flexion—have him perform normal forward bend actions, with the pelvis initiating the action and both the pelvis and lumbar spine contributing equally throughout the first half of the range of motion.

Teaching Points

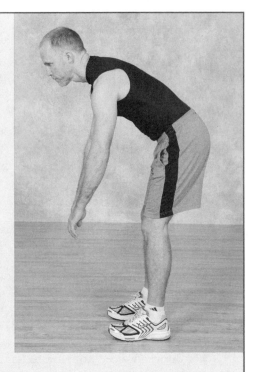

▶ Initially your client can perform this action in isolation.

▶ Make the action more functional by having him bend to pick up small, light objects from varying heights such as a table, stool, chair, and gym bench.

▶ If your client begins to bend too much from the spine, consider using taping along the length of the erector spinae to limit flexion range (chapter 5).

Sitting Pelvic Tilt Using Gym Ball

Goal: Teach anterior–posterior pelvic tilt control.

See chapter 10 for a more thorough discussion of gym ball exercises and for more advanced exercises. The ball used is a standard 65 cm ball. Instruct your client to sit on the ball with her knees apart, feet flat on the floor. Both hips and knees should be flexed to about 90°. She should then tilt her pelvis alternately in both anterior and posterior directions, making sure that her shoulders and thoracic spine remain inactive. At first, she should attempt only small ranges of movement; as she gradually works up to larger ranges, the ball should roll forward and backward slightly.

Teaching Points

▶ If your client finds the isolation of this movement difficult and her whole body moves, have her use her arms to stabilize her upper body.

▶ Have her sit in front of a high table and place her hands on the tabletop.

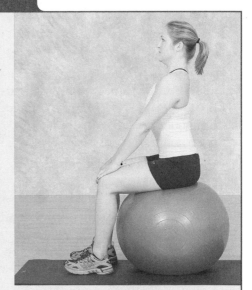

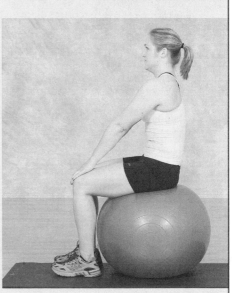

Sitting Lateral Tilt Using Gym Ball

Goal: Teach lateral pelvic tilt control.

Instruct your client to sit on the ball, as in the previous exercise, and to use lateral tilting to roll the ball from side to side, transferring her body weight from one ischial tuberosity to the other. Again, the shoulders should remain still throughout the action. The aim is to control the movement throughout the range using a smooth action and to avoid falling into the end-range position.

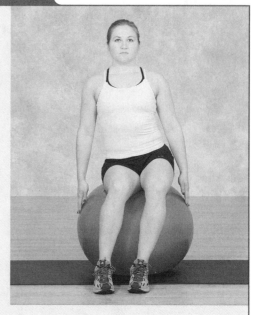

Teaching Points

▶ Upper-body fixation (see sitting pelvic tilt using gym ball, p. 149) may be used to assist the control of this exercise.

▶ A firm ball is easier to use in this exercise because it rolls easily.

▶ This exercise becomes harder with the hands placed over the head.

Reproduction of Passive Positioning (RPP)

Goal: Teach individuals how to maintain neutral position by improving the accuracy of body segment position.

Four-point kneeling is the best starting position for restoring RPP during back stability training. Have your client kneel, with her lumbar spine in neutral position. After you passively move her spine away from neutral, instruct your client to place her spine back into the neutral position. Initially, work with single movements from flexion back to neutral and then extension back to neutral; then progress to combinations of movements—flexion–extension and lateral flexion and then back to neutral, for example. The aim is to increase the precision of movements so that the individual is able to accurately reproduce the neutral position alignment after each movement away from this starting position.

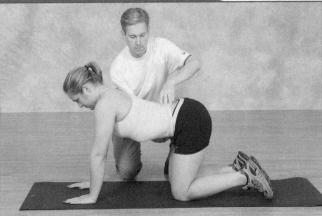

Teaching Points

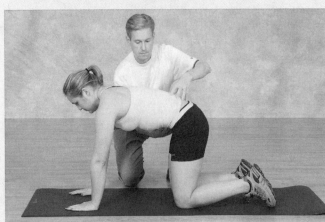

▶ Begin by gripping your client quite firmly to provide intense tactile feedback. As she improves, reduce your grip.

▶ After your client has mastered RPP in the four-point kneeling position, move to other positions—especially those common to daily activities, such as sitting and standing.

Reproduction of Active Positioning (RAP)

Goal: Teach individuals how to maintain neutral position by improving the accuracy of movement.

After your client has become proficient in passive positioning, she should initiate her own movements. Instruct her to begin in neutral position, move away from this position using single movements, and then move back into the neutral starting position. It sometimes works best if she begins RAP with a sitting or standing position—that way she can practice in front of a mirror, with her hands flat over her lower abdomen and sacrum to monitor pelvic tilt. Eventually, she uses no mirror and performs the movement without monitoring the action with her hands. Again, use a variety of movements from several starting positions.

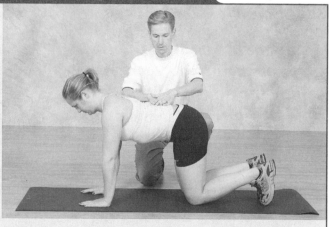

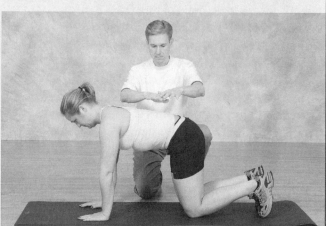

Teaching Points

▶ Demonstrate the action to your client or use a skilled model.

▶ Also use equipment such as a balance board or gym ball and have your client follow you, ensuring that she tilts her pelvis to the same degree.

Key point: When performing exercises to improve reproduction of passive or active positioning, your client should focus on precision of movement.

When your client has performed sitting pelvic tilt using gym ball and sitting lateral tilt using gym ball (pp. 149 and 150), have her repeat the assisted pelvic tilt while sitting and controlled forward bending (pp. 144 and 127). You should now find that these actions can be performed with greater precision.

Four-Point Kneeling Abdominal Hollowing

Goal: Isolate the transversus abdominis and internal oblique.

Because the transversus fibers are aligned horizontally, four-point kneeling allows the abdominal muscles to sag, facilitating stretch. Position your client with his lumbar spine in a neutral position, his head looking at the floor, not forward, and his ears horizontally aligned with his shoulder joint. His hip should be directly above the knee, his shoulder directly above the hand. The hands and knees are shoulder-width apart.

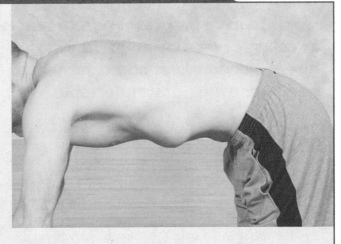

Instruct your client to focus his attention on his navel area, and to pull that region in and up while breathing normally. This action dissociates activity in the internal obliques and transversus from that of the rectus abdominis (Richardson et al. 1992). The exercise is thus useful for enhancing the stabilizing ability of the abdominals when the rectus abdominis has become the dominant muscle of the group.

Teaching Points

▶ If your client finds this position painful on his knees, place a folded towel beneath his knees.

▶ If the position is painful on the client's wrists, rather than taking weight through the flat hand, he should use an open fist instead.

▶ As repetitions progress, people tend to flex the spine. Monitor your client closely for this.

▶ This client has allowed his lumbar spine to flex. When you see this on a client, stop. Regain neutral position and restart the exercise.

Abdominal Hollowing: Standing

Goal: Teach a progression from four-point kneeling or provide an initial position for obese individuals or others for whom four-point kneeling is uncomfortable.

Some subjects find four-point kneeling difficult to control and tend to round their spines as they attempt abdominal hollowing. In this case, wall-supported standing is a more appropriate starting position. Your client should stand with his feet 6 in. (15 cm) from a wall and his back against the wall while maintaining a neutral spinal position *(a)*. An easy way to monitor neutral position is for your client to place one hand behind his back (over the sacrum) and the other in front of the abdomen, enabling him to monitor the position of his pelvis. He can also use his front hand to feel the contraction of the abdominal muscles as he initiates hollowing and draws the abdominal wall away from his hand.

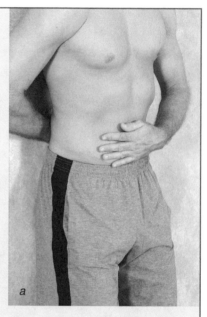

a

Teaching Points

▶ In an obese or poorly toned subject, the weight of the digestive organs will pull the abdominal wall out and down (visceral ptosis). If this occurs, position a belt below the client's navel *(b)*, instructing him to contract the lateral abdominals and to pull the abdominal wall in and up, trying to create a space between the abdomen and the belt.

▶ Because motor programming links lateral abdominal action and pelvic floor action as part of the intra-abdominal pressure mechanism, pelvic floor contractions are also useful to aid learning of abdominal hollowing.

▶ Instruct a female client to pull in the pelvic floor as though trying to stop herself from urinating. Tell male clients to use the imagery of lifting the penis.

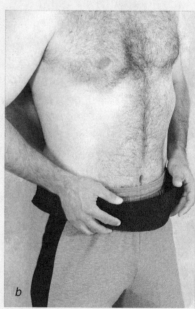

b

Sitting Abdominal Hollowing

Goal: Provide further practice for subjects who are already able to maintain the neutral lumbar position and control body sway.

Sitting on a stool or office chair is a useful starting position because clients can practice this exercise throughout the day. When your client is sitting on a stool, the upper part of his trunk is unsupported, so he will have to control body sway. Using an office chair supports the thoracic spine, but don't allow your client to slouch. He must be more active in controlling his upper trunk when it is unsupported, paying attention to the hollowing action as well as to the position of the lumbar spine (maintaining neutral position) and the position of his shoulders (avoiding body sway). Have your client pay close attention to movement of the rib cage, as well as to shoulder position, pelvic tilt, and maintenance of a neutral lordosis. Instruct your client to sit tall to facilitate correct alignment; this concept is also helpful in correcting whole-body posture while standing.

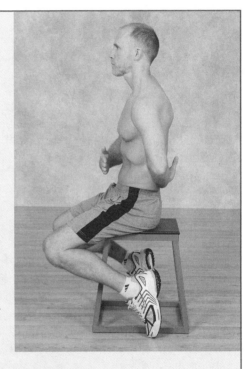

Teaching Points

► Make sure that your client sits tall and avoids a slouch sitting posture.

► Closely monitor him to ensure that he controls body sway.

► To avoid flexion in the lumbar spine, position his knee lower than his hip. This position reduces pull from the hip tissues, which would tend to posteriorly tilt the pelvis and flatten the lumbar lordosis.

► This client has posteriorly tilted his pelvis. This can encourage contraction of the lower rectus.

Prone-Lying Abdominal Hollowing

Goal: Provide further practice for lean individuals and those already able to perform hollowing.

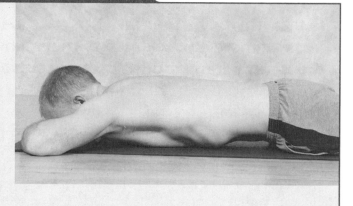

In prone lying, abdominal hollowing pulls the abdominal wall away from the floor—a practical cue for the beginner. Use of a pressure biofeedback unit can be very helpful (consult a medical supply catalog). The pressure biofeedback unit is useful only for assessment and not for continuing exercises. Place the bladder of the feedback unit below the client's navel, the lower edge of the feedback unit in line with the anterior superior iliac spines. As your client performs hollowing, the dial of the biofeedback unit will show a decline in his body's pressure on the bladder. Once your client has mastered this action, you can link it with hip extension movements, if you wish, to provide abdominal–gluteal co-contraction.

As an additional tactile cue to help your client understand the required action, place a belt beneath his abdomen below the umbilicus but about the waistband. Then pull on the belt gently and he will notice that his body weight is fixing the belt and preventing it moving. Have him perform abdominal hollowing, and as his abdomen draws away from the belt he will notice that you can pull the belt out from underneath him. Repeat this action several times until the client is familiar with the required muscle work.

Teaching Points

▶ Use a belt beneath your client's abdomen to familiarize him with the required movement.

▶ Use pressure biofeedback to measure the degree of abdominal hollowing.

▶ Make sure that your client does not hold his breath. Encourage him to breathe normally.

Supine-Lying Abdominal Hollowing

Goal: Teach self-monitoring of abdominal muscle contraction and pelvic position.

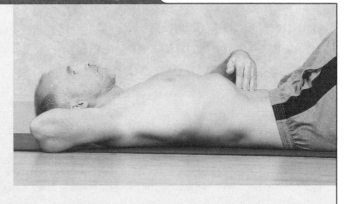

Abdominal hollowing in supine-lying position permits a person to feel the muscle activity of his abdominal wall and to monitor pelvic position. In addition, the movement is a precursor to the heel slide (p. 168). Have your client assume the crook-lying position, with his fingers flat against the lateral abdominals below his navel. Encourage him to gently press his fingers into his abdominals to feel their contraction. Make sure that this occurs as a "tightening the sheet" feeling (hollowing) rather than your client pushing outward against his hands (doming or bulging).

In addition, explain that no pelvic tilt should occur during lateral abdominal contraction—you can check this by palpating the anterior superior iliac spine. You can also use pressure biofeedback to monitor the depth of the lordosis: Flattening of the back (posterior pelvic tilt) shows as increasing pressure on the dial and indicates activity of the rectus abdominis; excessive hollowing shows as reduced pressure and indicates loss of stability associated with anterior pelvic tilt.

As your client performs abdominal hollowing, the pressure biofeedback unit should register no more than a 5 mmHg increase in pressure—at this level of pressure the internal oblique, the transversus abdominis, and the diaphragm are all recruited together. Higher values (up to 15 mmHg) will not increase the recruitment of the deep abdominals but will increase the activity of both the diaphragm and the rectus abdominis (Allison et al. 1998).

Teaching Points

▶ Place your client's hands into the correct position for him to feel his lower and lateral abdominals.

▶ Encourage your client initially to press his fingers into his abdomen and to tense his abdominal wall in response.

▶ As he improves he should gently monitor his muscle contraction only.

▶ Eventually have him place one hand over his lower abdomen to monitor muscle action and the other over his pelvic rim to monitor pelvic position.

▶ Note that this client's hand should be well below the navel to properly palpate his lower abdominals.

Prone-Lying Multifidus Contraction

Goal: Teach clients to learn to use the multifidus at will and separately from other muscles.

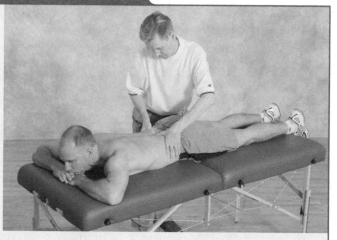

Your client begins in a prone-lying position while you palpate his low back medial to the longissimus at L4 and L5 levels. Identify the spinous processes and slide your fingers laterally into the hollow (paraspinal gutter) between the spinous process and the longissimus bulk. Palpate with your thumb and the knuckle of your first finger placed on either side of the lumbar spinous process at any one level.

Assess the difference in muscle consistency, and then determine your client's ability to isometrically contract the multifidus in a setting (muscle tightening) action. Ask him to bulge the muscles beneath your fingers and differentiate between erector spinae contraction (more lateral) and multifidus contraction (more central). Occasionally ask him to hyperextend his trunk to feel the erector spinae contracting, and instruct him that this is *not* the required contraction.

Teaching Points

▶ When you use this type of palpation, often what you do not feel is what's important.

▶ You should feel a slight muscle bulging or increased resistance to your palpation pressure in the spinal muscles but not from the erector spinae.

Side-Lying Multifidus Contraction Using Rhythmic Stabilization

Goal: Encourage your client to contract the multifidus and lateral abdominals simultaneously.

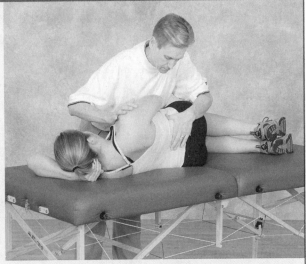

Rhythmic stabilization is a proprioceptive neuromuscular facilitation technique that involves alternating isometric contractions of the agonist and antagonist muscles, building up to co-contraction (Sullivan et al. 1982). The general idea is simple: First, you apply a resistance in one direction and your client contracts her muscle against the resistance. Once you feel that the contraction has reached a maximum, instantaneously apply your resistance in the opposite direction—at which point she contracts the antagonist muscle, with no momentary relaxation between the two contractions. In this way, the muscle pairs contract to gradually higher levels.

With your client in the crook side-lying position, palpate the intervertebral joints to ascertain the midpoint of the movement range at the spinal level where you have found pain or pathology (Maitland 1986). Remember that the multifidus muscle is unisegmental—that is, each fascicle stretches over only a single segment of the lumbar spine. Wasting of the muscle occurs at the same level as the segment of pathology (Hides et al. 1994). To place the relevant muscle fascicle at its optimum length, you must move the painful segment into its midrange. If you feel inadequate to do this, ask an experienced orthopedic physical therapist to work with you.

In this exercise, you push forward on your client's pelvis and backward onto the shoulder while your client resists the action. Then reverse the action: While you push backward on the pelvis and forward onto the shoulder, she continues to resist the action, not allowing herself to relax even for a second. The action can be more localized by an orthopedic physical therapist, who can palpate the specific spinal level that requires resistance to rotation. The client can perform general resisted rotation for the whole spine by having a partner help her use this exercise at home.

The exercise is repeated 5 to 10 times at each of three treatment sessions.

Teaching Points

▶ The motion change is very subtle; do not rotate your client's spine too far, no more than 2 in. (5 cm).

▶ Begin gently and build up pressure gradually. On a scale of 1 (least pressure) to 10 (most pressure), begin with a pressure of 1 and increase to 4 only.

Sitting Multifidus Contraction

Goal: Encourage your client to contract the multifidus and lateral abdominals simultaneously.

Have your client sit on the edge of a bench with his feet on the floor. Place his lumbar spine into neutral position. Palpate the multifidus and ask your client to perform abdominal hollowing to assess whether you can feel multifidus contraction. If you cannot, continue to palpate and reeducate the muscle, linking pelvic floor and abdominal hollowing actions with multifidus work. You may sit behind and slightly to the side of your client and have him lean his body weight back onto you. This relaxed and supported position is often easier for clients to use. If you can feel multifidus contraction, allow your client to self-palpate and continue the action for 10 repetitions, aiming to hold each for 10 s while breathing normally.

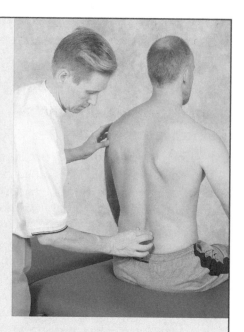

Teaching Points

▶ Do not allow your client to hold his breath; encourage him to breathe normally.

▶ When your client is self-palpating, tell him to place his thumbs together behind his back while you position his thumbs on a spinous process at L4-L5 level.

▶ Ask you client to part his thumbs by 1/2 in. (1.2 cm) and press into the tissue at the side of the spinous process. This is the position he must be able to find for self-palpation.

Forward Stride (Walk) Standing Multifidus Contraction

Goal: Encourage your client to contract the multifidus and lateral abdominals simultaneously.

Instruct your client to stand with one foot in front of the other. Have him self-palpate the L4-L5 level by placing his thumbs on a lower lumbar spinous process and moving them outward slightly (1/2 in. or 1.2 cm) into the spinal tissue. Tell him to place his weight onto his front leg and then onto the back leg alternately. Tell him to feel the muscles beneath his thumbs switching on and off. Encourage him to perform abdominal hollowing and at the same time increase the muscle swelling he feels beneath his thumbs.

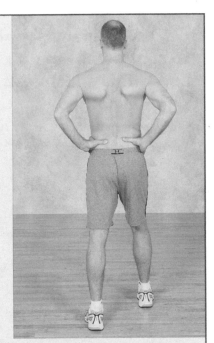

Teaching Points

▶ To differentiate between the erector spinae and multifidus, ask your client to move his thumbs farther apart (4 in., or 10 cm) and angle his body forward. He should now feel the erector spinae contract, a muscle action that he should aim to avoid as he contracts the multifidus.

▶ As an alternative to using both thumbs, he can leave one thumb palpating the spine and raise the other arm horizontally forward from the shoulder. This arm-raising action may help to fire up the multifidus muscle.

▶ Note that this client's thumbs are too far apart. They should be only one inch apart.

Side-Lying Multifidus Contraction Using Femoral Pressure

Goal: Encourage your client to contract the multifidus and lateral abdominals simultaneously.

Place your patient on side, lying on a treatment couch, knees and hips comfortably flexed. Stand in front of him at waist level and raise the couch to your hip level. Palpate his multifidus with the fingers of your left hand. Place your right hand and forearm on his upper femur. As he performs abdominal hollowing and multifidus contraction, gently press along the length of the femur toward him (approximation) and pull away from him (traction). Encourage him to resist your pressure using muscle contraction alone.

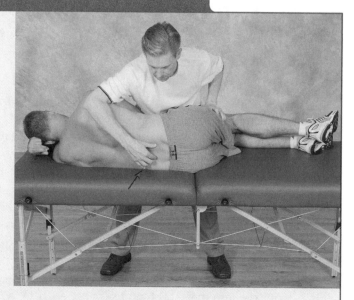

Teaching Points

▶ By palpating the multifidus, you are giving tactile feedback at the point where contraction should occur.

▶ Femoral pressure is used to challenge rotary stability and force the multifidus to contract.

Part III
Progressing Stability Training

If you bring a client through the assessments and exercises in the previous chapters, he or she should be posturally aware, should have a basically stable back, and should be experiencing little back pain. The demands of day-to-day living, jobs, and sport, however, mean that most clients will need more.

They need to be able to rely on their back not to give way when they do an unexpected movement. To give your clients a fully functional back, one that they don't have to guard or protect during the activities of daily living, you must help them to progress their stability training.

Chapter 8
Limb Loading

After your clients have used the procedures and exercises of previous chapters to achieve basic back stability, they are ready to build on that stability. By now they should have learned to control pelvic tilt; to automatically assume the neutral position; to maintain abdominal hollowing (at 30-40% of the maximum effort); or, in quantitative terms, to perform the basic procedures in part II. With your help, they should have begun correcting muscle imbalances using the approaches in chapter 6. They should have developed their abdominal strength using the exercises in chapter 7. They should be able to maintain proper posture as described in chapter 5. Many people who are relatively sedentary and whose back stability is rarely challenged through workplace or leisure-time activities may have little motivation to proceed with additional training. Others will want to go further, however, especially if they are involved in sports or if they face heavy physical demands on the job. In this chapter, I cover exercises for developing even greater back stability using limb loading.

Key point: When performing the exercises in this chapter, your clients should gently contract their deep abdominal muscles to perform abdominal hollowing and maintain this contraction throughout the exercise. In addition, they should begin all exercises in the neutral position.

SUPERIMPOSED LIMB MOVEMENTS

Each of the following exercises involves limb movements that are superimposed on a basically stable back, which the exercises in part II can create (i.e., in these exercises, an individual tightens his back stability muscles and then moves his limbs on the stable base). As your clients focus their attention

on limb movements, they will become more able to control their back stability muscles without conscious thought. This kind of automatic response occurs only with many repetitions of the exercises. You should find it surprisingly easy to observe the point at which your clients are exerting automatic control. If they perform a limb-loading exercise such as the standing single-leg raise or the crook-lying heel slide, for example, movement of the pelvis will reveal lack of back stability. In this case, you would retreat a couple of steps and have your clients practice the hollowing actions to enhance their ability to stabilize the spine. Once they have built up endurance of these muscles and can hold the abdominal contraction for 10 repetitions of 10 s each, you would once again try adding limb movements to the basic exercises. If clients can now successfully control limb movements while avoiding unwanted pelvic movement (maintaining the lumbar spine's neutral position throughout the action), you will know that they are gaining automatic control of the stabilizing muscles—they no longer have to focus their attention on these muscles and can now concentrate on accurate positioning of the limb.

Key point: Use of limb loading helps your clients stabilize their back automatically without conscious focus.

For the following exercises, your client should progress in a single session only to the point at which he can no longer maintain neutral position, correct pelvic tilt, or abdominal hollowing. Have him do the exercise daily for 4 days, rest 1 day, and then resume the pattern, gradually increasing the progression or the number of repetitions until he eventually can do the exercise in its most challenging form for 10 repetitions, holding (where appropriate) for 10 s each time. Obviously, all one-sided movements should be performed on both right and left sides, one being the mirror image of the other. The client should perform each exercise in a slow, controlled fashion, maintaining the neutral position of the spine throughout the exercise. Because limb leverage changes when arms and legs are bent and straightened, your clients will have to vary the amount of abdominal work they use to maintain the neutral position. This variation makes the difference (in terms of skill) between the holding exercises, such as abdominal hollowing, and these more advanced exercises that involve limb movements on the stable trunk base.

Key point: As your clients move their limbs, changing leverage forces mean that they must vary activity of the stabilizing muscles to continue to maintain a neutral lumbar position.

Determining the Starting Position

An individual's starting position depends on his physical characteristics and abilities. You should always be open, however, to changing the starting position if you perceive that your first choice may not have been the best—which will be the case if your client is not succeeding with an exercise. Some exercises are easier than others because they involve less muscle work. For example, in the heel slide movement, the ground partially takes the weight of the leg, whereas in the single-leg raise, the subject lifts the whole of the leg weight. The former exercise is therefore easier in terms of pure muscle work. Some movements may be more comfortable for certain subjects. Because lying positions are more supported than kneeling, for example, many people feel more secure in lying.

The program generally follows a neuro-developmental progression (i.e., the sequence that children go through when they learn to sit, stand, and walk). Here, we go from ground support to apparatus support and finally to increasingly complex free exercises.

Exercises in the Crook-Lying Position

 The crook-lying position, which was used to perform abdominal hollowing and pelvic tilting, is a good starting position for superimposed limb move-

ments. As a person straightens the leg or lowers it to the ground, the overload placed on the trunk becomes progressively greater—the person must therefore vary the intensity of muscular stabilization to maintain the neutral position. This variation in muscle contraction intensity increases the person's control rather than simply strength or endurance capacity.

Key point: The neutral position of the lumbar spine must be maintained throughout the exercises. If the pelvis tilts and neutral position is lost, the exercise must be stopped, and the client should revert to an earlier stage of the exercise in which the pelvic tilt was accurately controlled. Be certain also that your clients keep their abdomens hollowed throughout the exercises, avoiding any sign of abdominal doming.

Exercises in the Four-Point Kneeling Position

 The four-point kneeling position is initially stable because four symmetrical points (both hands and both knees) bear the weight. As one arm or one leg is lifted to reduce support to three points, the body is less stable and the stability muscles must work harder to maintain trunk alignment and stop the body from tipping.

Exercises in the Side-Lying Position

 We saw in chapter 7 that in the frontal plane, the gluteus medius may lack endurance and inner-range holding ability, leading both the tensor fasciae lata and iliotibial band and the hip adductors to tighten. With exercises in the side-lying position, we are attempting to work the gluteus medius and to stretch the adductors while maintaining stability of the pelvis and lumbar spine in the frontal plane. The stability is achieved by contraction of the lateral abdominals and the quadratus lumborum acting together. Each of the following exercises overloads the quadratus lumborum and the oblique abdominal muscles on the upper side of the body. The movements must be mirrored (right and left sides) to provide a symmetrical overload.

Exercises in the Standing Position

The standing position is clearly important for the activities of daily living. The aim of these exercises is to add limb and thoracic movements to the stable lumbar spine and to add whole spinal movements to the stable hip. You can monitor changes in the depth of the lordosis by having your client lean against a wall—his feet 4 to 6 in. (10-15 cm) forward of the wall, his buttocks and scapulae on the wall—while you place the bladder of a BFU between his lumbar spine and the wall.

Exercises in the Sitting Position

Incorrect sitting positions often cause or exacerbate low back pain, especially that of postural origin. But, while sitting at home or work, one can also conveniently practice the following exercises throughout the day. The first exercise uses the process of relative flexibility to overload the stabilizing system.

The sitting position used in these exercises must reflect the optimal alignment of body segments. The hips should be at 70° flexion; the knees should be below the hips and slightly wider than shoulder-width apart (bringing the knees together posteriorly tilts the pelvis through soft tissue tension). About 70% of the body's weight should rest on the ischial tuberosities, 30% on the pubis.

Key point: In a correct sitting position, about 70% of your client's body weight should rest on her ischial tuberosities, 30% on the pubis.

The gravity line for the upper body should pass from the center of the hip joint to the shoulder joint and ear canal, with the spine evenly distributed along the gravity line. Your instructions to hollow the abdomen and lengthen the spine will help bring about the correct alignment. You can monitor the depth of the lumbar lordosis with pressure biofeedback, placing the bladder of the unit between the lumbar spine and the chair back. (Note that the sitting position used in this case is not what most people use in everyday activities; they can have their backs against the chair for use with a pressure bladder by slightly straddling the seat with their legs, which, as you recall, are to be somewhat spread, with knees lower than hips.)

SUMMARY

- Once individuals have achieved basic back stability through the exercises in previous chapters, they can begin building greater stability and training their backs for sports or on-the-job lifting by using the advanced exercises in this chapter.

- Advanced stability exercises, with movement of limbs on the stable trunk, will greatly increase an individual's ability to maintain back stability automatically, without conscious thought.

See pages 182-187

See pages 188-190

Heel Slide—Basic Movement

Goal: Place minimal but progressive limb loading on the trunk.

Instruct your client to slowly straighten one leg, with the heel resting on the ground. This movement is easier if the heel is on a slippery surface (a cloth if you are on a polished floor or a piece of shiny paper if on carpet). The moment the pelvis anteriorly tilts and the lordosis increases, the client must stop the movement and draw the leg back into flexion.

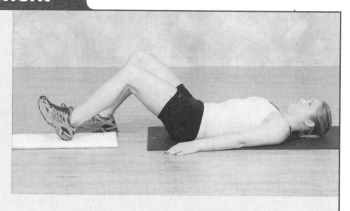

Teaching Points

▶ Have the client begin with the legs comfortably bent. If she bends her legs too much, the lumbar spine will flatten excessively.

▶ The crook-lying position is one of the most comfortable for those with back pain.

▶ Your client can self-monitor with her fingers on their pelvis (standing abdominal hollowing, p. 154).

Leg Lowering

Goal: Use limb loading as a progression from the heel slide.

Instruct your client to flex both her hips to 90°, so that her thighs are vertical to the ground, while keeping her knees relaxed. She should then slowly extend one hip and lower her whole leg until her foot touches the ground. Have her gradually extend the knee farther in subsequent repetitions, so that her foot touches the ground farther from the buttock, increasing the limb leverage and therefore progressing the resistance. She should perform the exercise daily for 4 days and then take a single day's rest. She should continue this sequence until she can perform the exercise with the leg almost straight.

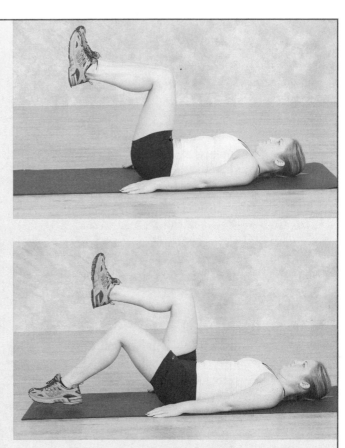

Teaching Points

▶ This exercise is far harder if your client has very heavy legs. If this is the case, place a strap or towel around her thigh and tell her to hold the strap with both hands, taking some of the leg weight.

▶ Dispense with the strap as the exercise progresses.

▶ Once she can perform the exercise with the leg almost straight, she can progress to single-leg raises.

Single Bent-Leg Raise

Goal: Progress from leg lowering.

Beginning in the crook-lying position, your client should lift one leg—still bent at the knee—while the other rests on the floor. He brings the knee up as far as he can without moving out of neutral position and then lowers it. Then he repeats with the other leg. As a progression on this action, have him begin lifting one leg just before the other limb has touched the ground so that momentarily both legs are off the floor at the same time. Finally, he should lift and lower both legs together, initially with minimal limb leverage (i.e., with knees well bent) and finally with increasing leverage (legs increasingly straightened). The maximum leverage will vary with each individual. For most well-conditioned individuals, 90° to 120° of knee extension is appropriate. At no time should the pelvis anteriorly tilt, and at no time should the abdominal muscles be allowed to bowstring or dome (bulge out-

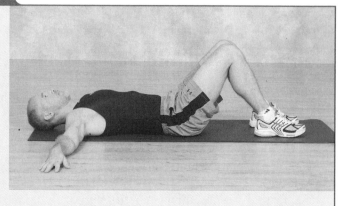

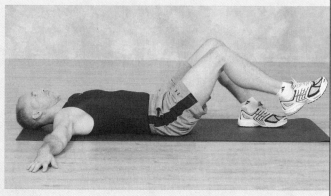

ward rather than maintain a flat or hollow contour). I do not recommend progressing all the way to bilateral straight-leg raises—the compression and shear forces imposed by the psoas muscle on the lumbar spine make this unsuitable for use in rehabilitation following low back pain.

Teaching points

▶ Clients often want to progress this exercise too fast. Slow them down and encourage movement precision.

▶ Even for strong athletes, the single-leg action is important because it teaches the subtleties of stability control.

Prone-Lying Gluteal Brace

Goal: Co-contract trunk stabilizers with gluteals.

Instruct your client to lie prone and then to dorsiflex one foot, with the toes bent up toward the knee. She should then slightly flex her knee (about 10°) and her hip (also about 10°). She then contracts her gluteal muscles to lift the femur into extension to the horizontal position (with the foot remaining on the ground), straightening the knee.

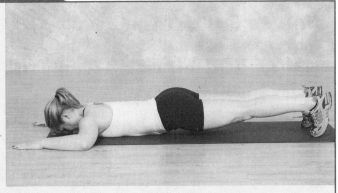

Teaching Points

▶ This exercise consists of muscle tensing rather than gross movement.

▶ The action is simply to tighten the abdominals and gluteals simultaneously and to hold the contraction while breathing normally.

▶ Those with poorly recruited gluteal muscles find this simple action extremely difficult.

Prone-Lying Bent-Leg Lift

Goal: Promote active movement of an unsupported leg on the stable trunk.

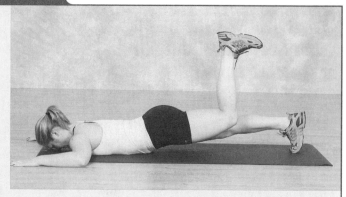

In the prone-lying position, your client should flex one leg to 90° at the knee. Instruct your client to set her abdominal muscles and contract the gluteals to lift the leg from the floor. To prevent passive anterior pelvic tilt, the maximum hip extension should be only 15°. This position places the hamstring muscles at a mechanical disadvantage, reducing the tension they can create and therefore throwing greater stress onto the gluteals. To increase the isolation of the gluteals from the hamstrings, have your client slowly flex her knee while maintaining hip extension—this causes the gluteals to act isometrically as hip stabilizers while the hamstrings act isotonically as prime knee flexors.

Teaching Points

▶ This exercise involves hyperextension of the hip, a range of motion that some clients find difficult.

▶ For such a client, begin the exercise in slight hip flexion. Have her lie on a gym bench with the exercising leg over the side, flexed at the hip and knee. Then she contracts the gluteals to bring the leg back to the horizontal (bench top) position only.

▶ When your client can perform 10 repetitions of this modified movement, have her return to the original exercise.

▶ This client has braced her straight leg and lifted her pelvis. Note that this is an advanced movement and is not required.

Bridge From Crook Lying (Shoulder Bridge)

Goal: Use leg power to lift the trunk while maintaining a neutral lumbar position.

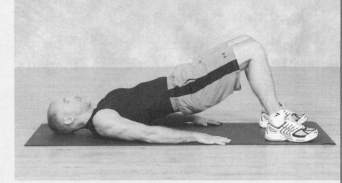

In a crook-lying position, your client should tighten his gluteal muscles and then lift his pelvis from the ground, aiming to form a straight line from shoulders to hips and then to the knees.

This exercise tends to induce movement in the sagittal plane (anterior–posterior pelvic tilt or lumbar flexion–extension). Lifting one leg (see next exercise) imposes an additional rotary stress, tending to cause movement within the transverse plane.

Teaching Point

▶ Clients fall into two categories with this movement: those who lift without their gluteals, using their hamstrings only, and those who arch up too high.

▶ For those who use only their hamstrings, facilitate their gluteals using tactile cueing and self-cueing or a surface electromyograph.

▶ For those who arch up too high, encourage them to form a straight line through the shoulder, hip, and knee at the end point of the exercise.

Bridge With Leg Lift

Goal: Progress from bridge from crook lying.

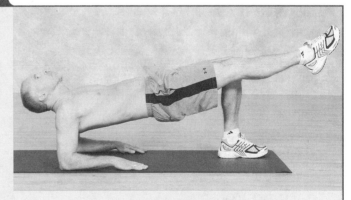

Instruct your client to assume the bridge position, starting from crook lying. Then he lifts one leg, avoiding the tendency to allow the pelvis to fall toward the unsupported side. Placing a stick across the anterior superior iliac spines of the pelvis gives useful feedback for keeping the pelvis level.

Teaching Points

▶ If your client has a very broad pelvis or is quite heavily built, the leverage forces acting across the pelvis may be too great for him.

▶ With these clients, place the weight-bearing foot closer to the center line of the body rather than keeping it at its original shoulder-width position.

▶ The client's head should stay in line with his spine. In this photo, the client has thrust is chin forward.

Four-Point Kneeling Body Sway

Goal: Learn to maintain neutral position as the limbs are moved.

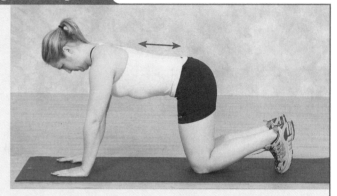

Your client begins in the standard four-point position. Instruct her to sway her body forward and back, moving at the shoulders and hips only. As she passes the critical point of 90° hip flexion, be sure that her lumbar spine remains in neutral position. As soon as she begins to lose the neutral lumbar position, she should reverse the movement back into full four-point kneeling. The aim of this action is to perform hip movement in isolation to lumbar movement.

Teaching Points

▶ To give tactile cueing of back position, place a hardcover book over your client's low back.

▶ Use only small movements so that your client appreciates the subtleties of movement.

Four-Point Kneeling Pelvic Shift

Goal: Unload the limbs before lifting them.

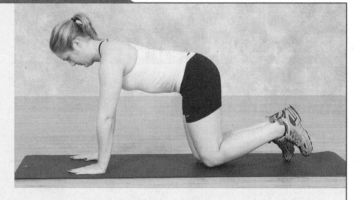

After assuming the four-point position, your client should shift to the side to take the weight off the far leg. She then barely lifts the leg on this side from the supporting surface, leaving only one knee in contact with the ground. Be sure that she lifts the leg a maximum of 2 in. (5.0 cm). Some people find the subtlety of this movement difficult and tend to lift the leg as much as 8 in. (120 cm), but this imposes an unwanted rotation on the spine and must be discouraged.

Teaching Points

▶ Placing a stick across the upper pelvis (level with the posterior superior iliac spines) is helpful.

▶ With the required subtle movement, the stick will stay in place. If the leg is lifted too far, however, pelvic rotation will cause the stick to fall.

Four-Point Kneeling Leg Movement

Goal: Control back stability in the presence of limb movement.

Your client should begin as for the previous exercise, shifting her weight to one leg. Instruct her to move the unloaded leg into flexion–extension and abduction–adduction while maintaining a neutral lumbar spine and keeping the lower leg parallel to the floor. She should use only small movements, the knee moving forward and backward and side to side by only 2 to 3 in. (5-8 cm). As with the prone-lying bent-leg lift (p. 172), your client is aiming to perform leg movements in isolation to lumbar movement.

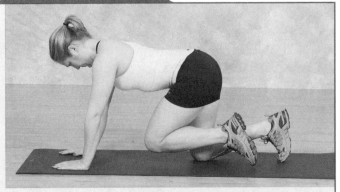

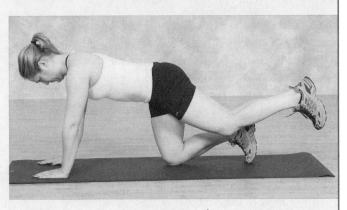

Teaching Points

▶ Larger movements will require greater changes in pelvic tilt and are more difficult to control.

▶ The movements should be slow to avoid excessive limb momentum—no more than one or two complete limb movements per second.

Four-Point Kneeling Leg Lift (Birddog)

Goal: Maintain stability during increasing complexities of leg movement.

From the basic four-point kneeling position, your client should extend one leg completely, keeping his foot on the ground *(a)*. The next step is to lift the leg until it is parallel to the floor *(b)*. Finally, instruct him to alternately flex and extend the raised leg at the knee, keeping the raised thigh parallel to the floor. The foot should remain in a middle (neutral) position, toes and foot neither fully pointed (plantar flexed) nor fully pulled up (dorsiflexed); holding the shin or calf muscles tight can cause muscle cramping.

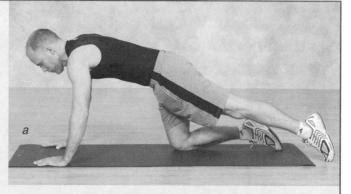

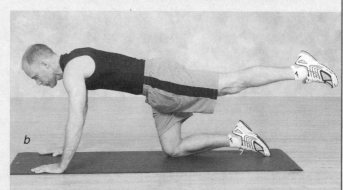

Teaching Points

▶ Several alignment faults are common in this final movement. First, while your client is focusing on the limb movement, he may forget to maintain contraction of the trunk stabilizing muscles—leading the abdominal wall to bulge because the hollowing action is lost.

▶ If this happens, the pelvis may anteriorly tilt, pulling the lumbar spine into excessive extension (back hollowing).

▶ Where the gluteals have poor endurance, your client may start to rely on his hamstrings to maintain the extended hip position: As the hamstrings begin to flex the knee, he loses the hip extension position and the leg drops below the horizontal. In each case, you should stop the procedure and return to the previous exercise.

▶ The client in these photos has an increased thoracic kyphosis (curve). To compensate, he has extended the cervical spine. When you see this, instruct your client to look at the mat level with his wrists.

Four-Point Kneeling Arm and Leg Lift (Full Birddog)

Goal: Increase the complexity of limb movements while maintaining back stability.

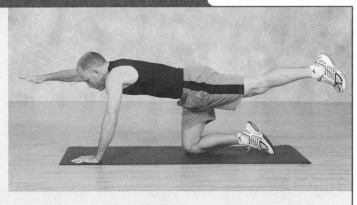

Have your client begin as with the four-point kneeling leg lift (p. 176). This time, once his leg reaches the horizontal, he should also lift the diagonally opposite arm. Make sure his shoulder does not sag or drop down on this side; the scapula should not move as the elbow bends to unload the arm. Once your client's hand has cleared the ground, he should lift the arm forward toward the horizontal.

Teaching Points

- ▶ This exercise is difficult because two limbs are lifting, which requires more muscle work and greater coordination.
- ▶ With strong athletes, don't allow them to lift their limbs with a vigorous swinging action. This can place excessive extension stress on the spine if stability control is poor.

Side-Lying Knee Lift (Clamshell)

Goal: Maintain trunk stability in the frontal (side flexion) plane during limb movement.

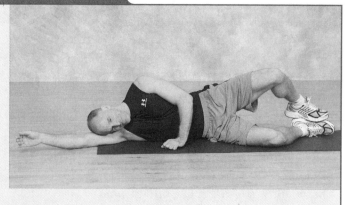

Have your client begin the exercise in side-lying position, and align his pelvis so that the line joining the two anterior superior iliac spines is vertical. He must maintain this alignment throughout the exercise. Do not allow lateral movement of the pelvis. Instruct him to bend both legs at the knee and hip. He should then lift the top knee by abducting and externally rotating his hip, keeping the foot in place. The action is like a clamshell opening. Palpate the posterior fibers of gluteus medius above and behind the greater trochanter to make sure they are contracting. Give your client feedback until he is able to tell when he is contracting these fibers as he lifts his knee. Once he is able to feel the appropriate contraction, have him attempt to lift to full inner range, but stop him immediately if the pelvis begins to move out of alignment.

Teaching Points

▶ Where tone of the gluteus medius is very poor, use knee lowering initially. Lift the upper knee for your client and instruct him to simply lower it back to the starting position by himself (eccentric muscle work).

▶ When he can achieve this, lift the leg and have him hold it in the upper position (isometric muscle work) for 1 to 2 s and then lower under control (eccentric muscle work).

▶ Finally, have him perform the whole movement, lifting (concentric muscle work), holding, and lowering (isometric and eccentric muscle work).

Side-Lying Leg Rotation

Goal: Maintain trunk stability and isolate pelvic control from hip rotation.

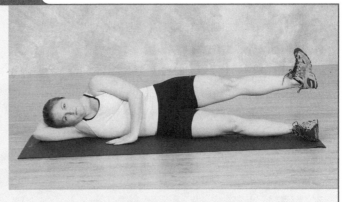

This exercise combines abduction ability and trunk stability while isolating hip movement from that of the pelvis. From the stabilized side-lying position, your client should hold her upper leg straight and abduct it to the horizontal. Tell her to then externally rotate the entire leg from the hip, turning the foot toward the ceiling and then back to pointing forward. Have your client perform three to five rotations before lowering the leg, unless she loses alignment of the pelvis—in which case she should lower her leg immediately.

Teaching Points

▶ This movement isolates hip motion from lumbar–pelvic motion and so develops segmental control.

▶ Where your client has a significant limitation to hip rotation range (e.g., from injury or joint replacement), the action is not appropriate.

Side-Lying Leg Abduction

Goal: Control hip abduction on a stable trunk.

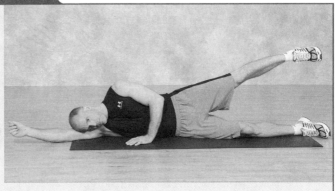

This exercise represents true abduction on a stable base. Have your client assume the stable side-lying position and then lift his upper leg into abduction while avoiding flexion and external rotation. Encourage him to lengthen his leg to avoid lateral pelvic movement and then to abduct his leg as high as he can without experiencing discomfort, up to a maximum of 45° from the horizontal. All the movement should be in the hip—tell him to avoid lumbar–pelvic movement. He may have to work up gradually to the 45° target.

Teaching Points

▶ You may use a pressure biofeedback unit (PBU) placed beneath the lower side of the body to monitor side flexion and lateral pelvic movement.

▶ Once the bladder of the PBU is inflated to fill the gap between the side of the trunk and floor, any movement of the trunk will alter the pressure reading on the machine dial.

Side-Lying Spine Lengthening

Goal: Control the quadratus lumborum and lateral fibers of the oblique abdominals.

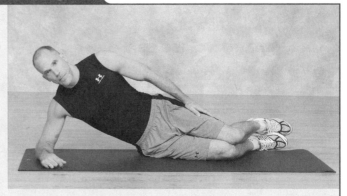

Side lying is also a useful starting position for strong co-contraction of the abdominal muscles with minimal compressive and shear forces on the lumbar spine (McGill 1997). Have your client lie on his right side, his thighs in line with his body but his knees flexed 90°, with his upper body supported on his right elbow to side flex the spine. He should then straighten his spine against the force of gravity, leaving the body supported on the forearm of the underneath arm and hip.

Teaching Points

▶ The action here is simply to change the curve of the side-flexed spine into a straight line.

▶ Use tactile cueing with your hands to encourage the correct action.

Side-Lying Hip Lift

Goal: Progress from side-lying spine lengthening.

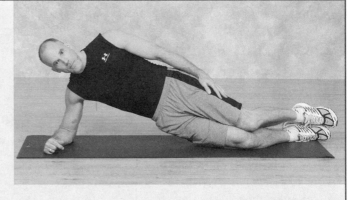

Have your client assume the position for the side-lying spine lengthening. Then have him lift his hips, leaving the body supported on the forearm of the underneath arm and the knees only.

Teaching Points

▶ Use a stick along the length of the spine from sacrum to head to guide your client's alignment.

▶ Some clients find that their knees run together painfully on this exercise. If this is the case, place a folded towel or small foam block between the knees.

Side-Lying Body Lift (Side Bridge)

Goal: Provide final progression for developing control of quadratus lumborum and lateral fibers of oblique abdominals.

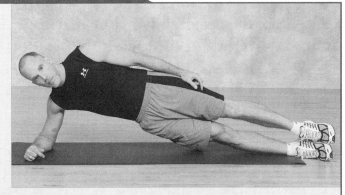

Have your client assume the position for the side-lying spine lengthening. Instruct him to straighten his knees and cross the upper leg in front of the lower leg. Then he should lift his body to the full side-support position, leaving the body supported on the forearm of the underneath arm and the feet. Encourage him to lengthen his body and to broaden his shoulders so they don't fall into scapular adduction—the aim is to form a straight line from the feet, through the pelvis, to the shoulders.

Teaching Points

▶ Some clients find the shoulder position of this exercise awkward and feel that their shoulders are bunched up.

▶ If this is the case, have them take their weight on the underneath hand and straighten the underneath arm. Although this increases the pressure on the wrist (take care!), the feeling of lengthening that it gives makes aligning the shoulders easier.

▶ By stacking the feet on top of each other instead of placing one in front of the other, all of the lower body weight is taken through the side of one foot. Note how this has forced that foot into inversion.

Standing Sternal Lift

Goal: Correct excessive thoracic kyphosis by extending the thoracic spine in isolation.

This exercise repeats the sternal lift action that your client may have practiced for postural correction if he had a kyphotic posture. The idea of the action is to teach your client to move the thoracic spine independently from the nonmoving, stable lumbar spine. Instruct your client to stand facing a table, his thighs pressed against the edge to prevent anterior shift of the pelvis into a swayback position. Have him lift the sternum up and forward while drawing the scapulae down. Suggest that he place one hand in front of his sternum to monitor the sternal lift action. The anterior upward movement and posterior downward movement work like two guide wires pulling a wheel with its axle in the chest. The action is to flatten the thoracic curve rather than simply expand the chest or extend the lumbar spine.

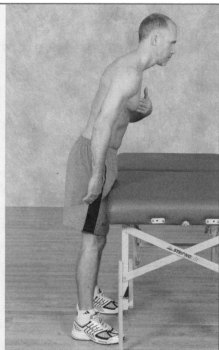

Teaching Points

▶ If your client finds it difficult to isolate the thoracic from the lumbar movement, have him try the same action while sitting—he should place his feet on a low stool to bring his knees above the level of the hips, thereby flexing the lumbar spine and reversing the lumbar lordosis.

▶ This action reduces the available extension in the lumbar spine and focuses the action to the thoracic area. After the client has mastered the action in a sitting position, have him work on it while standing.

▶ This client has flexed forward at the hip. Encourage your client to avoid this and isolate the movement of the thoracic spine.

Pelvic Shift With Unloading

Goal: Correct excessive thoracic kyphosis by extending the thoracic spine in isolation.

Initially your client should stand with his side to a wall for support (gripping wall bars is also ok). As he develops skill in the movement, he should do it in a freestanding position. Instruct him to lengthen his spine (tell him to grow taller); to shift his pelvis to the left while maintaining alignment *(a);* and then to unload the right leg by slightly flexing the knee and lifting the heel, while keeping the toe on the floor *(b).*

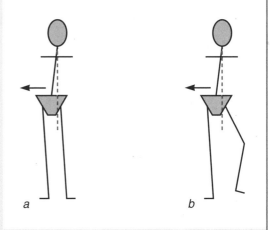

Teaching Points

▶ For tactile cueing, stand behind your client and place your hands over the sides (rims) of his pelvis.

▶ Move his pelvis sideways, keeping it horizontal, and ask him to follow the action.

▶ Gradually reduce your pressure from passive movement to passive guiding. Finally, allow your client to move independently.

Hip Hitch

Goal: Build pelvic control in the frontal plane

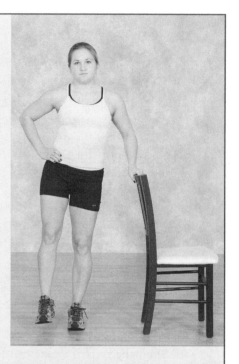

Initially, your client should stand side-on to a wall for support as in the side-lying hip lift (p. 180). As she develops skill in the movement, she should do it in a freestanding position and finally on a shallow step. Instruct her to shift her pelvis to the left, taking all of her weight onto the left leg. Keeping both legs straight, she should try to make the right leg shorter by hitching or hiking the hip upward. This action does not produce a lot of movement, perhaps only 2 to 3 in. (5-8 cm). Once she has mastered the action, have her hold the upper position for 5 to 10 s before lowering. This builds endurance of the hip abductor muscles on the weight-bearing (left) leg.

Teaching Points

▶ As your client performs repetitions of this movement, make sure she does not bend her legs.

▶ This exercise begins in the neutral position and pulls the abductor muscles into inner range.

▶ To progress from outer through to full inner range, have your client stand on a small (2 in., or 5 cm) block. She then begins the exercise with the hip hitched downward (abductor muscles on stretch, outer range), progresses to the neutral position (midrange), and then hitches upward (abductor muscles shortened, inner range).

Pelvic Shift With Leg Lift

Goal: Teach pelvic control and stability in single-leg standing.

Ask your client to shift her pelvis to the left, so that her body weight is over the left leg only (pelvic shift with unloading, page 183), and then slowly lift her right leg no more than 6 in. (15 cm) while maintaining alignment in all three planes; there should be no posterior tilt of the pelvis, no hip drop, and no spinal rotation. *(a)* Shows lateral pelvic tilt (incorrect!), and *(b)* illustrates anterior pelvic tilt (incorrect!). The action is one of pure hip flexion on a stable back: The supporting leg supports the pelvis, and the pelvis supports the back. The knee should be raised no more than 45° from the horizontal.

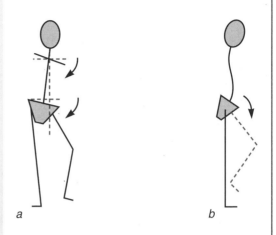

Teaching Points

▶ If your client finds the movement difficult to control, let her practice at first with her back supported by a wall.

▶ The sequence of pelvic shift, leg unloading, and knee lift are the same, but the back remains against the wall throughout the movement.

Standing Hip Abduction

Goal: Maintain stability in the frontal plane while performing hip abduction.

Your client begins by standing with her back 2 to 4 in. (5-10 cm) from a wall. If your client loses pure abduction as the movement progresses (i.e., if she uses any flexion or extension), she will know immediately because the leg will move closer to or farther away from the wall. Instruct her to shift her pelvis to the right, unloading the left leg (a). Then, maintaining alignment, she should abduct the left leg by 10° to 20° (b). Be sure that she

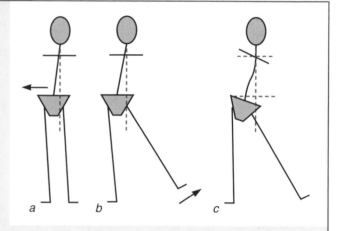

does not laterally tilt her pelvis or spine (c). She should gradually increase the abduction range to a maximum of 45°. Reduce the range or stop the exercise as soon as alignment is lost.

Teaching Points

▶ This exercise duplicates the Trendelenburg test (p. 141), which assessed stability of the hip and pelvis combined.

▶ If your client finds it difficult to keep her pelvis level (horizontal), use a pole placed across the top of her pelvis to augment tactile cueing.

Standing Hip Hinge With Table

Goal: Move the spine and pelvis as a single unit on the hip.

Have your client stand about 4 in. (10 cm) from a table. She may place her hands on the table only to help guide her movement, not to bear weight. Instruct her to bend from the hip, keeping her spine straight, until the spine is angled 30° to 45° from the vertical. It is often easier if your client focuses attention on her sacrum and imagines it moving from near vertical to near horizontal—tell her to push her tail away. Once she has mastered this movement, she should do it without table support.

Teaching Points

▶ Two kinds of feedback may be helpful. First, the client can monitor pelvic tilt by placing the flat of one hand over the lower (infraumbilical) abdomen and the back of the other hand over the sacrum *(a)*. The action is to tilt the pelvis while maintaining the relationship of the lumbar spine to the pelvis—the palm of the back hand should end up facing toward the ceiling.

▶ The second feedback method uses a long, straight stick. As your client places one hand over her sacrum and the other between her shoulder blades, she should grip the stick with both hands. She must keep her spine on the stick as she performs the hip hinge action *(b)*. Rounding the spine (a typical error) increases pressure of the spinous processes on the stick; hollowing the spine increases the gap between the spine and the stick.

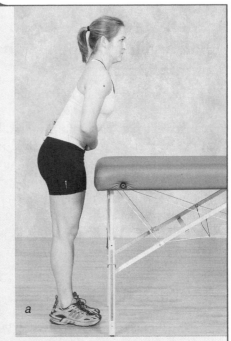

a

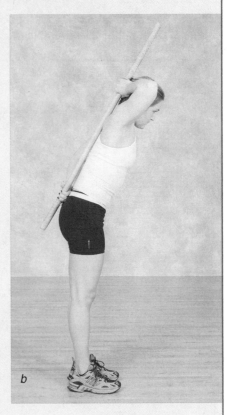

b

Sitting Hamstring Stretch

Goal: Maintain pelvic position against the pull of the hamstrings.

Begin sitting on a chair or gym bench. Instruct your client to straighten one leg to stretch the hamstrings while maintaining lumbar–pelvic alignment. As soon as the pelvis posteriorly tilts (to bring the ischial tuberosity forward and take the stretch off the hamstrings), stop the exercise, because alignment has been lost. Progress the exercise by gradually straightening the leg further (while maintaining alignment) until the knee can be locked fully with the hip at 70° flexion.

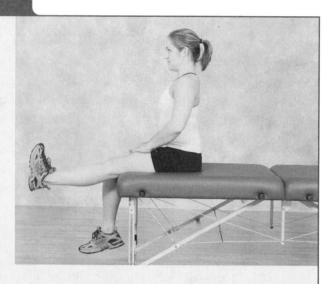

Teaching Points

▶ This exercise repeats the tripod test used to assess segmental control of the pelvis and lumbar spine.

▶ The action also stretches the sciatic nerve. If your client experiences tingling or burning through the thigh rather than a simple muscle stretch, have a physical therapist examine his neural tension.

Sitting Sternal Lift

Goal: **Perform active thoracic extension and isolate it from lumbar extension.**

Instruct your client to raise his sternum while drawing the scapulae down, as in the standing sternal lift on page 182. The movement is one of thoracic spine extension rather than deep inspiration. To assist the learning process, place the flat of your hand on your client's sternum and draw it up at the same time that you place the thumb and forefingers of your opposite hand on the inferior angles of the scapulae and draw it down.

Teaching Points

▶ If breathing control proves to be problematic, encourage your client to breathe out as he begins the sternal lift.

▶ Many people mistakenly extend the lumbar spine rather than the thoracic spine. If this occurs with your client, let him practice the exercise with his feet on a small stool to bring his knees above hip level—this position reverses the lumbar lordosis and throws the extension force high up the spine to the thoracic region.

▶ Once he has mastered the movement in this position, try the standard position again; see sternal lift exercise *(a)*, p. 103.

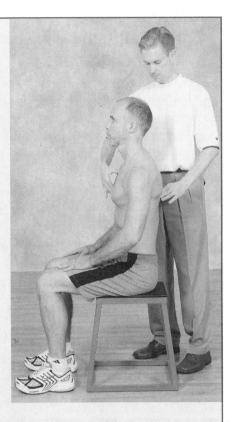

Sitting Knee Raise

Goal: Maintain pelvic position against the pull of the hip flexors.

In this exercise, we overload the stability muscles by using the pull of the iliopsoas to displace the lumbar spine. Instruct your client to raise one knee, in stages, to about 3 in. (8 cm) above the horizontal, while maintaining lumbar–pelvic alignment. Be sure that he avoids posterior pelvic tilt. Initially, he should gradually unload the limb by lifting just the heel. If he is able to maintain good alignment, have him lift the entire leg.

Teaching Points

▶ This exercise mimics the test used to assess lengthening of the iliopsoas muscles (p. 110).

▶ If the client's iliopsoas is excessively short or excessively tight, the exercise is not appropriate.

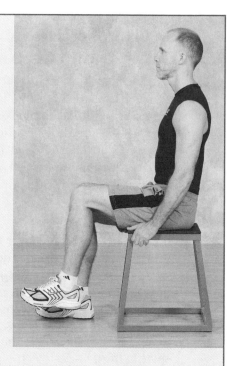

Sitting Knee and Arm Raise

Goal: Increase the complexity to challenge coordination.

Have your client flex one arm to 90°. Holding a small (7.5-10 lb, or 3-5 kg) dumbbell in the hand increases the overload; he should keep the dumbbell moving rather than holding it still. Combining alternate arm and leg movements is a useful progression—the right arm is lifted at the same time as the left knee to provide a diagonal stress on the body; this is then reversed with the left arm and right knee being raised.

Teaching Points

▶ This exercise can be practiced using resistance bands rather than dumbbells.

▶ Have your client sit on a gym ball (chapter 10) to increase the difficulty of the movement.

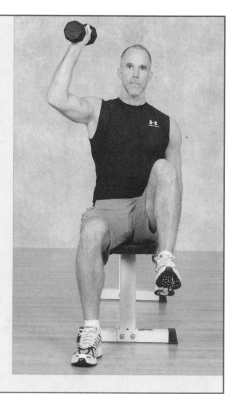

Chapter 9
Unstable Base

If your client's stabilizing muscles are not able to contract fast enough, your client can still be injured. Imagine what would happen if severe stress was imposed on your client's spine 0.25 seconds into the lift, but it took 0.5 seconds for their muscles to be fully active. The result is that all of their new found muscle strength is of no use to them. The damage is already done. In this chapter we work to train the stabilizing muscles to contract with the correct timing— neither too soon nor too late.

THEORY OF PROPRIOCEPTION

Because you need to know the underlying mechanisms behind the activities you prescribe for your clients, the next few paragraphs provide an overview of proprioception. Also, reread pages 131-132 for more information on this subject.

Movement Sense

Kinesthetic awareness, or movement sense, includes the detection of both joint displacement and change in velocity (i.e., acceleration). It is commonly assessed by measuring the threshold to detection of passive motion (TTDPM): Individuals simply state when they feel that movement has begun. One cannot act to correct imbalance until one is aware that there is an imbalance. The awareness can be conscious or unconscious, however, and the corrective action likewise can be intentional or automatic. The purpose of proprioceptive training is to help individuals learn both to detect and to correct imbalances without conscious awareness that they are doing so. Consciously performed joint-positioning activities, especially at end range, will enhance the development of automatic control and cognitive awareness (Lephart and Fu 1995).

Regulation of Muscle Stiffness

Dynamic joint stability (i.e., the body's ability to constantly make unconscious microcorrections to keep a joint stable) occurs via reflexes at the spinal level. Reflexes by definition are not conscious or intentional movements. A common illustration is the body's response when your finger touches a hot skillet. The incoming nerve stimulus (afferent, i.e., going toward the central nervous system) doesn't even make it to the brain—rather, it gets only as far as the spinal cord before it is processed and an appropriate outgoing signal (efferent, i.e., going away from the central nervous system) is sent to the muscles: "Move your hand!" In fact, you move your hand without thinking about it because your brain had nothing to do with the reaction—it all occurred in a closed loop of signals between your hand and your spinal cord.

The ideal situation for back stability is that you have such closed-loop efferent signals constantly going out to your stability muscles: The receptor nerves detect a slight increase in instability, they send messages to the spinal cord, and instantaneously outgoing efferent signals are sent out to tweak your stabilizing muscles. It all happens dozens of times a second without your even thinking about it.

Such is the goal of proprioceptive exercises. It is possible to train your nervous system to be more sensitive to incoming messages that tell you stability is weakening and to provide more automatic outgoing signals that instruct which muscles to change in which way. If such a fine-tuned system seems unimaginable, try this experiment: Open a water faucet at least halfway, hold a drinking glass under it, and keep the glass as perfectly level as you can. You'll find that you can keep it quite still. Now consider the complexity of the nerve signals involved in the task you just completed. Thousands of times per second, afferent signals left your hand with the message that the cup has just gotten heavier. And thousands of times per second, efferent signals returned from your central nervous system: "OK, tighten such-and-such muscles a bit more." But it all happens so fast, and the microadjustments are so smooth, that for the most part your hand is able to hold the drinking glass stable. This is a closed-loop system. Your brain isn't significantly involved. The signals go to your spinal cord, they are processed, and the return messages head immediately back to your hand.

Proprioceptive exercises involve sudden alterations in joint position to train the body's reflexes. To thoroughly follow an individual's progress, you theoretically can measure the precise onset of muscle contraction in relation to joint displacement; unfortunately, however, you most likely would need to refer your client to a physical therapy (PT) department or specialist biomechanics lab to make accurate measurements. Yet, with experience, you can assess onset of muscle contraction to some degree by palpating the muscle during an exercise. This type of examination, although not exact, can be useful for muscle reeducation. The aim is simply to note whether the muscles are able to limit joint displacement and effectively stabilize the joint.

BENEFITS OF TRAINING

Using TTDPM and reproduction of passive positioning (RPP), Barrack and colleagues (1983) found decreased kinesthesia with increasing age (i.e., the closed-loop system for stability works less well). Injury further reduces proprioceptive input because of prolonged inactivity and damage to proprioceptive nerve endings within the injured tissues. A number of authors have stressed the importance of proprioceptive training in rehabilitation following injury to the knee (Barrack et al. 1983; Beard et al. 1994), ankle (Freeman et al. 1965; Konradsen and Ravn 1990; Lentell et al. 1990), and shoulder (Lephart et al. 1994; Smith and Brunolli 1990).

The functional importance of proprioceptive training has also been emphasized during rehabilitation of the spine (Norris 1995a), although the use of proprioceptive training in spinal rehabilitation is less common than for other areas of the body. Differences in proprioception have been shown between patients with back pain and those who were pain free (Gill and Callaghan 1998), in terms of movement accuracy measured as deviation from a target. In addition, RPP has been shown to be worse in individuals with lumbar instability (O'Sullivan et al. 2003). Interestingly, proprioception has been shown to be worse in patients with low back pain than normal people in flexion but not extension. Using RPP, Newcomer and colleagues (2000) monitored lumbar proprioception using a 3Space tracker unit to analyze three-dimensional body position in a standing and bending task. These authors suggested that increased activation of mechanoreceptors in facet joints may have led to the proprioceptive improvement with extension.

Proprioception and accompanying reflexes may indeed be enhanced with training. Barrack and colleagues (1983) found enhanced kinesthesia in trained dancers, and Lephart and Fu (1995) demonstrated the same in intercollegiate gymnasts. Both types of athletes practice free exercise using body weight as resistance and using complex multijoint activities. This type of training appears appropriate for proprioceptive rehabilitation.

Key point: Proprioception and stabilizing reflexes may be enhanced by using training that involves complex multijoint activities.

The basis of proprioceptive training for the back is maintenance of stability against a rapidly applied force tending to displace the spine. In most cases, you can instruct your clients to practice one or more of the following exercises for at least 5 min a day, 4 or 5 days per week. The limiting factor is whether your clients can keep their spines stable (they should stop before they lose stability). They should do the most advanced exercises of which they are capable, as quickly as they are able. Remember, the idea is to train their reflexes to act with such extreme speed that maintaining spinal stability will be as smooth an operation as your holding the glass motionless as it fills under a tap.

Now, let's put theory into practice and begin to enhance proprioception. We start with some basic foundation movements, teaching your clients to stabilize their backs much more rapidly than they have been doing up to now.

Rapid Displacement Exercises

These exercises involve knocking your client off balance slightly, so there are safety issues to address. Explain to your client exactly what will be required of him—clear instructions will prevent misunderstanding later. Begin all the exercises slowly, and as your client's proprioception improves, speed the exercises up.

Repeated Pelvic-Tilting Exercises

Moving the pelvis beneath an immobile trunk is an excellent teaching method initially used to improve slow control of the neutral position. As the pace quickens, muscle reaction speed will be improved to further enhance stability. We can use both rocker boards (which move like a see-saw) and wobble boards (mounted on a hemisphere—move in any direction).

SUMMARY

- Proprioception includes both movement sense and regulation of muscle stiffness.
- Both threshold to the detection of passive movement (TTDPM) and reproduction of passive positioning (RPP) are used to retrain proprioception.
- Rapid displacement and repeated pelvic tilting exercises are suitable for retraining.

Rapid Displacement in Sitting

Goal: Develop muscle reaction speed for back stability.

Have your client sit on a stool with her spine optimally aligned. A training partner stands behind her and presses against her shoulders from multiple directions to flex, extend, and laterally flex the spine. Initially the pressure should be even, but gradually it should become varied in both direction and force. The aim is for your client to be able to rapidly stabilize her spine before the spine moves away from its neutral position. Instruct her to relax her trunk muscles between repetitions (which should last about a minute each), rather than hold them rigidly braced throughout the whole exercise.

Teaching Points

▶ If you have it available, use surface EMG to monitor changing muscle tone.

▶ As your client's reactions become more proficient, the movements should become faster—but she must always maintain good alignment.

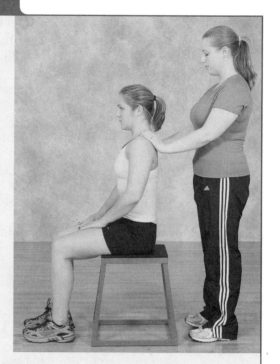

Muscle Reaction Speed Using a Mobile Platform

Goal: Further develop muscle reaction speed for back stability.

Instruct your client to assume a two-point kneeling position on a balance board and to align her lumbar spine into its neutral position. Then a training partner should push her off balance so that the platform tilts. The aim is to maintain lumbar stability as the board tilts while keeping the edges of the board off the ground. Your client will initially feel very insecure, as though she is going to fall off the board; reassure her that she is only 2 to 3 in. (5-8 cm) from the floor! With time, she will gain confidence.

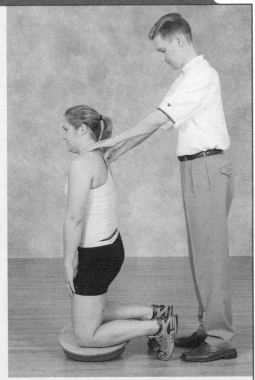

Teaching Points

▶ Start with a rocker board (allows single-plane motion), advancing later to a domed balance board (wobble board) that allows triplane motion.

▶ You may also want to use other mobile platforms such as the Fitter ski trainer (Fitter International Inc., Calgary, Alberta, Canada), the slide trainer (Forza Fitness Equipment, London, UK), or a mini-trampette (available in most large sports stores).

▶ Increase the speed of the movements as your client becomes more proficient.

Throwing and Catching on a Mobile Surface

Goal: Develop rapid-onset back stability.

Throwing and catching a basketball or medicine ball on a mobile surface will increase the challenge to the stabilizing system. The aim is to align the lumbar spine optimally while balancing on the mobile surface. As your client catches the ball, she must maintain spinal alignment despite the platform's motion. Instruct your client to increase the speed of the exercises as she becomes more proficient. She may either stand on the board (placed on the floor) or sit on it (placed on a secure bench).

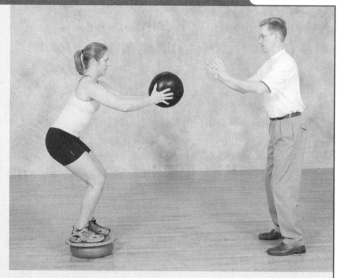

Teaching Points

▶ Use a light ball to begin with and throw and catch gently. Less force will displace the trunk less.

▶ Build up both the speed of throwing and catching and the force used by standing farther away from your client and swapping the light basketball for a heavier medicine ball.

Sitting Pelvic Tilt, Progressing to Balance Board

Goal: **Advanced control of pelvic tilt.**

Begin with a review of some points. Have your client sit in the optimal position (see p. 73) on a wooden bench or stool with her feet on the floor. Remind her how to tilt her pelvis alternately in the anterior and then posterior direction. Make sure she maintains the position of her shoulders and thoracic spine. The aim is to isolate the pelvis and lower lumbar spine from the thoracic spine and the shoulders from the upper lumbar spine. Progress the exercise by having your client perform it while sitting first on a rocker board, wobble board, or sit-fit cushion.

Teaching Points

▶ Sitting on a sit-fit cushion enables your client to subtly change pelvic position far more easily than she can on a normal chair.

▶ Encourage your client to try using this piece of equipment on her standard office chair—many people find this surprisingly comfortable.

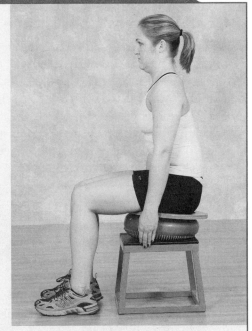

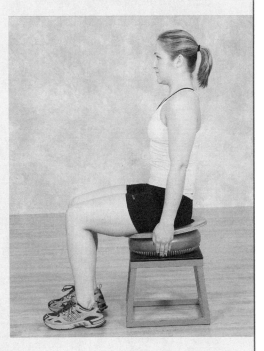

Pelvic Rock on Rocker Board

Goal: Progress from simple pelvic tilt.

Initially place the rocker in the frontal plane to facilitate anterior and posterior tilting of the pelvis. Changing the rocker orientation of the board to the sagittal plane will facilitate lateral tilting. In each case, the lumbar–pelvic movement must be isolated from that of the upper body. To begin working for muscle reaction speed, apply pressure on the shoulders to push your client off balance while she tries to stay upright on the rocker board.

Teaching Points

▶ Alternate the orientation of the board between frontal and sagittal planes.

▶ You'll know when to stop any given session when your client is no longer able to maintain neutral position or maintain abdominal hollowing.

▶ Build up to 2 min in both planes before progressing to the wobble board.

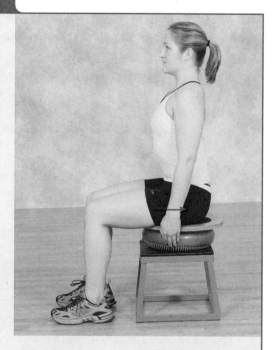

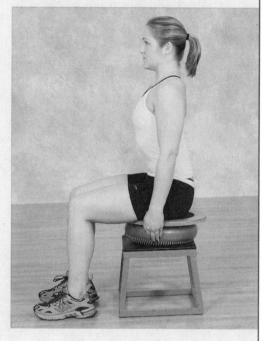

Pelvic Rock on Wobble Board

Goal: Develop multiplane (sagittal, frontal, and transverse) stability in sitting.

Initially, have your client merely sit on the wobble board and attempt to maintain the optimal sitting position. Have her progress to single plane actions (flexion–extension and lateral flexion). Once she has mastered these actions, instruct her to tip the board around a clock face (i.e., to tilt to 1 o'clock and then back to neutral, to 2 o'clock and back to neutral, to 3 o'clock and back to neutral, and so on).

Teaching Points

▶ Initially, encourage your client to use slow, deliberate movements, taking perhaps 2 to 5 s to reach each position of the clock.

▶ As she improves, build the speed and complexity of the task by using rapid movements, combining movement directions.

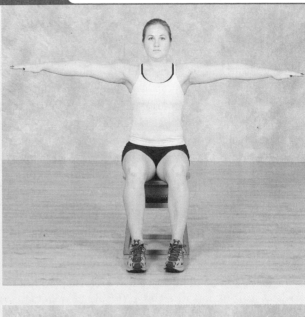

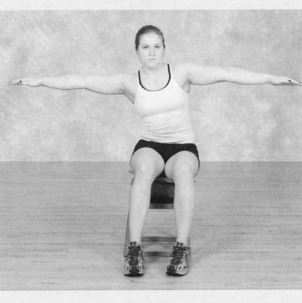

Neutral Position Maintenance

Goal: Build stability reaction speed in sitting.

Try to knock your client off balance while she maintains the neutral position on a wobble board. Initially use slow-onset pressure, working gradually up to rapid pressure from a variety of directions. Have your client close her eyes to facilitate anticipatory muscle action and muscle contraction speed.

Teaching Points

▶ The progression here is one of time. Initially, try to prolong the movement for 30 s and then 60 s, stopping each time when alignment is lost or your client loses her balance.

▶ Ask your client to try this exercise with her eyes closed. Because she is unable to anticipate the movements as well, the action becomes more difficult.

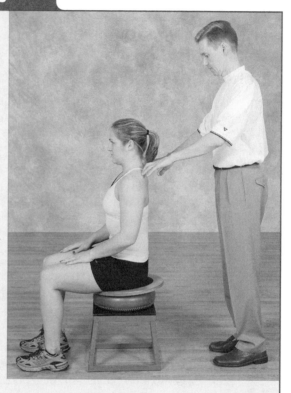

Sitting Hip Hinge

Goal: Move spine and pelvis as a single unit on the hip.

The final exercise is the sitting hip hinge (compare it with the standing hip hinge, p. 187). As in all these sitting exercises, be sure your client begins in the optimal sitting position, with the knees astride to facilitate pelvic tilt (see description under Exercises in the Sitting Position, p. 167). Have him tip the whole of his upper body forward as a single unit, moving the pelvis and spine on the fixed femur. He should initiate the action by leaning his whole body forward to change the sitting weight distribution. In optimal sitting, approximately 30% of the body weight is taken on the pubic bones and 70% on the ischial tuberosities. As your client leans forward, he takes weight from the ischial tuberosities and places it onto the pubic bones, ending with 70% to 80% of his weight on the pubic bone. To lean back, he reverses the weight transference.

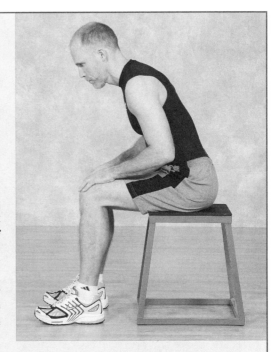

Teaching Points

▶ To facilitate the action, suggest that your client initially perform this exercise while sitting on a rocker board.

▶ In this exercise, the pelvis and spine should move as one unit, avoiding any change in lordosis.

Chapter 10
Gym Ball

In chapter 9 we looked at muscle reaction timing and its importance to stability training. Now, we will use the commonly found gym ball to train this feature. The gym ball is an ideal piece of equipment for home stability training especially. It is low in cost, comes in different sizes to match your client's body dimensions, and is fun to use. Draw your clients' attention to the safety aspects of gym ball training, however, because injury can occur through poor technique.

GYM BALL EXERCISES

See pages 205-218

Your clients can obtain advanced levels of stability using exercises with gym balls (also called stability balls or Swiss balls). These exercises require quite complex movements and will help increase the stability already obtained through previous exercises in this book. They also can strengthen stability muscles that otherwise might not be exercised.

At first your clients should use the ball under your supervision, but later they can use it at home—it is an inexpensive and effective apparatus for back stability. Gym ball exercises have become popular in exercise classes and for exercise forms such as Pilates. Exercises taught in this way are useful to increase your exercise vocabulary, but be certain that the movements you choose are suitable for a client who has suffered from back pain.

A 26 in. (65 cm) gym ball provides the optimal sitting position for most people. Your clients should be able to sit on the ball with their femurs horizontal and their hips and knees both at 90° to 100° of flexion, so that their knees are slightly below their hips. Feet should be shoulder-width apart and flat on the floor to enable free pelvic tilting and provide a wide base of support. The ball should be inflated so that it feels firm but will give slightly when a person sits on it. Use higher infla-

tion pressures for heavier clients. Deflating the ball slightly will increase the base of support.

You can reduce the ball's tendency to roll by setting it on a collar, which is a plastic ring on the floor. When you need to increase your clients' confidence or provide support, place the ball between two chairs: With either position, the chair backs toward the ball so that your clients can lightly touch the chair with arms outstretched at shoulder level, or, for even more support, position the seats toward the ball so your clients can place the flats of their hands on the seat surface.

As with all exercises, your clients should warm up before engaging in any of the more intense exercises. During all exercises clients should return to the neutral position of their spine when the exercise is complete and keep their abdomens hollowed when stress is imposed on the spine. Clients should perform mirror images of any one-sided exercises, so the body is worked symmetrically.

The progression with stability ball exercises is similar to that for previous exercises: Begin with 8 to 10 repetitions, for example, and then increase to 12 to 15. The gym ball introduces balance as an additional variable. Even if your clients are not fatigued, if they lose alignment or lose their balance and become unstable (and therefore are likely to slip off the ball), they must stop, rest, and start again using a lower number of repetitions.

At first have your clients use a slow count of 4 or 5 to move into the holding position; hold the designated position for a count of 5, and then use a count of 4 or 5 to move back into the starting position. Clients can progress by adding reps or by adding to the holding time. Determine the limits for a given exercise by observing the point at which your clients just begin to lose spinal alignment or abdominal hollowing or begin to lose their balance—then instruct them to stay just below that level of timing or rep number for at least a week before trying to add holding time or reps. They should always stay just a little bit within their maximum capacity, as determined by their ability to maintain alignment and abdominal hollowing.

You will probably want your clients to use gym ball exercises as part of a general back stability program. For those clients who want to use gym balls as their only exercise, they should incorporate the back stability exercises into a more general conditioning program based on the ball. I do not recommend daily exercise on the gym ball because it can be too intense and not varied enough. The maximum would be three to five sessions per week, allowing the weekend as a rest period to recover.

SUMMARY

- The gym ball should be the right size to allow your client to sit with his hip slightly above his knee.
- Deflate the ball slightly to increase its contact area.
- Begin with simple actions and progress to more complex movements.

Sitting Knee Raise On Gym Ball

Goal: Maintain stability in the presence of hip movement on a reduced base of support.

While sitting upright on the gym ball, your client should lift a single knee from 90° hip flexion to 120° hip flexion. He must make the action slow and deliberate, maintaining his body position throughout and avoiding the temptation to fall toward the lifting leg.

Teaching Points

▶ Have the client begin by lifting one leg and placing it back on the floor before lifting the other leg.

▶ Have him progress to lifting one leg as the other is lowering, leaving a split second period when both legs are off the ground.

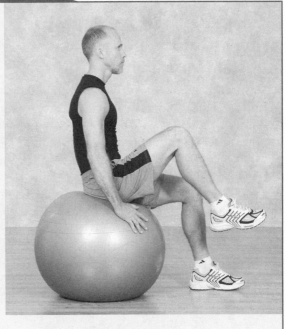

Abdominal Slide

Goal: Control the action of the rectus abdominis while moving.

Instruct your client to tilt his pelvis backward from a sitting position on the ball and then roll back until his spine rests on the ball. The action is to roll through the spine—the ischial tuberosities begin on the ball, but the weight is transferred to the coccyx and sacrum and eventually to the lumbar spine. The final holding position is with the trunk slightly flexed and the abdominal muscles contracted in a half-sitting position. He should hold this lower position and then return to sitting using the same curling action in reverse.

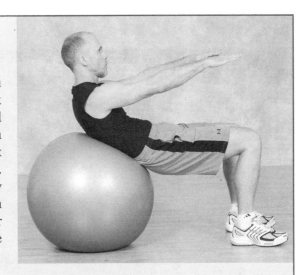

Teaching Points

▶ Make sure that your client begins with abdominal hollowing and holds the hollow (flat contour) abdominal position throughout the movement.

▶ Ensure that you client does not hold his breath during this exercise.

Half-Sitting Arm and Leg Movements

Goal: Maintain stability while moving arms and legs in an unstable position.

Have your client perform the abdominal slide action just described but maintain the position when his trunk is at 45° to the horizontal. Then he should raise one arm while lowering the other. Once he can do this in a controlled fashion, with the trunk remaining in alignment, have him rest his arms and then lift one leg while lowering the other. He should try to keep the thigh of the leg being raised parallel to the ground (i.e., only the lower leg should move). Finally, he should perform arm and leg movements together—the right arm and left leg lifting together, and vice versa.

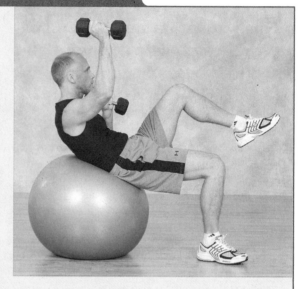

Teaching Points

▶ To make the exercise even more challenging, suggest that your client hold small dumbbells in his hands as he does the movements.

▶ Tell your client to avoid a vigorous swinging action because this will build too much momentum and make the action difficult to stop.

Lying Trunk Curl Over Ball

Goal: Strengthen upper rectus abdominis muscles.

Instruct your client to begin with his thoracolumbar spine supported on the ball, his arms at his side. He should move from this slightly flexed position to spinal extension, relaxing over the ball. He then performs a curling movement while performing abdominal hollowing and pressing his lumbar spine onto the ball surface.

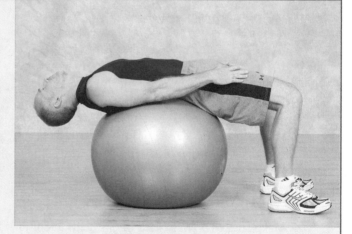

Teaching Points

▶ Once your client can perform the basic exercise well, increase the difficulty by having him hold his arms by the side of his head or even completely overhead.

▶ Increase the work on the lower abdominal by combining the curl with posterior pelvic tilting.

Lying Trunk Curl With Leg Lift

Goal: Strengthen upper and lower abdominals.

From the position that was used for the lying trunk curl over ball, your client should lift one leg while maintaining the stable position, trying to keep the thigh parallel to the other thigh. The movement is easier if the ball rests closer to his shoulders with his waist at the ball's edge rather than at the ball's center. Lying over the ball, in fact, is an excellent way to stretch the whole spine into extension as part of postural correction of a flat-back posture.

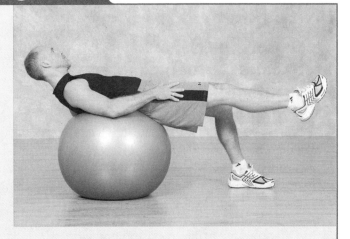

Teaching Points

▶ Taller clients will find this exercise harder because of the longer lever length of their legs.

▶ If your client finds that the ball wobbles too much, place the side of the ball against a wall.

Basic Superman

Goal: Strengthen the spinal and hip extensors.

Have your client lie prone with her abdomen on the ball and her feet astride and flat against a wall. She should tighten her abdominal muscles to form a firm surface pressing against the ball and retract her head (tuck her chin in without looking down). She should retract and depress her shoulders to draw her arms downward and back and then extend her thoracic spine to bring her chest off the ball. Have her hold the inner-range position for 5 to 10 s.

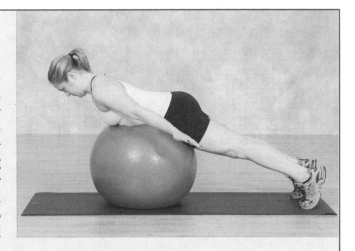

Teaching Points

▶ Spinal extensor muscle endurance is a vital component of back health. The superman exercise is a classic movement to work this.

▶ This exercise can also be performed with the feet on the ground and the ball closer to the chest.

Superman With Arms

Goal: Strengthen spinal extensors; help shoulder retractors contribute more to movement.

From the basic superman movement, instruct your client to extend first one and then both arms overhead to increase the overload for both trunk and shoulders. Holding a light ball or balloon between her hands can help give her the feeling of lengthening her body. Observe carefully to make sure that your client doesn't lose alignment and hyperextend her spine.

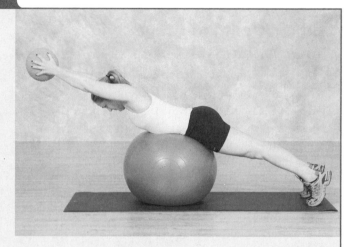

Teaching Points

▶ There should be a straight line through your client's heels, knees, hips, shoulders, and hands.

▶ This action is excellent for improving thoracic spine extension ability as well.

Bridge

Goal: Simultaneously strengthen both hip extensors and spinal extensors.

Have your client lie with her shoulders and upper back on the ball and her feet flat on the floor, knees apart. Place a small stool under her buttocks and instruct her to raise and lower her body from the stool using hip extension force. Once she is able to hold the raised position, remove the stool. Instruct her to hold the position, making sure that her lumbar spine is in its optimal position.

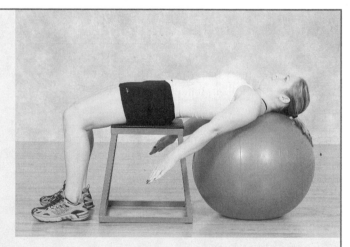

Teaching Points

▶ Your client should gradually build up the holding time to 30 s.

▶ With clients who find recruiting their gluteals difficult, use isolated gluteal contractions (p. 89w) first.

Bridge With Pelvic Tilt

Goal: Strengthen back and hip extensors while improving control of pelvic tilt.

While your client holds the bridge position, have her perform a pelvic tilt. She can intensify the bridge movement by combining an anterior tilt with lowering her buttocks onto the floor and a posterior tilt with lifting herself back into the bridge position. This exercise helps teach the subtleties of muscle control involved in minor adjustments in pelvic tilt.

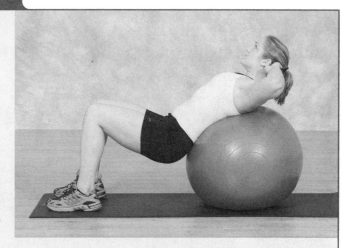

Teaching Points

▶ This exercise is especially helpful to clients who can only perform a tilt as an all-or-nothing movement using maximal force to bring about a full tilt.

▶ To vary the exercise, ask your client to stop the pelvic tilt action at various points and hold each position for 2 to 3 s.

Bridge With Leg Lift On Gym Ball

Goal: Increase overload—especially of lower abdominals—during bridge.

Have your client perform the standard bridge exercise; once he is in the high position, he should lift one knee to bring his foot off the ground. Be sure that he maintains spinal alignment, avoiding the temptation to tip the pelvis toward the lifted leg.

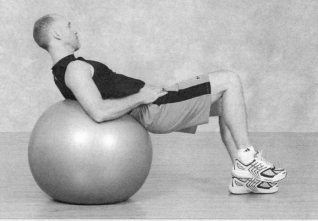

Teaching Points

▶ If your client finds it difficult to keep his pelvis level, place a stick across the front of the pelvis just below the level of the anterior superior iliac spines. If the pelvis tilts too far, the stick will fall off!

▶ An alternative to using the stick is placing a hardback book flat across the lower abdomen and pelvis.

Bridge With Leg Lift and Extension

Goal: Strengthen lower abdominals while increasing leg control.

Have your client perform the standard bridge and lift his right knee so that his right foot clears the floor, avoiding the tendency to allow the pelvis to tilt to the right. At the high position, he should gradually straighten the right leg until it is completely in line with the spine. After maintaining this position for 2 to 3 s, he slowly bends the leg and lowers it until his foot is back on the ground.

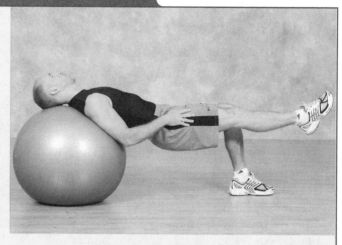

Teaching Points

▶ Ensure that your client forms a straight line between his foot, knee, hip, and shoulder. Do not allow the leg to sag.

▶ It is common for clients to have asymmetry and to find that lifting one leg easier than the other.

Bridge With Therapist Pressure

Goal: Strengthen hip and trunk stability muscles by challenging stability with continuously variable overload from multiple directions.

While your client performs the standard bridge, kneel at his side. Push against his pelvis from above and below and side to side. Rapid pushes will decrease muscle reaction time, training the muscles to contract more quickly without loss of intensity.

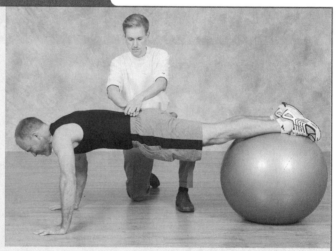

Teaching Points

▶ This exercise trains proprioception (see p. 191).

▶ Begin with slow predictable presses and then progress to faster presses moving in an unpredictable manner.

Reverse Bridge

Goal: Strengthen back and hip muscles while increasing leg motion control.

Your client should place her feet and calves on the ball with her trunk on the floor. Instruct her to abduct her arms to about 30° to aid balance. Then she should lift her hips to make a straight line from the shoulders to the hips and feet.

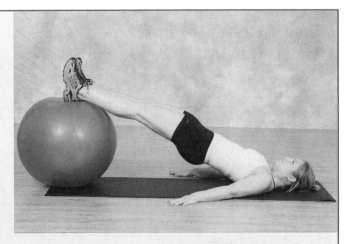

Teaching Points

▶ Initiate the movement with a gluteal contraction to ensure that the gluteals rather than the hamstrings are used intensely.

▶ If your client finds that the ball moves too much, place it on a collar or hoop to stop it rolling.

Reverse Bridge and Roll

Goal: Strengthen back and hip muscles while increasing leg motion control.

Once your client is in the high position of the reverse bridge movement, she should roll the ball toward herself by flexing her knees and hips and then roll it away by extending her legs again.

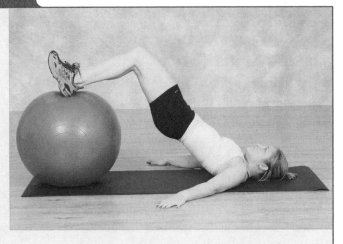

Teaching Points

▶ Your client can also roll the ball from side to side to work her trunk side flexors.

▶ Encourage her to begin with small amounts of motion and progress to larger movements when she is able.

Heel Bridge

Goal: Increase overload in the bridge position.

Instruct your client to assume the high position of the reverse bridge, with this difference: Only her heels should be on the ball. Instruct her to push each heel alternately into the ball—this entails pushing down with the whole leg to activate the hamstrings and gluteals, rather than simply flexing the knee to work the hamstrings alone.

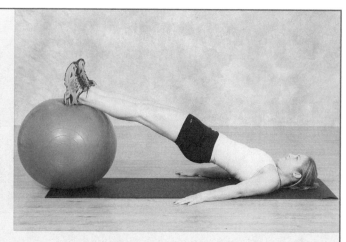

Teaching Points

▶ This exercise relies on leverage to provide overload. Consequently, it is harder for taller clients.

▶ If your client finds the control of this movement difficult, have her practice initially with her heels on a gym bench before progressing to the ball.

One-Leg Heel Bridge

Goal: Provide maximal overload in the bridge position.

Your client's trunk should be on the floor, and only her heels should be on the ball. Have her lift one leg and hold it away from the ball. Then have her perform a single-leg heel bridge by pushing her heel into the ball and lifting her buttocks off the floor. She should hold the position for 5 to 10 s and then lower her body to the starting position in a controlled manner.

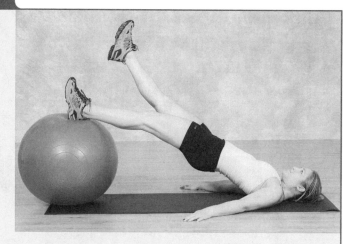

Teaching Points

▶ It is common for clients to have one leg that is stronger than the other.

▶ To correct symmetry, work harder on the weaker leg.

▶ To work the trunk side flexors, have the client move the ball from side to side.

Prone Fall

Goal: Provide co-contraction for the hip and trunk muscles.

Have your client place his thighs on the ball, with his legs together and his hands on the floor. He should lengthen his body to achieve a neutral spine and retract his head to maintain cervical alignment. He should begin with the ball close to his pelvis and then walk his hands forward so that the ball moves down his legs toward his knees. Shifting the body's center of gravity farther from the center of the ball increases the leverage effect.

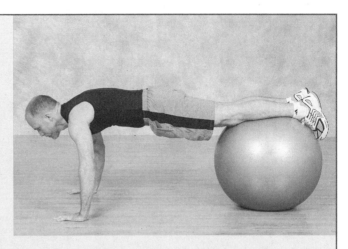

Teaching Points

▶ Ensure that your client maintains a straight body position.

▶ If he begins to sag, only allow him to roll the ball toward his knees as far as he can while maintaining optimal alignment.

▶ If your client finds that this exercise hurts the wrists, he can take his weight through his forearms instead.

Prone Fall With Arm Lift

Goal: Increase overload in prone fall.

Have your client begin with the prone fall movement. Then he should lift one hand about 0.5 in. (1.3 cm) from the floor without allowing the shoulder girdle to dip down. He then lifts the arm first to the side and eventually forward, pointing the hand and lengthening the whole body.

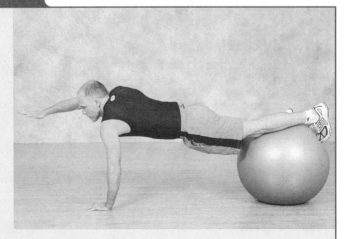

Teaching Points

▶ This exercise provides intense work for the shoulder stabilizer muscles as well as the trunk stabilizers.

▶ The push-up position also works the pectoral muscles, which may be tight in a kyphotic client (one whose thoracic spine is flexed). If your client is grossly kyphotic, do not choose this action.

Prone Fall With One-Leg Lift

Goal: Increase overload (especially for gluteals) in prone fall while training for abdominal–gluteal co-contraction.

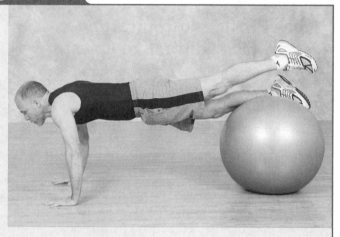

Have your client begin with the prone fall movement and then lift one leg to 15° hip extension, keeping the knee locked. Instruct him to perform alternate single-leg lifts.

Teaching Points

▶ To train for speed as well as strength, have your client gradually increase the speed of the lifts.

▶ Eventually he should perform the lifts as fast as he can without losing correct alignment.

Wall Sit

Goal: Prepare the body for lifting while strengthening the legs to provide power for the lift.

Your client performs the following exercise with the ball sandwiched between his back and a wall. This has two main advantages over simply leaning against the wall. First, vertical movement is easier because the rolling of the ball removes the friction between the person's back and the wall. Second, these exercises require more control because the subject is leaning on a mobile object rather than a fixed wall. The greater degree of control builds more automatic stability (i.e., the person need not focus so much on the stability muscles to keep stable).

While your client stands with his back toward the wall, his feet about 2.5 ft (0.75 m) from the wall, place the gym ball between the wall and the lumbar region of his back. Instruct him to lower his body to the sitting position while rolling the ball down the wall. Once he achieves 90° hip and knee flexion (a), he should hold the position for 5 to 10 s and then roll back up to the starting position. He can then progress to the single-leg wall sit (b), straightening on leg at the knee.

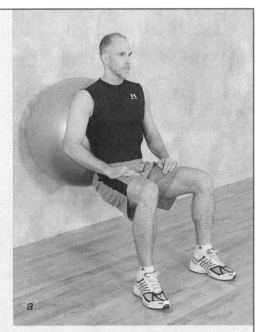

a

Teaching Points

▶ Ensure that your client maintains optimal lower-limb alignment throughout this exercise.

▶ The knee should be over the foot (avoid a knock-kneed position), and the weight should be toward the center or outside of the foot (avoid a flat foot position).

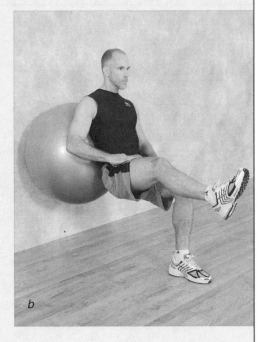

b

Free Squat

Goal: Teach whole-body control during vertical movement.

Place the gym ball on a collar to prevent it from rolling. Have your client stand in front of the ball, feet astride. She should slowly squat, keeping her back aligned, until she sits on the ball, and then slowly stand up again.

Teaching Points

▶ This exercise is excellent for promoting optimal alignment in the squat.

▶ Begin using the ball for a hip hinge action.

▶ Once this has been perfected, progress the exercise to the full free squat.

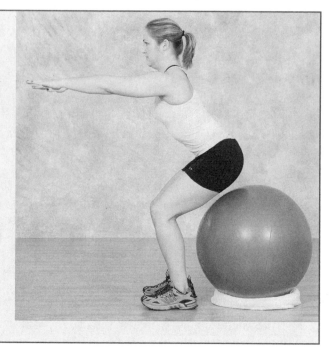

Four-Point Kneeling Arm Lift

Goal: Increase overall stability during shoulder movements.

Decrease the ball pressure for kneeling actions so that the ball will fit comfortably under your client's abdomen in four-point kneeling. Once your client is kneeling over the ball, instruct her to lift first one *(a)* and then both arms to the horizontal. Tell her to lengthen her body through the arms and hold the fully extended position for 5 to 10 s. The next progression is for the client to extend her spine and lift her arms behind herself to the horizontal *(b)*.

Teaching Points

▶ If your client finds the gym ball too unstable, she can perform the same exercise kneeling over a gym bench.

▶ Some clients may not like direct pressure on their abdomen. If this is the case with your client, do not use this exercise.

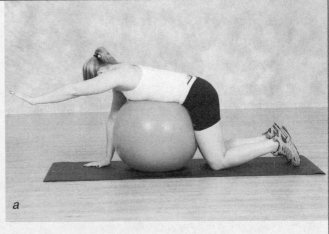

a

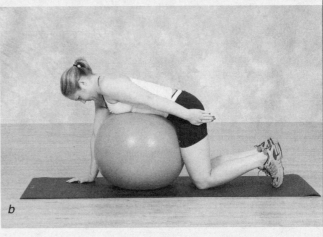

b

Two-Leg Raise

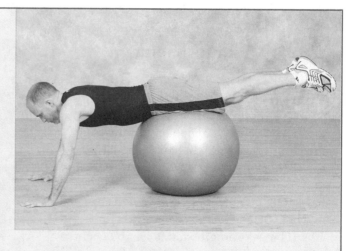

Goal: Increase strength of hip and spine extensors while promoting trunk stability.

Your client begins as with the previous exercise but with the ball lower down the body toward his hips. Have him first lift one leg to the horizontal, maintaining good body alignment throughout the action. He can then progress to lifting both legs. If your client's legs are especially heavy, his arms may lift from the floor during this exercise. To prevent this, he should hold onto a low object such as the legs of a heavy gym bench. He should hold the fully extended position for 5 to 10 s.

Teaching Points

▶ Your client will have to angle his body downward slightly to balance the weight of his legs.

▶ To reduce the work of the hamstrings but increase that of the gluteals, have your client bend his legs and cross his feet or shins lightly.

▶ If your client does bend his legs while lifting them, don't let him hyperextend his back markedly.

Chapter 11
Foam Rollers

Foam rollers enable your client to combine two important aspects of stability training—proprioception and function. As an unstable base, they will help your client work on muscle reaction speed and timing. In addition, as standing and walking exercise and balance can be used, your client is able to practice the same techniques (e.g., lifting) they would use in daily life.

PRINCIPLES

Foam rollers are commonly used within physical therapy for rehabilitation and during exercise classes such as Pilates and Feldenkrais. They are normally 3 ft (1 m) long and either 3 or 6 in. (7.6 or 15.2 cm) in diameter. Rollers may be either full rolls (circles) or half rolls (D-shaped), made of polyurethane or similar materials, which are durable and suitable for weight bearing up to 350 lb (159 kg). Because the rollers are narrow, their contact area with the floor is quite small, making them ideal as an unstable base of support. Because they are firm but forgiving, they are especially useful for exercises that require direct body contact. Foam rollers have the advantage over wooden wobble boards in this feature.

Providing your client does not have any foot skin pathology (e.g., plantar warts, athlete's foot), advise him to use bare feet if possible for these exercises. This will enhance his sensory awareness from the feet and speed the development of proprioception. Wipe the foam roller with a sanitizing wipe after your client has finished. Make sure that the wipe does not react with the foam, however. Each exercise should be performed for 10 repetitions or 5 reps to each side (10 in total) if using single-sided movements. Because these are balance exercises, they may be progressed through timing and complexity. Slowing the exercise down will require your client to balance longer during a movement, which makes the exercise harder. Using a number of movements together (e.g., moving the arms and legs rather than just the arms) increases the complexity of the movement. Closing the eyes removes visual input and means that tactile input must increase to compensate.

SUMMARY

- Foam rollers are commonly used within physical therapy for rehabilitation and during exercise classes such as Pilates and Feldenkrais.

- Foam roller exercises are better practiced barefoot to enhance sensory feedback.

- The firm but forgiving nature of rollers makes them especially useful for exercises that require direct body contact.

See pages 220-224

Standing Squat

Goal: Develop balance in the squatting action.

Have your client stand on a 6 in. (15.2 cm) D roll with her feet shoulder-width apart. Initially she should face a wall and place her flat hands on the wall for balance. Ask her to gently hollow her abdomen and bend her knees to squat down. Stop the action just above 90° flexion at the knee. The client should maintain good spinal alignment throughout the action and avoid flexing the thoracic spine.

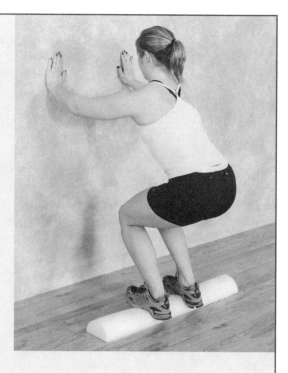

Teaching Points

▶ Initially ask your client to place her hand fully on the wall for support.

▶ As her confidence builds, she may use just her fingertips and eventually no contact at all.

▶ Placing the foam roller round side down increases the surface movement, making the balance harder.

Balance Beam Walk

Goal: Develop balance and stability while walking.

Line up three 3 ft (1 m) D-shaped foam rollers with the flat side on the floor. Ask your client to walk slowly over these, getting her balance after each step. As her balance improves, turn the roller over so that the convex side is on the floor and repeat the movement.

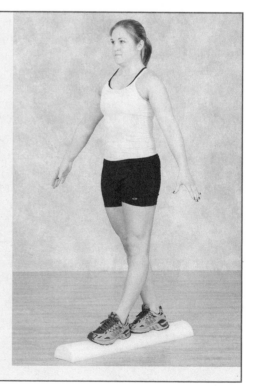

Teaching Points

▶ Make sure that your client stands tall and pulls her abdomen in slightly during this exercise.

▶ The exercise is harder if your client pauses after each step.

▶ If your client finds this action very difficult, have her walk along a line on the floor initially and later progress them to the foam roller.

Supine-Lying Leg Lift

Goal: Develop back stability in an unstable lying position.

Ask your client to lie along the length of the flat surface of a D-shaped foam roller, with the roller along the length of her spine. She should bend her legs into crook-lying position and place her hands on the floor to her sides at 45° to her body. From this position she lifts one leg from the hip, keeping it bent in a crook position until the shin is horizontal. She should pause briefly in this position and then lower the leg before repeating with the other leg.

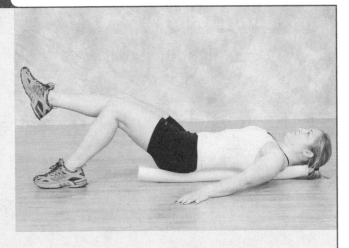

Teaching Points

▶ Lifting the arms off the floor makes the exercise more difficult in terms of balance.

▶ Make sure that the leg remains bent throughout the exercise to reduce leverage.

Four-Point Kneeling Arm and Leg Lift on Foam Roller

Goal: Develop back stability on an unstable platform.

Before practicing this exercise, your client must be able to perform 10 repetitions of the four-point kneeling arm and leg lift (full birddog) (p. 177) with optimal alignment. Begin with your client kneeling with both hands on a single foam roller and both knees on a single foam roller. Ask him to practice this until he is able to hold his balance for 30 s. Ask your client to raise one leg, hold the position, and then lower. He should repeat this action with each leg five times.

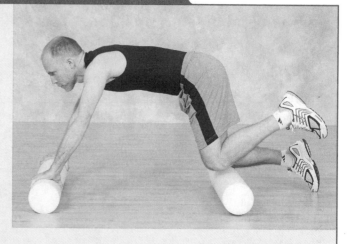

After your client rests, ask him to lift his right leg and left arm toward the horizontal. He should pause in the upper position and then lower the leg and arm under control. Repeat the movement using the left arm and leg.

Teaching Points

▶ This action is simply a repeat of the four-point kneeling arm and leg lift, but this time it uses an unstable platform, which increases the balance demands of the movement.

▶ If your client finds this hard, begin with just the knee on a roller, hands flat on the floor, and use alternate leg lifts. Once he is familiar with the balance of this movement, progress to using both rollers.

Two-Point Kneeling Balance

Goal: Improve body alignment and balance reactions in two-point kneeling.

For this exercise, your client will need a foam roller to kneel on and another placed vertically with its end resting on the floor. Begin with your client kneeling on one foam roller with her toes on the ground. Use the other roller as a strut for balance. Instruct her to perform abdominal hollowing and lengthen her spine to kneel as high as possible. When she can perform this action, get her to take her toes off the ground so that she is balancing only on the roller itself.

Teaching Points

▶ You can progress this exercise in two ways. First, tell your client to release her hand from the vertical roller to see if she can maintain balance with her knees alone.

▶ Second, instruct your client to lean onto one leg and unload the other while still holding the vertical roller. She should hold this position for 3 to 5 s and then reverse the action.

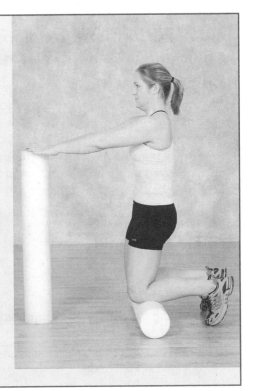

Bridge With Heel Raise on Roller

Goal: Develop spinal extensor and gluteal muscle endurance on an unstable platform.

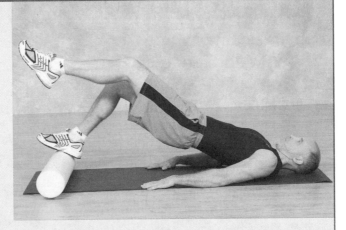

Before teaching your client this exercise, make sure he can perform 10 repetitions of the bridge from crook lying exercise (p. 173) maintaining optimal alignment. Have your client lie on the floor in crook-lying position with his feet on a roller, arms 45° to his sides and flat on the floor. Instruct him to lift into a bridge position keeping both feet in contact with the roll. Once he is in this position, instruct your client to lift one foot off the roller and maintain his optimally aligned position. He should pause with his foot off the roller and then lower his leg back onto the roller and repeat the action with the other leg.

Teaching Points

▶ Heavier clients may find it difficult to keep their pelvis level.

▶ Have a heavy client bring the weight-bearing leg closer to the center body line, shifting it medially by 4 to 6 in. (10-15 cm).

Gym Ball Bridge on Roller

Goal: Perform progression on bridge with heel raise on roller.

Ensure that your client can perform the bridge exercise on a gym ball (p. 209) before beginning this exercise. Have your client lie on a roller with the roller along the length of her spine. Place her heels on a gym ball, arms on the floor at 45° to her body. She should lift into the bridge position until her shoulders, hips, and heels are in line. Have her hold this high position for 3 s and then lower.

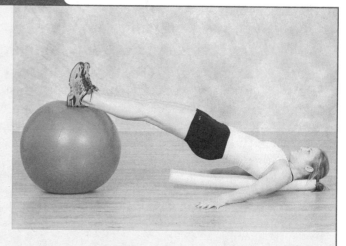

Teaching Points

▶ Lifting the arms from the ground increases the balance requirement and stability intensity of this exercise.

▶ Your client can increase the intensity still further by taking one foot off the gym ball once in the high bridge position.

Prone Tuck on Roller

Goal: Develop whole trunk strength and range of motion.

Have your client lie in a press-up start position with her thighs on a foam roller. Keeping the hands fixed, she draws her legs up beneath herself, flexing at the hips and knees and rounding the spine. Her legs will roll over the foam roller, and she should stop the movement when her shins reach the roller. She should then reverse the action, rolling back again and straightening her body into the press-up position once more.

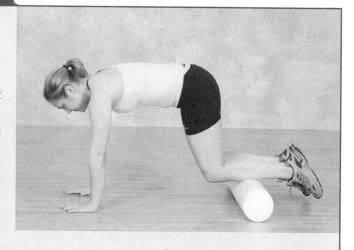

Teaching Points

▶ Instruct your client to begin with small movements, rolling from the thighs to the knees until she is confident.

▶ She can progress to the full movement when she is able to perform 5 repetitions of the limited range action.

Part IV

Building Back Fitness

Much of the back stability program involves working on the abdominal muscles. Especially for your clients who want to take abdominal training further (to enhance performance rather than merely build stability), you must offer training that is both safe and effective. First I discuss currently popular abdominal exercises and assess their effects on the muscles and tissue. Then I present modifications to improve the safety and effectiveness of these exercises.

Chapter 12
Faults With Traditional Abdominal Training

Abdominal training can be dangerous, whether for competitive sport or for general fitness. Sit-up exercises performed at speed, for example have caused spinal cord injury (Dickerman et al. 2005), stroke, and spinal epidural hematoma (Uber-Zak & Venkatesh 2002). These same exercises have been shown to produce low back compression levels close to the maximum recommended by the U.S. National Institute for Occupational Safety and Health (NIOSH) (McGill 2002). Athletes often adhere with almost religious fervor to these traditional but potentially harmful training methods. In the general population, fashion often dictates which movements are in favor—yet many popular exercises lack reliable scientific foundation. Before you can prescribe the most appropriate trunk exercises for your clients, you must understand what the traditional exercises actually achieve. I begin by briefly analyzing the two major categories of abdominal exercises: the sit-up and the leg raise.

SIT-UP

In the sit-up, an individual comes from a supine-lying to a long-sitting position using hip flexion, usually combined with trunk flexion.

In a classic sit-up, the rectus abdominis shows activity as soon as the head lifts (Walters and Partridge 1957), and as a consequence the rib cage is depressed anteriorly. This initial period of flexion emphasizes the supraumbilical portion of the rectus; the infraumbilical portion contracts later, with the internal oblique (Kendall et al. 1993). As the internal oblique contracts, it pulls on the lower ribs, increasing the infrasternal angle by causing the ribs to flare out.

Fixation of the pelvis is provided by the hip flexors, especially the iliacus through its attach-

ment to the pelvic rim. The strong pull of the hip flexors is partially counteracted by the pull of the lateral fibers of the external oblique and the infra-umbilical portion of the rectus abdominis, which tend to tilt the pelvis posteriorly. Action of the external oblique, if powerful enough, compresses the ribs and reduces the infrasternal angle once more (Kendall et al. 1993).

Problems Resulting From Poor Conditioning

Initiation of the sit-up action sometimes leads to bowstringing in poorly toned individuals. For the superficial abdominals (rectus abdominis and external oblique) to pull flat, the deep abdominals (transversus abdominis and internal oblique) must be able to pull on the rectus sheath to hold the abdominal wall down. Many people, however, have lost the ability to coordinate contraction of both the superficial and deep abdominals, which this action requires—the two sets of abdominal muscles are imbalanced, with poorly recruited deep abdominals and dominant superficial abdominals. When this is the case, the abdominal wall appears to bowstring, or dome, and the athlete may lift the trunk with the lumbar spine extended or flat rather than flexed (figure 12.1).

Key point: Weak deep abdominal muscles cannot hold the rectus abdominis down as it contracts, leading to doming of the abdominal wall.

Poorly conditioned subjects also tend to use the hip extensors to momentarily tilt the pelvis posteriorly at the beginning of a sit-up,

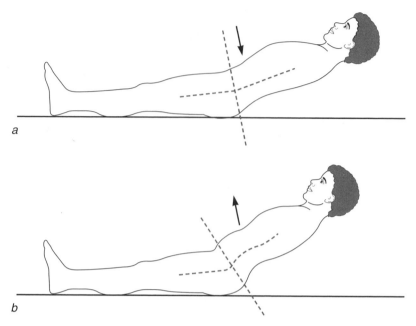

Figure 12.1   Trunk alignment during a sit-up exercise. *(a)* Strong deep abdominals flatten the abdominal wall. *(b)* Weakened deep abdominals allow abdominal wall doming, while lengthened superficial abdominals allow anterior pelvic tilt and hollowing of the back.

Reprinted from *Sports injuries: Diagnosis and management,* 2nd ed., C.M. Norris, page 176. Copyright 1998, with permission from Elsevier.

prestretching the hip flexors. This gives the hip flexors a mechanical advantage before hip flexion occurs and reduces both the work required of the abdominals and the conditioning effect of the exercise on the abdominals.

During this phase, the abdominal muscles work eccentrically (Ricci et al. 1981).

Effects of Foot Fixation

If a person attempts a sit-up from the supine position without allowing trunk flexion, the legs tend to lift up from the supporting surface—this occurs because the legs constitute roughly one third of total body weight, whereas the trunk contributes two thirds.

The upper body's center of gravity moves toward the hip as the abdominal muscles flex the spine, reducing the lever arm of the trunk and enabling the subject to perform the sit-up without lifting the legs (figure 12.2). As the center of gravity moves, there is a critical point at which maximum trunk weight must be lifted (Cordo et al. 2003). If the trunk muscles are able to flex the trunk sufficiently to reduce the lever arm and

pass through this critical point, the sit-up can be completed.

When the abdominal muscles are weak and lengthened, maximum spinal flexion does not occur because the muscles are unable to pull the lumbar spine into full inner range—the lever arm of the trunk remains long, and the legs lift. The point at which this occurs in the movement depends on a subject's weight and height.

If the feet are fixed, however, the hip flexors can pull powerfully without causing the legs to lift. The act of foot fixation itself, in fact, may facilitate the iliopsoas (Janda and Schmid 1980). To pull against the fixation point, one must use active dorsiflexion—which simulates the gait pattern at heel contact, increasing activity in the tibialis anterior, quadriceps, and iliopsoas (a pattern known as flexor synergy during gait) (Atkinson 1986).

Key point: The hip flexor muscles contract powerfully in a traditional sit-up. Fixing the foot causes the hip flexors to work even harder, without significantly increasing the work on the abdominal muscles.

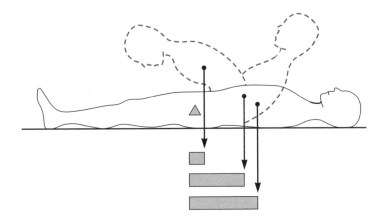

Figure 12.2 As the trunk flexes, the center of gravity of the upper body moves caudally.

Reprinted from *Sports injuries: Diagnosis and management*, 2nd ed., C.M. Norris, page 177. Copyright 1998, with permission from Elsevier.

STRAIGHT-LEG RAISE

The bilateral straight-leg raise (SLR) creates only slight activity in the upper rectus, although the lower rectus contributes a greater proportion of the total abdominal work in this exercise than with the sit-up (Lipetz and Gutin 1970). The rectus works isometrically to fix the pelvis against the strong pull of iliopsoas (IP) (Silvermetz 1990). The IP contracts with maximum force when the lever arm of the leg is greatest (near the horizontal) and reduces as the leg is lifted toward the vertical. Two muscle synergies occur: (a) high levels of rectus abdominis and external oblique activity with low levels of internal oblique activity and (b) low rectus abdominis activity with high external oblique and high internal oblique activity (Shields and Heiss 1997). The former synergy, with lower levels of internal oblique activity, is seen in the poorly conditioned client.

Electromyographic recordings of this exercise (Juker et al. 1998) demonstrate the problem well. If we compare contraction intensity with maximum (100%), IP contraction in the straight-leg raise is 35% but in the trunk curl exercise only 7%. However, contraction of the rectus abdominis (the target muscle) is 62% in the trunk curl and 37% in the SLR. So in the SLR the client believes that he is working intensely, but the work intensity and pain come from contraction of the IP, which is working as hard as the abdominal muscles themselves (figure 12.3)

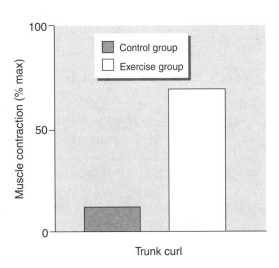

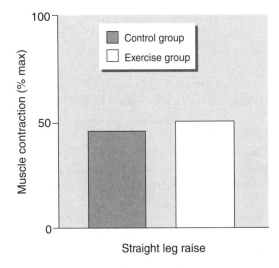

Figure 12.3 Muscle activity during trunk exercise.

Problems Resulting From Poor Conditioning

In subjects with weaker abdominals, the pelvis tilts and the lumbar spine hyperextends during the SLR. This forced hyperextension dramatically increases stress on the facet joints, especially those in the lumbar spine. The movement is likely to be limited by impaction of the inferior articular processes on the laminae of the vertebrae below (see chapter 2) or, in some cases, by contact between the spinous processes (Twomey and Taylor 1987). Rapid action of this kind can damage the facet joint structures. Once the facet and lamina are touching each other, further loading causes axial rotation of the superior vertebra (Yang and King 1984); the superior vertebra then pivots, causing the inferior articular process to move backward, overstretching the joint capsule.

Effects of Arm Fixation

When the legs are lifted in an SLR, the body position is less secure because its base of support is smaller. People tend to rock toward the side of the lifted leg (where one leg is lifted) or to struggle to keep their backs on the floor (where both legs are lifted). Fixing the arms by holding onto an overhead object (e.g., gym bench) or by pressing down with the flats of the hands with the arms by the side improves the security of the starting position.

The disadvantage of fixing the arms, however, is that people can pull harder with their hip flexors without realizing that they have lost their lumbar alignment. This is especially true of the bilateral leg raise action. At the beginning of this action, the leverage from the legs is maximal, because they are horizontal. Without fixing their arms, poorly conditioned subjects may be unable to lift their legs at all—thereby self-limiting potential stress on the lumbar spine. With arms fixed, however, they may be able to lift their legs by rapidly pulling with their arms and jerking their legs up with a rapid contraction of the hip flexors. Once the legs move toward the vertical, their leverage is reduced and the movement can be continued—leading people to believe (wrongly) that because they completed the action, they must have performed it correctly. The jerking action is extremely dangerous, how-

ever, because of the compression and shear forces it imposes on the lumbar spine.

For SLRs, then, permit your clients to fix their arms only when they will perform the exercises in a slow and controlled fashion and only after you have chosen the exercise most appropriate for their specific body condition. Straight-leg actions are inappropriate for poorly conditioned subjects or for those with a history of back pain.

Key point: If your client is poorly conditioned, do not allow her to fix her arms unless her technique is excellent. Fixing the arms can allow a client with poor technique to think that she is performing the exercise well.

POTENTIALLY DANGEROUS EXERCISES

Some exercises are best avoided unless you are sure that your clients' back stability technique is exceptional and that the exercise in question provides them with an action that is specific to their sporting requirements. If you do select a potentially dangerous exercise, always look at the risk and benefit. Ask yourself what is being achieved by using the exercise and whether you could gain the same benefit using a safer, modified movement.

Leg Lowering With Dumbbell

This is a popular exercise seen in more traditional bodybuilding gyms and in training for certain sports such as boxing and the martial arts. It is popular because it gives an intense overload to the abdominals and rapidly makes the muscles burn, convincing clients that they are going to get rapid results. The exercise is performed holding a small dumbbell gripped between the feet. To stabilize the trunk against this weight, the client normally holds onto a piece of gym apparatus and lifts and lowers both legs simultaneously. The most dangerous point of the action is when the straight leg is close to the floor. Here, the combined weight of the legs and dumbbell acting on a long lever arm cause the IP to contract intensely.

To prevent the pelvis from tilting, the abdominal muscles will contract intensely as well, but if you look closely at this exercise you will often see an underlying fault. The intensity of the movement is such that as the client becomes tired, his pelvis tips and his low back hyperextends, leaving the floor or bench surface. This action jams the facet joints against each other, dramatically increasing compression and shear forces acting on the joints. These forces are accompanied by an increase in intradiscal pressure attributable to psoas contraction pulling one vertebra downward against the other.

Leg Lowering From Gym Bench

This exercise is traditionally practiced on a weight-training gym bench with the client holding onto the top of the bench overhead and lifting and lowering the legs from this position. The features of the muscle work are very similar to those described for leg lowering with a dumbbell. However, now there is an additional, more sinister factor. The length of the bench is such that with the arms stretched overhead, as the legs are lowered, the feet go down below the horizontal. The end of the bench acts as a fulcrum for the lumbar spine, forcing the spine into loaded hyperextension and maximally stretching the abdominals. The stress placed on the lumbar spine with this action is immense. Quite apart from the dangers of the movement, the abdominal muscles are placed on stretch, so the aim of the exercise (giving the client a flat stomach) is unlikely to be realized. The high cost of this action and the relatively few benefits make it contraindicated for all but the competitive gymnast or dancer.

Medicine Ball Stomach Drop

This is a traditional exercise used in boxing and martial arts. It involves tensing the abdominals and allowing a training partner to drop a medicine ball onto the abdominal region. In terms of training specificity, there is some justification for this action because in combat sports a blow to the abdomen is common, so training must reflect this. The problem is that the movement is often performed by those wanting to harden their abdominals, often before they have trained the body region with any intensity.

This movement should not be practiced unless your client is actively involved in competitive combat sports—in other words, unless he is likely to receive a blow to the area. Do not allow teenage bodybuilders to use the exercise in the belief that it will give them a six-pack or washboard stomach. This type of muscle development requires a combination of diet and resistance training. If your client is involved in combat sports, the exercise like any other should be built up progressively. The client should perform intense abdominal training after having perfected stability work. He must be able to perform abdominal hollowing quickly, and muscle reaction timing may be reduced simply using palpation. Instruct him to perform abdominal hollowing to high intensities (80-90% of maximum voluntary contraction) in response to your tactile cue of pressing his abdomen. Having performed this well, he can begin the medicine ball drop with a light plastic football and progress to a basketball and light medicine ball. Also, he should perform the action while standing in a fighting stance to be totally specific. In this position, initially use palpation and progress to a light blow using a gloved hand.

Sit-Up With Hands Behind Neck

The sit-up exercise has traditionally been practiced with the hands interlocked behind the head or neck. Fortunately, as a result of intense education and awareness campaigns by sporting bodies, this movement is now less common. However, it is sometimes practiced and can be extremely serious. Dickerman and colleagues (2005) described a 14-year-old male wrestler who presented with acute paresis of the upper extremities and progressive weakness of the lower extremities immediately following an abdominal training regime involving this type of sit-up. Injury (which resolved within 3 months of rest and anti-inflammatory medication) had occurred through extreme hyperflexion. Buckling of the ligamentum flavum was proposed as a pathology. Alteration in spinal cord diameter had caused acute ischemia through repetitive microinjury to the cord.

Athletes generally use this action because they are unable to shorten their abdominal muscles sufficiently to reduce the lever arm of their spine. By placing the arms behind the head, they can pull themselves through the sticking point.

If your client is performing a sit-up action, make sure that her hands are not in contact with her head, so she is unable to create cervical hyperflexion.

Key point: Loaded hyperflexion of the cervical spine must be avoided at all costs. If this movement is allowed, spinal cord injury may occur.

SUMMARY

- Traditional abdominal training has many hidden dangers for your client.
- The sit-up and straight-leg raise form the basis of most traditional movements.
- Several traditional exercises have additional dangers.

Chapter 13
Abdominal Training Using Stability Concepts

Your clients will find it easier to learn modifications of exercises they already know than to learn totally new procedures. Such modifications also may be more acceptable to experienced trainers than if you try to convince them to change their ways completely. In every case, your clients should begin with their abdomens hollowed and the lumbar spine in neutral position. Except where otherwise noted, have your clients perform 8 to 10 reps of each exercise once a day, 3 days per week. The initial movement of each exercise should take about 2 to 3 s; your clients should hold the position for 1 to 3 s and then should perform the reverse movement in 2 to 3 s. Note, however, that these are mere guidelines. If at any time your clients are not working hard enough, increase the overload by slowing down the exercise or increasing the number of repetitions. If your clients are working too hard, reduce the overload.

As your clients become more proficient at a given exercise, they can increase the number of repetitions, perform the movements more slowly, or increase the time for the holding period. Emphasize to your clients that when moving slowly, they must breathe normally (no holding their breath!). The limiting factor is not how many times people can superficially perform an exercise (quantity) but rather how well they can do it while still maintaining proper spinal alignment and abdominal contour (quality).

Key point: Quality rather than quantity is the important feature of abdominal exercise. Instruct your client to stop as soon as movement quality degrades. Do not complete the set!

MODIFICATIONS OF THE SIT-UP

See pages 236-239 Bending the knees and hips to alter the starting position of the sit-up affects both passive and active actions of the hip flexors and the biomechanics of the lumbar spine. Supine lying stretches the iliopsoas, aligning it with the horizontal (figure 13.1). As the muscle contracts in this position, trunk lifting is at a mechanical disadvantage and vertebral compression is at its greatest—the ratio of lifting to compression is approximately 1:10 (Watson 1983). Flexing the knees pulls the iliopsoas more vertically, reducing the ratio of trunk lifting to vertebral compression to 2:5 in crook lying and 1:1 in bench lying.

If flexion has in the past exacerbated a client's back pain (consult with her physical therapist), she can use fewer repetitions (2 or 3) while increasing the exercise timing (8-12 s in each direction). This schedule reduces the number of flexion movements but maintains the overload on the muscle.

With 45° hip flexion, tension in the iliopsoas is 70% to 80% of its maximum; with the hips and knees flexed to 90°, the figure reduces to 40% to 50% (Johnson and Reid 1991). However, the iliopsoas develops passive tension attributable to elastic recoil. Because the iliopsoas is not fully stretched when the hips are flexed, the iliopsoas cannot passively limit the posterior tilt of the pelvis. Instead, to fix the pelvis and provide a stable base for the abdominals to pull on when the hips are flexed, the hip flexors contract earlier in the sit-up action. This contraction has reduced

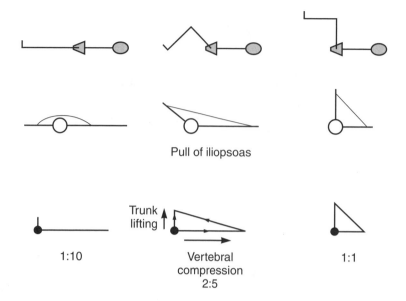

Pull of iliopsoas

1:10

Trunk lifting

Vertebral compression 2:5

1:1

Figure 13.1   Flexing the hip lengthens the moment arm of the iliopsoas, enabling the muscle to complete the sit-up action with less force. Thus, vertebral compression is reduced.

Reprinted from *Sports injuries: Diagnosis and management,* 2nd ed., C.M. Norris, page 177. Copyright 1998, with permission from Elsevier.

intensity, however, because of the length–tension relationship of the muscle.

With the legs straight in the traditional sit-up position, the iliopsoas are stretched and can passively limit posterior tilting of the pelvis. The stretched position also enables the iliopsoas to exert greater force during hip flexion, which means that if the abdominal muscles are too weak to maintain the position of the pelvis, the stronger hip flexors will hyperextend the lumbar spine and cause the pelvis to tilt forward, thus lengthening the abdominals and hyperextending the lumbar spine. This type of action is therefore unsuitable for postural reeducation if the aim is to shorten lengthened abdominal muscles.

MODIFICATIONS OF THE STRAIGHT-LEG RAISE (SLR)

See pages 240-242

Because none of the abdominal muscles actually cross the hip, these muscles are not prime movers for the SLR. The SLR is nevertheless important for abdominal training because it enhances the pelvic stabilizing function of the infraumbilical portion of the rectus abdominis and lateral external oblique.

Several modifications of the bilateral straight-leg raise can help reduce stress on the lumbar spine.

AB ROLLER EXERCISES

See pages 243-245

The ab roller can help your clients reeducate their muscles for the trunk curl action (spinal flexion), as distinct from the sit-up movement (straight spine moving on a fixed femur). The frame allows only trunk flexion, while the subject's lumbar spine remains in contact with the ground.

TESTING MIDSECTION MUSCLE ENDURANCE

See pages 246-248

We saw in chapter 3 that endurance of the erector spinae muscles is often a deciding factor in the development and continuation of low back pain. In addition, endurance of these muscles is a predictor for susceptibility to low back pain. The classic Biering-Sorensen test (Biering-Sorensen 1984), described next, is a reliable measure of spinal endurance in both symptomatic and asymptom-

Table 13.1   Normative Values for Midsection Muscle Endurance

Test	Men	Women	Ratio (compared with extensors)
Back extensor, s	146	189	1.0
Bent-knee sit-up, repetitions	144	149	0.79
Side bridge, s	94	72	0.47

Data from Liebenson 2007.

atic individuals and so is a vital screening test for your clients. Two further tests are useful for screening athletes especially: the bent-knee sit-up and the side bridge. Normative data for these tests have been established (Liebenson 2007; McGill et al. 1999), quoted in seconds or repetitions (table 13.1), and the ratio of trunk flexor and side flexor muscle endurance is compared with that of the back extensor muscles, with these latter muscles given the ratio of 1:0. Reduced muscle endurance ratios in comparison with those of the back extensors indicate muscle imbalance requiring rehabilitation.

SUMMARY

- Popular abdominal exercises can be only moderately effective, or they can even be dangerous, for some people with low back injuries.

- Poorly conditioned people tend to place emphasis on the wrong muscles to perform straight-leg raises and sit-ups; modified versions of these exercises force people to use the correct muscles.

- Poorly conditioned subjects, or those with a history of back pain, should avoid straight-leg abdominal exercises altogether.

- It is generally more productive for you to introduce your clients to modifications of exercises they already know than to try to teach them totally new movements.

Bent-Knee Sit-Up

Goal: Develop rapid-onset back stability.

Have your client begin with the crook-lying position, knees flexed to 90° and hips flexed to 45°. He should lift his trunk, moving from the hip alone, and either at the same time or slightly later flex his hips. Suggest that he imagine himself as a hinge pivoting on the hip joint. The action must be slow and controlled, without strain. A pure bent-knee sit-up requires keeping the spine straight, moving it around the fixed hip, and reducing the action of the hip flexors. Tell your client that if he feels his back muscles straining instead of his abdominals, he should stop the exercise and perform abdominal hollowing before resuming the exercise.

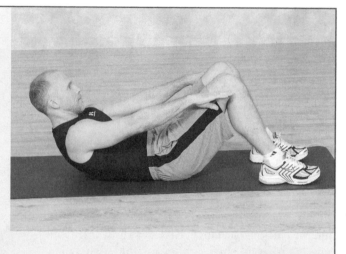

Teaching Points

▶ This exercise has both good and bad points. On the positive side, spinal forces are reduced because of changing leverage. On the negative side, however, the iliopsoas is contracting in a shortened position, so repetition may shorten an already tight muscle.

▶ Following this exercise, encourage your client to stretch his iliopsoas using the Thomas test stretch on p. 118.

Trunk Curl

Goal: Shorten and strengthen the rectus abdominis.

In this exercise there is no hip flexion; the lumbar spine remains in contact with the supporting surface. Have your client assume the crook-lying position, knees flexed to 90° and hips flexed to 45°. Instruct him to roll through his spine, performing cervical flexion until his chin comes toward his chest, followed by thoracic flexion, until only the lumbar spine remains on the supporting surface. He then should reverse these actions, first lowering the thoracic spine from bottom to top and finally releasing the cervical spine so that his head is gently lowered back onto the supporting surface.

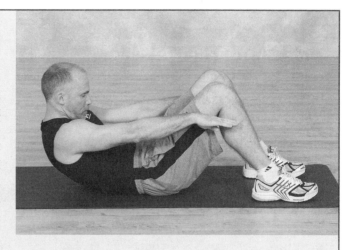

Teaching Points

▶ This exercise is an alternative to the sit-up but will not completely shorten the rectus abdominis because no pelvic tilt is involved. If your client has a lordotic posture and you want to shorten the rectus, use the modified trunk curl (p. 88).

▶ Because this movement is quite slow, clients tend to hold their breath. This must be avoided, because it is likely to raise blood pressure.

Bench Curl

Goal: Strengthen the upper abdominals (supraumbilical portion of rectus abdominis with the lateral fibers of external oblique) while reducing the pull of the hip flexors and lessening the stresses on the lumbar spine.

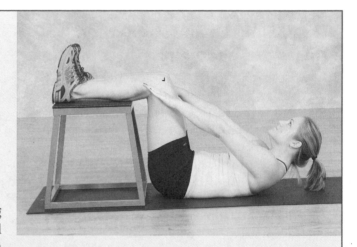

The bench curl is performed from a starting position of 90° flexion at both the hip and the knee, with the calves supported on a bench or chair. Because shortening the hip flexors in this way reduces their ability to contribute to the movement, hip flexor action does not obscure the action of the abdominals. Instruct your client to roll through her spine, just as in the trunk curl.

Teaching Points

▶ This action has a limited range of motion, but discourage your client from performing it with a vigorous pumping action.

▶ The action should be controlled and continuous.

▶ Ensure that your client stretches her iliopsoas periodically (two or three times per week) when using the bench curl action regularly.

Full Heel Slide

Goal: Statically overload the abdominal muscles, increasing the emphasis on the deep abdominals.

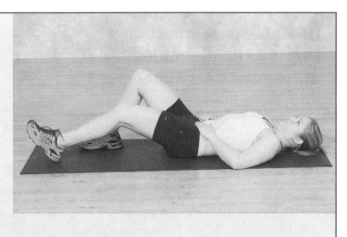

Have your client assume a crook-lying position and then straighten one leg while keeping her heel on the ground and sliding the leg into extension. Instruct her to place her hands over her lower abdomen on either side of the navel, her fingertips 5 to 6 in. (12-15 cm) apart. She should perform abdominal hollowing and keep the abdominal muscles tight beneath her hands as she slowly performs the leg action over a period of about 3 to 5 s (see pp. 133-137).

Teaching Points

▶ This is a classic stability exercise and as such is often frowned on by strength athletes, who see it as too easy.

▶ Done correctly, however, the heel slide is an intense movement.

▶ Emphasize to your client that she must maintain optimum alignment and perform the action slowly.

Bilateral Straight Leg Lowering

Goal: Increase the static overload on the abdominal muscles while maintaining a neutral spine.

Instruct your client to lie supine with his hips flexed to 90° but with the knees extended so that the straightened legs are vertical. Tell him to slowly lower his legs until his pelvis begins to tilt. As soon as this occurs, he should raise his legs again to 90° hip flexion. Each cycle should take about 3 to 5 s. The advantage of this exercise over the standard straight-leg raise is one of changing leverage. With the standard leg-raising action, the subject starts with maximum leverage on the leg, forcing the hip flexors and abdominals to work maximally from the very beginning. With leg lowering, the starting position provides minimum leverage. As the legs are lowered away from the vertical, leverage increases—but the subject is able to control the descent of the legs and avoid the position of maximal leverage that would cause the spine to hyperextend.

Teaching Points

▶ Should your client find the leg-lowering action difficult to control, tell him to bend his knees to reduce leverage on the leg.

▶ Alternatively, have him perform the exercise close to a wall, so he cannot fully lower the legs.

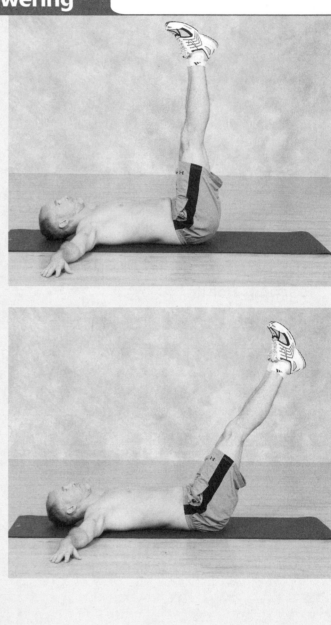

Lying Pelvic Raise

Goal: Strengthen the abdominal muscles, especially the lower (infraumbilical) portion of the rectus abdominis.

Instruct your client to lie supine and flex both hips and knees 90°—a position she will maintain throughout the movement. She should place her arms by her sides, hands flat on the table or floor. Have her lift her buttocks from the ground by flexing her lumbar spine, while keeping her legs relatively inactive.

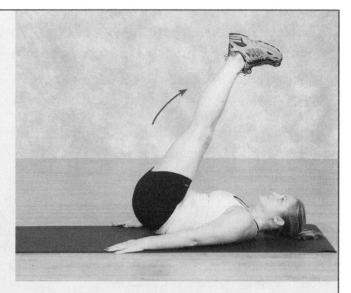

Teaching Points

▶ Although in this movement the lumbar spine is flexed, as with the trunk curl, the movement occurs from below and moves upward, with the L5-S1 joint moving first followed by flexion of each successively higher lumbar segment.

▶ The trunk curl provides the reverse movement (above downward).

Wall Bar–Hanging Leg Raise

Goal: Strengthen the lower rectus, with increasing leg leverage, while providing traction for the lumbar spine.

Performing leg raises while hanging from a wall bar considerably reduces the leverage forces on the lumbar spine and provides traction. Explain to your client that he must hold a neutral pelvic position throughout all versions of this exercise, preventing anterior tilt of the pelvis and (except in the last variation) pressing the small of his back into the wall bars. There are three forms of the exercise:

1. Instruct your client to stand with his back against the wall bar, place his arms overhead, and hold onto a bar above head height. Then, avoiding any jerking action, he should slowly take his weight onto his arms and, keeping his legs straight, raise his feet slightly off the ground *(a)*. Tell him to feel the stretch through the whole of his spine and tighten his abdominal muscles while pressing his lower back into the wall bar and breathing normally. Instruct him to hold this position for 2 to 3 s and then release it slowly.

2. The action then progresses to include hip and knee flexion. For this exercise, instruct your client to bend his knees and raise them until he has achieved 90° hip flexion (i.e., knees level with hips), while still keeping the lumbar spine in contact with the wall bars. Be sure that he doesn't jerk his knees up—the movement should be slow, lasting about 3 to 5 s. Suggest that he focus his attention on his abdominal muscles, pulling them in as he moves his legs. After holding the 90° flexed position for 2 to 3 s, he should slowly lower his legs to the starting position.

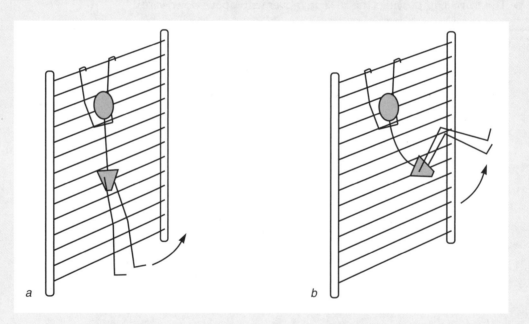

a   b

(continued)

3. The final progression of this exercise requires flexing the lumbar spine to lift the back away from the support of the wall bars. This action, while working the abdominals hard, also strengthens and possibly shortens the hip flexors. Once your client has reached the 90° flexed position as in the previous exercise, instruct him to round his spine to slowly lift his tailbone away from the wall bar *(b)*. Emphasize that in the reverse movement, your client must not allow his body to fall and strike his tailbone hard onto the wall bar.

Teaching Points

▶ This is a very old exercise traditionally used in bodybuilding and physical education after World War II. As such, it is sometimes performed too quickly and with little control.

▶ The key to this movement is control. At no time should your client feel that he has lost control and that his legs are swinging and stressing the spine.

Basic Crunch

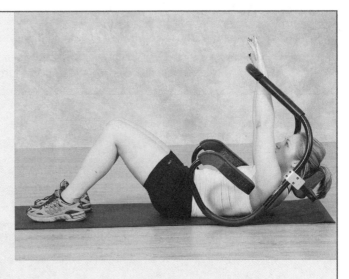

Goal: Work the abdominal muscles in general, with increased emphasis on inner-range activity of the upper abdominals.

Instruct your client to lie on her back with her knees bent and feet flat on the floor (crook lying), her head and neck on the neck rest of the machine. She should either grasp the centers of the curled handles at the sides of the device's arms or hold her arms straight with her wrists against the horizontal piece that connects the handles—whichever is more comfortable for her. Tell her to curl her trunk (basic crunch), keeping her head on the pad and gently assisting the movement by extending the shoulder. Her focus should be on pulling the abdominal wall in (hollowing). There is a tendency with this exercise for people to rapidly pump the movement—an error that adds considerable momentum to the spine and may forcibly overstretch the posterior tissues.

Teaching Points

▶ Make sure that the exercise is slow and controlled, with each movement lasting 2 to 3 s.

▶ With time, your client will gain sufficient control to rest her elbows on the machine pads and press down with her elbows (shoulder extension), gripping only lightly with her open hand on the machine frame.

Reverse Crunch

Goal: Provide intense strengthening for the lower rectus abdominis.

This action emphasizes the lower portion of rectus abdominis. Instruct your client to raise her legs (one at a time) into a vertical position and maintain this position throughout the exercise. The exercise action is to vertically lift the leg as though trying to reach the toes to the ceiling, while keeping the upper body still. In so doing, she will lift her sacrum from the floor, a movement that combines posterior pelvic tilt with lower lumbar flexion.

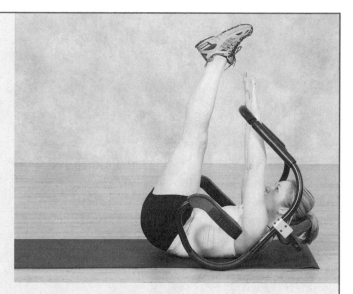

Teaching Points

▶ The movement must be slow and controlled with no lunging or bouncing.

▶ Ensure that as your client becomes tired she does not allow her legs to sag toward a horizontal position because this will increase stress on the lumbar spine.

Double Crunch

Goal: Strengthen the upper and lower rectus abdominis.

The double crunch movement combines the actions of the trunk curl and the leg raise, working both the upper and lower portions of the rectus abdominis. Because two body areas work together for this exercise, it requires a greater degree of coordination than the other crunches. The starting position is the same as that of the basic crunch. Instruct your client to simultaneously raise her knees toward her chest, posteriorly tilting the pelvis, and raise her upper body (as in the basic crunch) to flex the spine. The lumbar spine remains on the floor, while the shoulders and sacrum both lift off the floor. She should perform the action slowly and precisely, avoiding the excess momentum on the spine that rapid pumping actions cause.

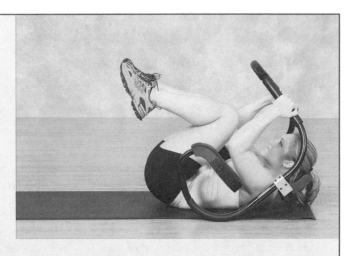

Teaching Points

▶ Make sure that your client neither holds her breath nor hyperventilates (breathes too rapidly).

▶ If she does hyperventilate, she should rest on her side and not attempt to stand up until the light-headedness has passed.

Side Crunch

Goal: Strengthen the oblique abdominals while also working the rectus abdominis.

Have your client begin in the basic crunch position and then lower her knees to one side; she should raise her arms up straight and cross them, her wrists resting on the horizontal bar as in one version of the basic crunch. Instruct her to perform, from this altered starting position, the same actions as in the basic crunch—to curl her trunk, keeping her head on the pad.

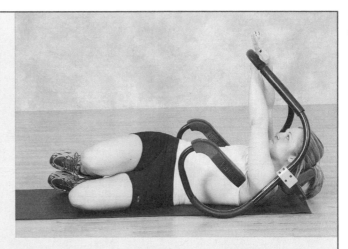

Teaching Points

▶ Because asymmetry is common in this body region, your client may find that one side is stronger or more flexible than the other.

▶ As she continues with this exercise (assuming she uses correct form), the asymmetry should resolve and both sides should perform equally.

Back Extensor Endurance Test (Biering-Sorensen Test)

Goal: Assess spinal extensor muscle endurance.

The subject lies prone over the end of a treatment couch or gym bench, with her anterior superior iliac spine supported on the bench edge. Her ankles are fixed by the therapist or using a fixation belt, and the client keeps her hands by her sides. The client maintains the horizontal position for as long as possible, beginning timing when the horizontal unsupported position is achieved and ending when she drops below the horizontal plane. The duration of holding is measured in seconds, up to a maximum of 240 s.

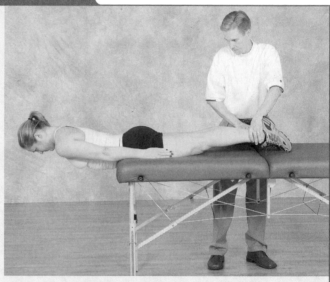

Teaching Points

▶ The test is stopped if the client reports low back pain rather than intense muscle work.

▶ The test is stopped if the client reports leg muscle cramping.

Bent-Knee Sit-Up Endurance Test

Goal: Assess trunk flexor muscle endurance.

The client sits on a mat in crook-lying position with his knees flexed to 90°. He sits up and places his hand (thenar portion) over the patella and then curls back to the supine lying position, taking 2 to 3 s to do so. Have him sit back up using trunk muscle power only and repeat the movement. Count the number of repetitions achieved to a maximum of 50.

Teaching Points

▶ The movement should be controlled, requiring a minimum of 2 s to repeat each action.

▶ Emphasize to your client that because the total number of repetitions is counted, a rapid ballistic action gives him no advantage.

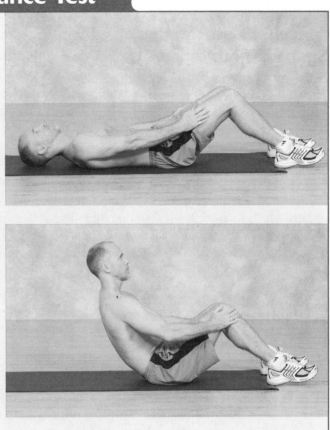

Side Bridge Endurance Test

Goal: Assess side flexor muscle endurance.

Your client lies on a mat on her side with her feet slightly apart (9-12 in., or 23-30 cm), the top leg forward. Her hip is on the mat, and she takes her upper body weight on her forearm with her elbow bent and hand facing forward. She lifts her pelvis to establish a straight line through her feet, hips, and shoulders and holds this aligned position. Test the time (in seconds) that she is able to hold the aligned position. Test each side and compare values. Muscle imbalance is indicated with a side to side difference (ratio) greater than 0.05 (McGill 2002).

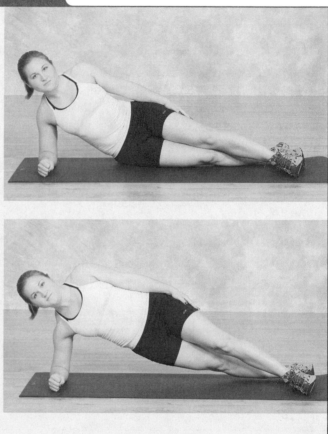

Teaching Points

▶ The client fails the test if she is unable to maintain the aligned position (i.e., she side flexes).

▶ The client fails the test if she cannot raise her hip to the aligned position at all.

Chapter 14
Resistance Training for Core Strength

If your client's goal is merely to develop adequate back stability, special equipment is unnecessary. People with sport and occupational injuries, however, require limb strength in addition to back stability to complete their rehabilitation—especially if they are to resume on-the-job lifting tasks or sports activities in which the body works against resistance.

Weight training has several important advantages for those with low back problems. First, it can increase the limb strength needed for lifting, pushing, and pulling actions. Second, it can further enhance trunk muscle strength and stability to the level often required in sports—especially contact sports where abdominal strength can have a protective function for the internal organs. Third, weight training may help to guard against further back injury.

When we use weight training for back stability, we are strengthening muscles on an already stable base—weight training is appropriate only for individuals who have already reeducated and built up endurance within the stabilizing muscles. Weight training takes the process further, adding greater resistance both to strengthen muscle and to challenge the stability system itself. The target muscles are those of the trunk, the limb muscles attaching to the trunk, and the limb muscles that provide the power for lifting.

Key point: Weight training for back fitness should only be used for clients who have already developed good back stability using exercises described earlier in this book.

WEIGHT TRAINING

As you move your client on to weight training, it is appropriate to add a word of caution. Injuries in weight training and weightlifting (free weights) range in severity from simple muscle strains to death (Risser 1991). Examples of injuries include discal prolapse and spondylolisthesis to the low back, fractures to the lower limb, meniscal injuries to the knee, impingement pain to the upper limb, and dislocation of the shoulder.

Looking at 354 adolescent athletes using weight training, Risser and colleagues (1990) tabulated injuries that resulted in 7 or more days of missed participation. These investigators demonstrated a 7.6% general incidence of injury, with the most common injury type being strain (74.1%) and the most common site the low back (59.3%). The most common cause was loss of form when lifting heavy weights, and fewer injuries occurred in carefully supervised programs.

Key point: Weight training injuries normally occur with loss of form (technique and alignment) when using heavy weights. Fewer injuries occur with carefully supervised programs.

Emphasize to your clients that the weight training you are providing is part of a back stability program, and therefore the activities will be somewhat different from those they may see other people doing in the weight rooms. Tell your clients that they must follow your instructions, resisting the temptation to emulate the practices of other exercisers.

Before You Start

Before introducing any of these weight-training exercises, give your clients the following instructions: (1) They must keep the whole spine correctly aligned and the lumbar spine in neutral position. (2) They should perform abdominal hollowing to gently tighten the stabilizing muscles to provide a stable base on which the limbs can move, when the spine is loaded. (3) They should exhale when lifting a weight, rather than holding their breath, and should take care that deep breathing does not lead to hyperventilation and associated dizziness.

Weight training involves three types of muscle work. The weight is lifted through concentric muscle action, held steady by isometric action, and lowered under control by eccentric action. Your clients should use all three phases. Remind them that the common practice of lifting the weight rapidly and then dropping it minimizes eccentric and isometric action, both of which are vital to stability work. A ratio of lifting for a count of 3, holding for a count of 2, and lowering for a count of 4 will emphasize each type of muscle work.

Your clients should feel comfortably challenged during these exercises rather than excessively strained. Their breathing rates will increase, but they should be able to talk normally at all times; if they are fighting for breath, the exercise intensity is too great for rehabilitation and you should stop the exercise. Individuals may sweat lightly and experience mild reddening or darkening of the skin; but excessive red coloration and bulging of veins in the face and neck are indications that the exercise intensity is too great and the exercise should be stopped. See that a therapist or trainer supervises your clients during the initial stages of weight training, until both parties are confident that the exercise techniques are correct.

Safety Check

All exercise equipment has risks that must be minimized (see Safety Checklist for Weight Training). The risks fall broadly into two categories: those associated with moving machinery and those associated with the lifting action itself. Here are the rules you should present to your clients and the explanations you should provide for why the rules are important:

• Control the weights. Moving weights carry considerable momentum. Unless the weights are kept under control throughout the full range of motion, there is considerable risk to joints and body tissues. When a limb reaches the end of its motion range, the ligaments and muscles surrounding it become tight and limit further movement. Movements that are too rapid lead to loss of control—the joint stops moving at the end of the motion range, but the inertia of the weight forces the joint further against the tightening support tissues, causing severe trauma or overuse injury. With a traumatic injury, tissues are suddenly torn and function is lost—the athlete sometimes feels the body part tear or give. Bleeding and swelling result. Overuse injuries are more insidious. The tissues undergo microtrauma as they are continually pulled further than their normal range allows. The resulting low-grade inflammation in some

Safety Checklist for Weight Training

❑ Always warm up before training.
❑ Check machinery before use.
❑ Set up machinery to suit your height and weight.
❑ Tie back long hair and be careful with loose clothing.
❑ Remove jewelry.
❑ Wear serviceable footwear—no flip-flops!
❑ Use correct exercise techniques and keep the weight under control.
❑ Watch your body alignment—keep a neutral, stable spine.
❑ Keep abdomen hollowed during exercises.
❑ Practice good back care—lift correctly.
❑ Train within your own limitations.
❑ Never train through an injury—see a physical therapist.

Adapted, by permission, from C.M. Norris, 1995, *Weight training: Principles and practice* (London: A & C Black).

cases gives rise to formation of scar tissue and in others may actually pull a tendon attachment away from the bone. When this happens the bone membrane (periosteum) may be lifted and the area may calcify, giving a cloudy appearance on X ray. In either case, the message is clear: When using weight-training apparatus, your clients must always move the weights in a controlled fashion.

Key point: When using weight-training equipment, your clients must move the weights in a controlled, slow manner. Tell them, "Make sure you control the weight; don't let it control you!"

- Wear appropriate clothing. Even though most machines have guards, fingers and especially hair and clothing can be trapped in the moving weight stack with severe results. Instruct your clients to tie back long hair when they use machine weights and to keep loose clothing well away from the machines. They should remove watches, large rings, and dangling jewelry. Good sports shoes will help protect their feet—the weight gym is no place for beach shoes or flip-flops! Toes can be stubbed and free weights dropped onto feet. As well as giving your lower limbs better alignment, sports shoes offer the first line of defense against foot injuries.

- Adjust the equipment. Most good weight-training machines allow users to adjust the unit for the shape and size of their bodies. Make sure that the machine is set up before it is used and that the user knows exactly how the machine works before beginning the exercise.

- Know your limits. Remind your clients to train well within their limits. An old adage says, Never sacrifice technique for weight. Lifting a weight that is too heavy can impair both technique and body alignment and increase the risk of injury.

- Listen to your body. Your clients must not train with an injury unless they are following a structured rehabilitation program. The key is to listen to the body, especially pain. Never allow someone to exercise through increasing pain. If a movement hurts and is continued slowly, the pain may diminish—in which case the person is probably suffering from stiffness that is working loose. If pain increases, however, the movement must stop. Some rapid, repeated actions may reduce pain simply because the exercise hurts more than the

injury! Alert your clients to this possibility, and remind them to stop such movements immediately if they even suspect a masking effect.

Key point: Never exercise through increasing pain.

Machine Exercises

See pages 255-264

A major advantage of machine exercises is that they usually allow only single-plane motions and are therefore easy to coordinate (pulleys are an exception—because they allow motion in three planes, they require more complex coordination). Have your clients use pyramid training to begin with. With this training, the first set of repetitions is light and your clients use a greater number of reps, let's say 15. They then rest to recover until their breathing becomes normal and use a heavier weight for fewer reps (12). After another rest period, have them perform 10 reps with a heavy weight. For experienced clients, you could even give a fourth set of reps with a maximum weight to fatigue (failure). Pyramid training of this sort allows your clients to become familiar with the exercise technique using a lighter weight. Once they have rehearsed the movement technique with the first sets, the weight gets heavier.

Key point: With pyramid training, 3 or 4 sets are performed with the weight increasing as the number of reps is reduced.

Inexperienced clients in particular should use slow repetitions to make the movement exact and light resistances to build endurance. Obviously, they should do all exercises using both left and right sides of their bodies—they should simply follow mirror-image instructions for any one-sided exercises described in the next section.

Once your clients have mastered the basic movements for any of these exercises, using fairly light weights, prescribe a progressive program similar to the following, taking your clients' individual needs into account:

- For each machine, determine the weight with which the clients can perform 15 full repetitions and still have enough energy left to do 3 or 4 more before reaching exhaustion. Prescribe 12 to 15 reps per exercise session, three sessions per week, skipping at least 1 day between sessions.

- After 2 weeks, they can increase the weight, again according to how much they can lift using 15 full reps and not quite be at the point of exhaustion.

- Let them follow this program—12 to 15 reps per session, three sessions per week, for at least 10 weeks, never increasing the weights past the point where clients can do 15 reps and still believe that they can do several more.

- Remember, this is not a program of building photogenic bodies—it is a program designed to further increase back stability and help prevent back problems.

You can prescribe higher numbers of repetitions (20-25) to enhance muscle endurance rather than strength. Although 12 to 15 repetitions will increase both muscle strength and muscle endurance somewhat, higher numbers of reps are required for muscle endurance with minimal joint loading. This is relevant for clients whose clinical conditions preclude their handling larger weights. Those with high blood pressure or severe osteoporosis, for example, may require higher numbers of repetitions with very little resistance. This type of workout will help your clients learn the proper movement without overloading the joints.

The weight your clients lift should always feel comfortable and lightly challenging. If a weight feels too heavy, it will lead to poor exercise technique—and body alignment will suffer. If you see this happening, reduce the weight.

Key point: Use higher numbers of reps with lighter weights for endurance and fewer reps with heavier weights for strength.

Free Weight Exercises

In the context of a back stability program, free weights are mainly for people whose bodies have heavy demands for strength and speed—people who perform medium or heavy manual handling on their jobs or who are involved in strenuous sports. However, free weights are also helpful in late-stage

rehabilitation because of the complexity of skills they require (compared with machine weights).

It is best if before beginning this stage, your clients have mastered the machine weight exercises just described, because those exercises help build the strength needed in these more complex free weight movements. Clients must perform the exercises in this section only under strict supervision until they have perfected the actions. Give special consideration to clients younger than 18 or older than 60 years of age, because their skeletons and joint structures are generally more prone to injury that those of other people. Clients of these age groups should exercise only under the supervision of a physical therapist or trainer who is specially trained to teach these groups.

Key point: Individuals must demonstrate good stability, segmental control, and whole-body alignment before beginning late-stage rehabilitation exercises.

Special Concerns Regarding Free Weights

Because free weight exercises combine both speed and weight, they expose the body to high levels of momentum (the product of mass multiplied by velocity). It's easy to stop a fast-moving arm if you are holding a pencil, but if your arm is moving at the same speed and you're holding a 20 lb (9 kg) weight, tissues in your hand can be torn if the movement is not controlled. Your athletic clients—whether they swing objects such as rackets or move their bodies quickly—must learn to control momentum forces. The same is true for clients involved in moving or lifting heavy objects on the job. Table 14.1 lists special concerns specific to the squat exercise.

Before allowing clients to begin free weight exercises, establish the following ground rules:

- Your clients must have good stability and alignment. They must be able to maintain a neutral spinal position against limb resistance, as illustrated by good performance on the heel slide (p. 168). They must be able to maintain good alignment throughout the free weight–training program, keeping their lumbar spines in or near the neutral position at all times—the thoracic spine should be at its optimal position for each

Table 14.1 Common Errors When Performing a Squat

Error	Technique modification
Knees come inward (knock-kneed position).	Foot may be hyperpronating; client should consider more supportive footwear. Have her practice a knee-bend position onto a bench in front of a mirror.
Knees stay behind feet throughout movement.	Check whether dorsiflexion range is limited in the ankle, and use a wooden block beneath the client's heels. Have her practice sitting onto a bench, pressing her knee forward onto your hand.
Back angles are too far forward.	Have the client press her knee forward and keep her spine vertically aligned. She should practice the basic squat motion side-on to a mirror.
Spine flexes in thoracic region.	Ensure that adequate thoracic extension range is available, and have the client practice the sternal lift motion in isolation. Help her strengthen her shoulder retractors and stretch her shoulder protractors (p. 102).
Anterior pelvic tilt is exaggerated and lumbar lordosis increases.	Have the client strengthen her abdominal muscles, and check for tightness in the hip flexors (p. 118). She should practice back flattening (p. 92) against a wall.
Heel lifts.	Ensure that the weight of the bar is taken through the center of the foot, not through the toes. Check for adequate dorsiflexion range in the ankle, and use a wooden block beneath the heel.
Bar dips to one side.	Have the client practice the squat in front of a mirror, and use a horizontal line drawn on the mirror to line up the reflection of the barbell.
Client bounces in the low position.	She should practice squatting onto a bench or stool, lowering gradually into the final position.

client, with shoulders held back comfortably (but not rigidly braced) and the chin held in.

• Participants must have good stability endurance. They should be able to perform 10 repetitions of each of the exercises in chapter 4, holding each rep for 10 s.

• Your clients should have mastered all the machine weight exercises in the previous section of this chapter.

• Participants must warm up and stretch lightly before each weight session. First, they should lightly exercise (treadmill, stationary bike) until they just begin to sweat. Second, they should perform light stretching exercises that take every major joint (hip, knee, shoulder, and spine) through its full range of motion. Third, they should rehearse each exercise by performing the first set at a light weight before adding further resistance.

• Clients must cool down adequately after each weightlifting session. This will flush fresh blood through the worked muscles and limit postexercise soreness.

• At the beginning, a qualified trainer or conditioning specialist should supervise all free weight exercises, until both client and trainer are satisfied that the exercise technique is good.

• Your clients should perform all free weight exercises progressively—using light weights, taking a rest period, progressing to medium weights, taking another rest period, and finally using heavy weights.

• Free weight exercises as part of a stability program are not competitive; they are intended to progressively develop your clients' abilities to perform work against a resistance at speed. Clients should not compete with each other to see who can lift the most weight.

Basic Free Weight Exercises

Have your clients go through all the following exercises in a single session. These exercises are appropriate for most individuals who fulfill the preliminary requirements just described. All the movements should be slow and well controlled. In the next section, I describe more advanced exercises for people who need a great deal of explosive power for the exercises in chapter 15.

The exercises are designed to build adequate strength, not bulk. Because free weight exercises require more balance and coordination than do machine exercises, less weight should be used. Prescribe about 10 to 12 repetitions for each exercise, using a final weight that is comfortable for that number of reps (i.e., if the participant can perform 20 repetitions, the weight is too light; if she can perform only 5 reps, the weight is too heavy). For each exercise, your client should perform 2 or 3 sets of 10 to 12 repetitions: Use a moderate weight (perhaps half the final weight) for the first set, three fourths of the final weight for the second set, and the full weight during the third set. This allows the muscles to gradually become accustomed to handling the weight. Your clients should rest after each set until their breathing rates and heart rates return to normal—never

let them start a fresh set while their hearts are pounding or they are out of breath. Explain to your more impatient clients that this type of training is designed to encourage strength adaptation, not force it. Training should be slow and controlled rather than fast and furious.

Prescribe 2 or 3 sets for each exercise, three sessions per week, skipping at least 1 day between sessions. After 2 weeks, clients may increase the target weight, again according to how much they can lift comfortably. Let them follow this program—2 or 3 sets of 10 to 12 reps, three sessions per week—for at least 16 weeks, never increasing the weights to the point where they feel exhausted.

Exercises described for just one side should be done on both sides; the instructions for the side not described are, of course, the mirror image of the instructions given.

Key point: Allow your client to recover between sets. Never let her begin a new set when she is out of breath or her heart is pounding.

SUMMARY

• Weight training is only used for clients who have good stability.

• Perform a safety check with your client before beginning.

• The weight being lifted should feel comfortable and lightly challenging. If it feels too heavy, exercise technique and body alignment will suffer.

• Free weight exercises combine both speed and weight to subject the body to potentially high levels of momentum.

Lateral Pulldown

Goal: Strengthen the latissimus dorsi (which tensions the thoracolumbar fascia, an essential component of stabilization).

For the lat pulldown, lower the bar either behind the shoulders or to sternal level on the chest. Either position can be used, and both have advantages and disadvantages. Pulling the bar behind the neck will increase your client's shoulder mobility, because that position requires a higher degree of external rotation at the shoulder than pulling the bar to the chest. Because external rotation is often limited, this is a desirable form of mobility training. Remember, however, that the seventh cervical vertebra has a very prominent spinous process (the point of bone pressing out through the skin), and your clients must take care not to strike this point with the bar. To lessen the likelihood of this happening, they should pass the bar behind the head by 2 to 3 in. (5-8 cm) rather than letting it brush the hair. In this way, the bar will miss the cervical spine and come to rest across the shoulders. People unable to adopt this position should pull the bar to the upper chest.

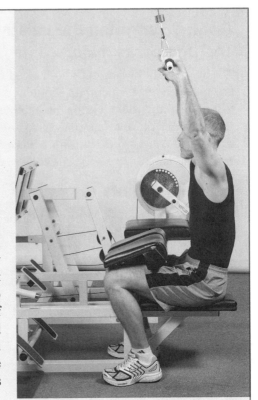

The action is a smooth pull downward, placing the bar (in the first case) behind the neck and across the shoulders. The head should be tilted forward slightly, and the bar must not strike the cervical vertebrae but rest across the middle fibers of the trapezius. The lowering action of the weight pulls the bar up again. Instruct your clients not to permit the weights to rest together at the end of the movement, so that useful traction will be maintained in the latissimus dorsi and the thoracolumbar fascia.

Teaching Points

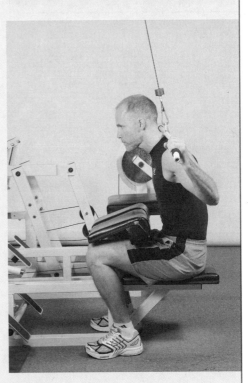

▶ Bringing the bar in front of the body to the top of the sternum reduces the range of external rotation and extension at the shoulder and is especially useful for less flexible individuals and those with a history of shoulder subluxation or dislocation.

▶ Permit your clients to use whatever grip seems most comfortable—wide, narrow, pronated, supinated, or midposition.

▶ A narrow grip either on a standard wide bar or a box frame (with elbows in pronated or midposition) will allow the elbows to pass close to the sides of the body as the bar is pulled down. Keeping the elbows in is traditionally said to thicken the latissimus dorsi rather than broaden it. Using a supinated grip reduces the emphasis on the latissimus dorsi and emphasizes the biceps brachii.

Cable Crossover

Goal: Strengthen the latissimus dorsi and pectoralis major.

The movement begins with both arms abducted. The feet are apart, slightly wider than shoulder width. The action is to exhale and pull both arms into adduction to the sides of the body. An alternate approach is to pull the arms forward across the chest—this technique increases the adduction range and emphasizes the pectoralis major.

Teaching Points

▶ The elbows should be slightly bent throughout the movement to reduce stress on the elbow joint.

▶ The exercise can also be performed unilaterally (single arm), a useful modification where one side of the body is significantly stronger than the other. Work more on the weaker side until symmetry is restored.

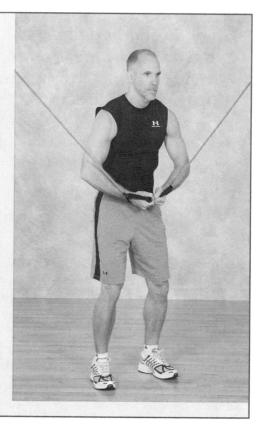

Back Extension (Machine)

Goal: Strengthen the erector spinae (full range).

The back extension machine can help rehabilitate and strengthen the back extensors but can cause problems if faulty technique is used. It requires close supervision. Permit clients to use this machine only after they have mastered the hip hinge (p. 147) and pelvic tilt (p. 99). Have your client adjust the machine so that knees and hips are bent to 70° to 80° and the pivot point of the machine is aligned with the hip joint axis. The movement begins with a posterior tilt of the pelvis, moving the seat contact point from the ischial tuberosities back onto the sacrum. The action is movement of the pelvis on the stationary femur, with the back stabilized and immobile throughout the early part of the movement. Only when the second half of the movement range begins should the spine move into extension.

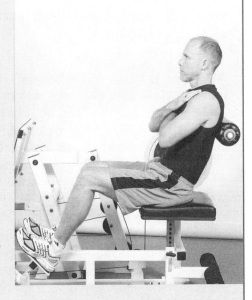

Teaching Points

▶ Flexing the knees and hips further will flatten the lordosis and degrade low back alignment on this exercise.

▶ Ensure that your client lowers her weight under control with this movement. It is common to see users allow the weights to drop and, in so doing, rapidly push their spine into flexion.

Back Extension (Frame)

Goal: Strengthen the erector spinae (limited range).

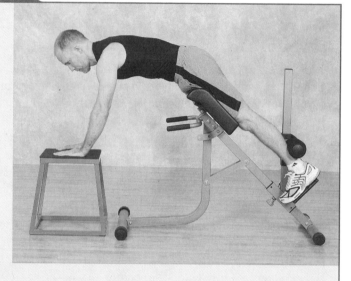

The back hyperextension frame is useful in both the early and advanced stages of training but can be dangerous if used incorrectly. The exercise position is similar to the superman (p. 207). Quality supervision is vital. Be doubly sure that your client maintains the neutral position at all times during this exercise and performs abdominal hollowing. Place a bench or stool in front of the machine, level with your client's shoulders. He should place his hands on the stool in a push-up position, with his legs locked onto the machine pads. He lifts first one hand and then both hands from the stool, placing his arms by his sides. Have him perform this action 10 times, resting his arms on the stool between each movement.

Once your client can perform this action in a controlled manner, add spinal extension. He should begin in the neutral position (with or without stool support), move into extension, lifting the shoulders about 2 to 3 in. (5-8 cm) above the hip only, then back to neutral, and finally down into flexion. Avoid full inner-range extension, to reduce loading on the lumbar facet joints.

Teaching Points

▶ This action can place excessive stress on the spine if a client has poor stability. At the beginning of the movement, if the abdominal muscles are relaxed, the pelvis will anteriorly tilt and the lumbar spine will hyperextend, compressing the lumbar facet joints without sufficient intra-abdominal pressure to reduce the loading.

▶ Back stability and good alignment control are essential for performing this exercise.

Seated Rowing

Goal: Strengthen scapular retractors (middle trapezius, lower trapezius, serratus anterior) and glenohumeral extensors (triceps) bilaterally.

Instruct your client to perform this exercise with his knees bent to relax the hamstrings and allow the pelvis to anteriorly tilt sufficiently for his lumbar spine to remain in neutral position. The action is upper-arm extension, keeping the elbows close to the sides of the body. The scapulae should adduct, and the thoracic spine should extend in the sternal lift action (chapter 7). When lowering his weight, he should not allow it to pull the thoracic spine into flexion.

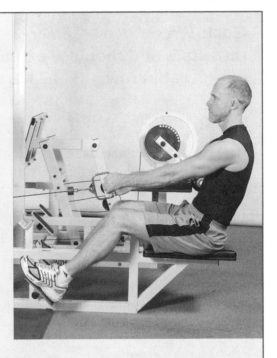

Teaching Points

▶ The action should be to pull the scapulae down and inward. Your client should avoid the tendency to shrug his shoulders as he pulls.

▶ For inner range work alone, he should perform the last part of the movement only, beginning with the upper arm vertical and moving into shoulder extension.

One-Arm Pulley Row

Goal: Strengthen scapular retractors and shoulder extensors (as in seated rowing) unilaterally.

Because this exercise combines back extension and rotation with shoulder extension, it offers a significant challenge to the stabilizing system of the back. Have your client stand in a lunge position to the left of the pulley, with his left foot forward and the D handle of the low pulley gripped in the right hand. He should place his left hand on his left knee for support and angle his body forward (trunk on hip) at 45°. He then pulls the right arm into extension at the shoulder, and, as the pulley hand approaches his chest, he slightly rotates his trunk to the right and extends his thoracic spine *(a)* (sternal lift action, see chapter 7). Using a low pulley position (pulley at midshin level) requires the exerciser to lean over slightly, increasing the workload on the spinal extensors *(b)*. This is suitable only where alignment is good and the client can keep his spine straight throughout the action.

Teaching Points

▶ Placing the pulley at waist height negates the requirement to lean forward, taking the workload off the spinal extensors and reducing leverage on the spine.

▶ Use the waist-high position if your client's alignment is poor.

▶ Combining this action with trunk rotation also works rotatory stability.

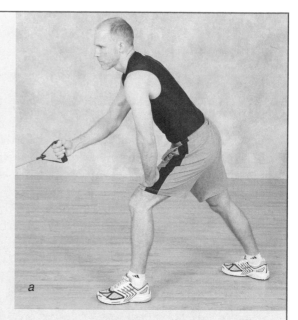

a

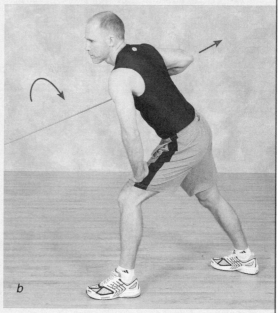

b

Low Pulley Spinal Rotation

Goal: Strengthen oblique abdominals.

One can perform spinal rotation exercises in lying, sitting, or standing positions. For the lying exercise *(a)*, have your client assume a half-crook-lying position perpendicular to the direction of pull, flexing her leg closer to the pulley. Attach the cable of the pulley to the flexed knee with a leather or webbing strap. The action is to rotate the spine so that the bent knee passes over the straight leg and onto the floor.

Your client sits on a stool *(b)*, facing perpendicular to the pulley, with her left side about 18 in. (0.5 m) from the pulley. She should flex her right arm 90° at the elbow, holding it across her body. After adjusting the level of the lower pulley so that it is level with her elbow, she should grip the D handle of the pulley with her right hand. The action is to rotate her trunk to the right, keeping her hips, legs, and arm immobile so the weight of the pulley unit is lifted by the trunk action alone.

The standing exercise is similar to the sitting. She again adjusts the pulley to elbow level and folds the outer arm across her body, her feet apart to maintain a wide base of support.

Teaching Points

▶ Make sure that the force for the movement comes only from trunk rotation and your client does not begin to pull with her arms or legs.

▶ It is common to have asymmetry of the oblique abdominals, with your client able to move more easily or further in one direction than the other. Focus on the weaker or stiffer side until you establish trunk muscle symmetry.

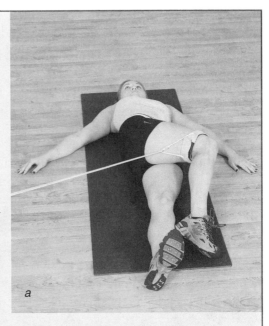

a

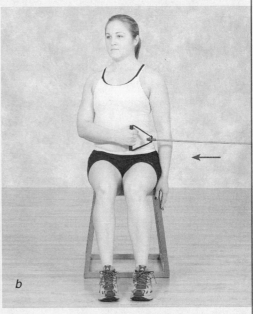

b

Rotary Torso Machine

Goal: Strengthen oblique abdominals while avoiding end-range movements.

Position the rotation lock to allow full rotation range but not to overstretch the spine. If rotation is painful or the range is limited, set the lock of the machine to avoid the painful end-range position. The action is a smooth rotation into full muscular inner range. Have your client hold the position and then slowly release it, avoiding the temptation to drop the weights rapidly and spin the machine. Reset the machine for the opposite rotation, remembering that range and strength are not necessarily symmetrical.

Remember also that the full inner-range position into which an individual's muscles can pull (physiological inner range) is generally less than the full inner range into which she can be taken passively (anatomical inner range).

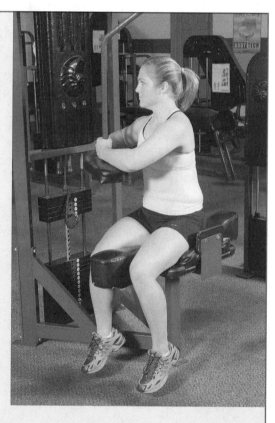

Teaching Points

▶ If the motion is smooth and not too fast in this exercise, your client is in no danger of overly stressing the facet joints of the spine.

▶ If the motion is too rapid, however, the momentum of the machine can take the spine past physiological inner range and into anatomical inner range, loading the facet joints unnecessarily.

Abdominal Machine

Goal: Strengthen the rectus abdominis.

Several abdominal machines are available on the market, but most provide resistance to trunk flexion, emphasizing the supraumbilical portion of the rectus abdominis. Some provide additional resistance for the hip flexors, working the infraumbilical portion of rectus abdominis as well. If possible, align the pivot of the machine with the center or lower portion of the lumbar spine rather than the hips. The rectus abdominis must not bulge outward or bowstring during the action, but abdominal hollowing (practiced in all these exercises) will alleviate this potential problem. Have your client grip the machine arms, holding his elbows in throughout the action. Instruct him to roll into flexion, keeping his back on the backrest and avoiding the tendency to lean forward. The movement begins by pulling the sternum down rather than forward. The eccentric component of the movement is important, so lowering the weight has to be slow and controlled.

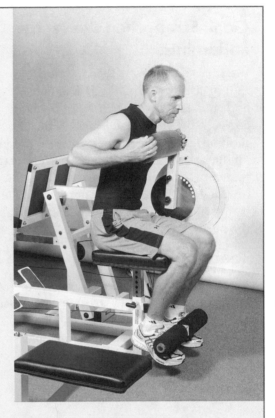

Teaching Points

▶ Ensure that your client practices some form of spinal extension exercise in parallel with this movement to ensure equal development of the spinal flexors (abdominals) and spinal extensors (erector spinae).

▶ Remember that training with weights (resistance) will cause a muscle to hypertrophy and get thicker. This may increase your client's waist measurement if he was particularly lean to begin with.

Trunk Flexion With High Pulley (Pulley Crunch)

Goal: Strengthen the rectus abdominis.

Instruct your client either to kneel (two-point kneeling) or to sit holding the D handle of the machine in both hands behind or in front of the neck (either is correct—the client should choose the most comfortable position). He should shuffle forward until he has taken up the slack in the machine cable. The action is to flex the trunk alone rather than the trunk on the hip (hip hinging), with the movement pointing the head downward toward the knees rather than forward in front of the knees.

Teaching Points

▶ This action must be slow and controlled, and the client must avoid any pumping action, which can leave the movement uncontrolled.

▶ Very little movement is available, so the machine cable must be tight before the action begins, to take up any slack in the cable.

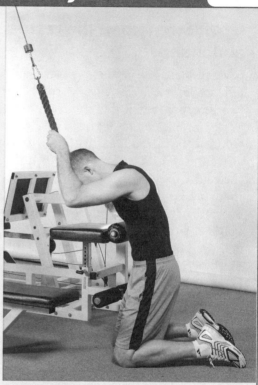

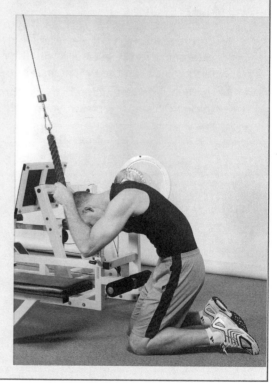

Lying Barbell Row

Goal: Strengthen shoulder retractors and increase thoracic spine extension (correct kyphotic posture).

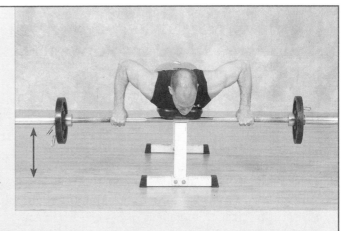

Instruct your client to lie prone on top of a gym bench, with a light barbell (about 22.5-32.5 lb, or 10-15 kg) beneath the bench. He should grip the barbell at arm's length and lift it until it touches the underside of the bench. He may hold his elbows either close to the sides of his chest or with arms abducted to 90°—the narrow position places greater work on the latissimus dorsi, whereas the wider grip emphasizes the posterior deltoids and scapular stabilizers.

Teaching Points

▶ Clients who have poor scapular stability might retract the scapulae too far so that they actually touch.

▶ If you see this type of alignment, have clients perform the exercise first using only a stick and encourage them to broaden their back, fixing their scapulae in optimal alignment and moving more from the shoulder joint.

Dumbbell Row

Goal: Correct asymmetry between the shoulder retractors (middle and lower trapezius, serratus anterior).

You can recognize asymmetry by your client's inability to lift the same amount of weight, or to perform the same number of repetitions, with each arm. Have your client assume the half-kneeling position on a gym bench, his left arm and left knee on the bench and his right leg straight with his right foot on the ground. He should grip a dumbbell (whatever weight feels comfortable to him) with his right hand and then pull (lift) it toward him, brushing the side of his body with his elbow. He should stop the movement when the dumbbell approaches his chest. As he pulls the upper arm into extension, the scapula is adducted; he should hold the inner-range position for 2 to 3 s before lowering the weight.

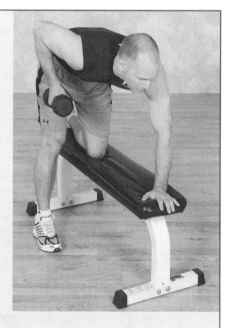

Teaching Points

▶ Avoid excessive trunk rotation with this exercise. Some clients try to lift a heavier weight by rolling the trunk rather than keeping the trunk stable and working from the shoulder.

▶ Resting the dumbbell on the floor between each repetition will enable the client's muscles to relax and blood to flow through them (muscle perfusion). On the other hand, not touching the floor maintains muscle tension and allows lactate build up, which may be beneficial in sports that require muscle endurance, such as rowing.

One-Hand Dumbbell Side Flexion

Goal: Strengthen the quadratus lumborum and external oblique.

Your client begins standing with her feet shoulder-width apart, with a light (5 lb, or 2.3 kg) dumbbell in her right hand. Place your client's left hand behind her head and instruct her to stand upright while she opens her chest and draws her left elbow backward slightly. Instruct her to side bend to the left, pointing her left elbow to the floor and keeping her right arm locked at her elbow. She should pause at the inner range position (maximum left side flexion) and then bend to the right, allowing the dumbbell to pull her trunk into right side flexion while she reaches her right hand toward the floor. She should perform 8 to 10 repetitions and then repeat the exercise holding the dumbbell in the left hand.

Teaching Points

▶ This exercise is sometimes performed holding a dumbbell in each hand, but doing this allows the weight of the lowering dumbbell to cancel out that of the raising dumbbell.

▶ Make sure that your client controls the lowering portion of this exercise and does not allow her body to be pulled into side flexion unexpectedly.

▶ Ensure that your client performs pure side flexion and does not angle her body into combined flexion–side flexion.

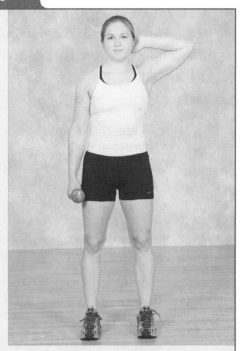

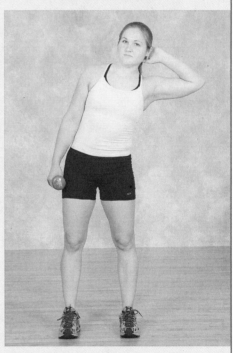

Good Morning

Goal: Work the spinal extensors statically and the hip extensors dynamically.

This is basically a hip hinge action (several variations are in chapter 7) performed with a weight. Instruct your client to stand with his feet just wider than shoulder-width apart. His knees should be unlocked to relax the hamstrings slightly and allow free pelvic tilt. With a light barbell (about 22.5 lb, or 10 kg) across his shoulders, he should tilt his pelvis anteriorly (always maintaining the alignment of the spine to the pelvis) so that his trunk angles forward to 45°. He should pause in this angled position and then return to standing.

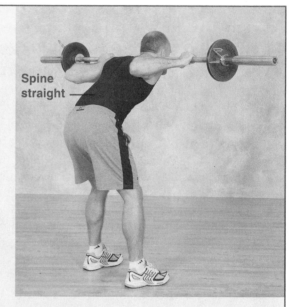

Spine straight

Teaching Points

▶ Be sure your client does not allow his spine to flex, moving the axis of rotation from the hip joint to the middle of the lumbar spine.

▶ Flexion of this type stresses the spine considerably and can increase intradiscal pressure significantly.

Squat

Goal: Teach correct spinal alignment and strengthen the quadriceps, hamstrings, and gluteals.

Have your client practice the correct form and movement using a light wooden pole (e.g., broom handle) until he has perfected the technique. The beginning weight should be 10% to 30% of body weight, depending on body build—stronger clients can use the larger value. Instruct your client always to use a squat rack, so he can take the bar in the standing position. His feet should be shoulder-width apart, toes turned out slightly. He should step under the bar, his hips directly under his shoulders, and, gripping the bar with hands slightly wider than shoulder width, place it across the back of his shoulders (over the posterior deltoids and trapezius). He should perform a sternal lift action and straighten both legs to lift the bar off the rack—then take a small step backward to clear the bar from the rack.

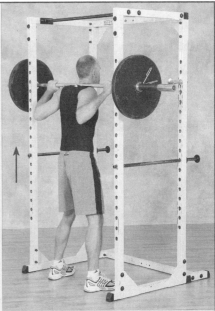

Throughout the movement, your client should look up and keep his spine nearly vertical. The action is to flex hips and knees simultaneously, keeping the weight of the bar over the center of the foot rather than the toes. Instruct him to lower the bar under control until his thighs are parallel to the ground. After a momentary pause in this lower position to assist balance (but no bounce!), he reverses his actions to lift the bar.

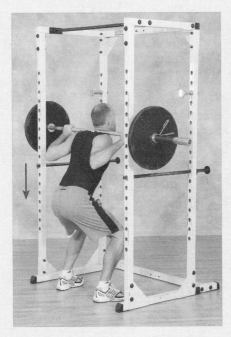

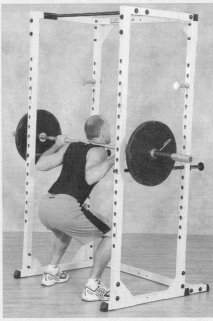

Teaching Points

▶ Be sure that your client's upward movement is controlled (no increase in speed toward the end of the action).

▶ Ensure also that his knees stay over the foot rather than moving apart or together.

▶ Before instructing your client, familiarize yourself with table 14.1, which lists common errors associated with the squat.

▶ Your client should look forward rather than up in the lower position to avoid hyperextending his cervical spine.

Barbell Lunge

Goal: Help improve spinal alignment and leg power but with less spinal compression than in a squat.

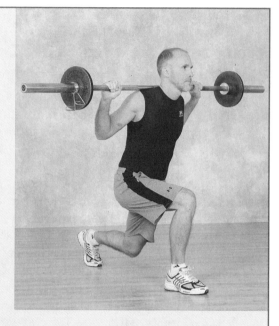

The start position is with the bar across the shoulders as for the squat. Because only one leg leads the movement, less weight (less than half) is used than in a squat—and so less spinal compression is created. Have your client stand with feet shoulder-width apart, the feet marking the end of an imaginary rectangle on the floor in front of him (shoulder-width wide and twice shoulder-width long). As in the squat, he should perform a sternal lift action while maintaining spinal alignment. Instruct him to step directly forward with his right leg (as though placing his foot along the long edge of the rectangle) and then bend his knees so that the knee of the leading leg obscures the foot and the knee of the trailing leg moves toward the ground, stopping when it is 2 to 4 in. (5-10 cm) above the floor. The side of the trailing knee should be 6 to 14 in. (15-35 cm) from the inner edge of the heel of the leading foot. To stand up again, he pushes off the leading leg, bringing the leading foot back to its shoulder-width start position.

Teaching Points

▶ The client must not fall into the lower position or jump into the upright position. Ensure that his rate of movement is uniform throughout the exercise.

▶ Throughout the movement, your client should look up and forward, to avoid rounding his spine.

▶ The bar should remain horizontal and should not tip to one side. If it does so, stop your client, correct the bar angle, and then continue.

Chapter 15
Speed and Power in Core Training

For most recreational athletes, almost any kind of training with rapid movements (such as those in the free weight exercises in chapter 14) will improve speed. For clients who participate in higher levels of sports competition, however, or who simply want greater fitness gains after mastering the exercises provided thus far, proceed to the following plyometric and power-based movements. These exercises can boost both reaction time and response time to high levels.

There is no simple formula to help you and your clients decide whether they should do the exercises in this section in addition to the weight-training work just described or instead of the weight-training exercises. Together, you must weigh your clients' precise needs and goals. The main considerations will probably center around your clients' needs either for quick, strong reactions (e.g., hockey goalies or rodeo athletes) or for simple strength that must be explosive but not necessarily blinding in its speed (e.g., football players or iron workers). If your client has the time and inclination, prescribe both kinds of exercise; if he has neither but still wants to do more advanced work, choose either weight training or plyometrics.

Key point: Speed and power training requires advanced stability. Build up your clients' back fitness before attempting the exercises in this chapter.

THEORY OF POWER THROUGH SPEED TRAINING

To explain the physiology behind the exercises, I need to present a bit of theoretical background. First, a few definitions: Power is the rate at which work is performed (work/time). Kent (1994) defined power, within the context of sports, as the ability to transform physical energy into force at a fast rate. Speed is simply the rate of movement. Reaction time is the time from the presentation of a stimulus to the initiation of a response. In terms of muscle work for stabilization, muscle reaction time is the time between the onset of a passive movement that disrupts stability and the initiation of muscle contraction to restabilize the joint (movement time). Response time combines both reaction time and movement time, the latter dependent on a variety of factors such as energy availability, nerve conduction, and actin–myosin coupling. Good muscle reaction time is vital to improving joint stability. Following ligamentous injury to the ankle, for example, the reaction time of the supporting peroneus muscles is the deciding factor for the return of full function—not just the strength of the muscles (Freeman et al. 1965; Konradsen and Ravn 1990). Following knee injury, the important factor for rehabilitation is the reaction time of the hamstring muscles to resist anterior displacement of the tibia—not the strength of those muscles (Beard et al. 1994). Each of these conditions requires proprioception, and you should revisit chapter 9 to review proprioception before beginning exercises in this section.

Key point: The response time of an exercise is a combination of reaction speed and movement speed.

The stretch–shorten cycle is important for anyone who trains for power and speed. Normally, the muscle supplies force through purely chemical means as actin and myosin filaments bond to cause the muscle to shorten. When an eccentric contraction (controlled lengthening) precedes a concentric action, however, force increases dramatically. This type of contraction is described a concentric–eccentric coupling. Observe how a batter swings his arms back immediately before swinging at a baseball. Or compare a squat jump (jumping from a static squatting position) with a countermovement jump (standing, dropping into a squat position, and then jumping). The height gained with the latter is greater than that from the former. Enoka (1988) measured average heights of 32.4 cm for squat jumps but 36.4 cm for countermovement jumps—more than 12% greater. The increased height comes from two sources: release of stored elastic energy and additional chemical energy through a preload effect.

Elastic energy results from passive stretching of the elastic components of the muscle. The muscle membranes (endomysium, epimysium) are noncontractile, but they are elastic and will recoil when released from a stretch, as will muscle tendons. The combined recoil of membranes and tendons provides a significant amount of energy.

It takes time for actin and myosin coupling to occur. Chemical energy increases in a countermovement, because when the muscle is contracted eccentrically before it is contracted concentrically, the additional time permits more coupling—which leads to release of more chemical energy. Providing extra time to allow chemical reactions to occur creates the preload effect. Think of elastic energy as the muscle's springing back or recoiling like an elastic band—it is passive and physical; preload is like giving the muscle a running start on the chemical processes that lead to earlier contraction—it is active and chemical.

Key point: In a countermovement, the extra energy gained relative to a standard movement comes from the release of stored elastic energy within the muscle and from the preload effect.

Three factors are important to energy release during concentric–eccentric coupling (Enoka 1988):

1. Time. If there is a delay between stretching the muscle and concentric contraction, some of the stored energy is dissipated. During the delay, actin and myosin filaments become detached and reattach farther along the muscle fiber under less stretch.

2. Magnitude. If the stretch magnitude is too great, fewer cross-bridges are able to remain attached, and less elastic energy is available.

3. Velocity. A more rapid stretch (greater velocity) creates more elastic energy.

To create maximum power with concentric–eccentric coupling, an exerciser must be warmed up, and a rapid eccentric movement must be followed immediately by a rapid concentric movement with no rest between the two phases. Any standard exercise can be performed in this way, and the exercises created are known as plyometrics. Yet not all exercises should be included in a plyometric workout because leverage forces and momentum acting on the spine can be dangerous: Beware especially of rapid end-range motion on the spine and long lever movements.

Before You Start

Before progressing to the following plyometric exercises, your clients must demonstrate the following:

- Good basic stability: Clients must be able to perform the heel slide (p. 168) 10 times and in general must be able to adequately perform the exercises in chapter 8.
- Good power and control in the trunk: Clients must be able to perform gym ball exercises, including the superman (p. 207) and bridge (p. 208).
- Good overall general fitness: The client must have participated regularly in moderate to intense exercise for at least the previous 6 weeks. The exercise intensity should have been sufficient to raise the heart rate above 100 beats/min. Each exercise session should have lasted for a minimum of 20 continuous minutes, with three periods of exercise per week.

Plyometric Exercises

 See pages 274-278 A number of exercises are useful. Be certain that your clients are supervised during all of the exercises until both subjects and trainers are satisfied that your clients have learned the proper technique. Have your clients perform each exercise (for both right and left sides if the exercise is asymmetrical)

a maximum of 20 times per session, stopping earlier if they lose alignment or abdominal control. They should aim for one to three sessions per week for at least 8 weeks, gradually increasing the speed of their movements as they are able. After the 8-week period, your clients may stop using plyometrics unless they are competitive athletes who require explosive strength to aid performance—in which case their strength coaches should prescribe the advanced plyometric exercises, tailoring them to the athletes' particular sports or events.

Free Weight Exercises for Explosive Power

 Because of unusually heavy demands at work or in strenuous sport activities, some people require a high degree of explosive strength: that is, movement against a resistance (the weight) performed at speed (rapid resisted movements).

A variety of free weight exercises can help develop explosive power in the late stages of a sport-specific or workplace-specific back stability program. To perform these exercises, your clients must have progressed through the full back stability program and have good segmental control and spinal alignment. They should have mastered the machine exercises and basic free weight exercises in the previous section of this chapter. Have them rehearse all of the power movements using a wooden pole.

Although you should still prescribe 2 or 3 sets of 10 to 12 reps, the first set should be with an empty bar so you are sure that the technique is correct and to train the muscles in the correct movements. Your primary guide for subsequent sets must be spinal alignment rather than the amount of weight the client can comfortably lift. If alignment is degraded, stop the exercise and reduce the weight, even if the client believes that the resulting weight is too light. The aim here is rehabilitation, not competitive weightlifting or body sculpting.

Key point: For advanced free weight exercises, determine the amount of weight not according to how much your client can lift but rather according to how much your client can lift and still maintain correct alignment of the spine.

SUMMARY

- Clients must have good stability before they attempt these exercises.
- After your client has attained basic back stability using exercises presented earlier in this book, he can progress to exercises using machines, plyometrics, and basic free weights.
- Advanced free weight exercises are appropriate for those whose jobs or sport activities are extremely demanding and require explosive strength.
- Plyometric exercises are particularly useful for people who need very fast reaction times along with strength in their movements.
- Because the material in this chapter is specifically designed for people with a history of low back pain, the exercises may differ from those you might prescribe for other clients.

See pages 279-281

Plyometric Side Bend Using a Punching Bag

Goal: Develop power and speed of the trunk side flexors while maintaining back stability.

Instruct your client to stand with his left side toward a punching bag, feet shoulder-width apart, with his left arm abducted to 90°. He should flex his trunk to the left and push (not hit) the bag with his straight left arm. As the bag swings back, he takes its weight with his straight arm and then side flexes to the right to decelerate the swing of the bag (stopping short of full range). The left side flexion begins the motion again. The action is reversed with the subject standing with his right side toward the bag.

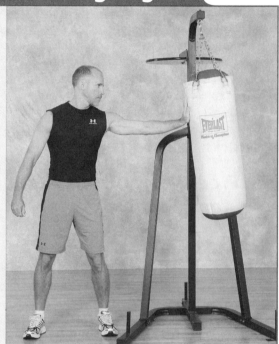

Teaching Points

▶ There are two parts to this exercise. The first is *force acceptance*—that is, the trunk muscles absorb the force of the punching bag as it swings toward your client. The second is *force production,* when your client swings the bag using his own power.

▶ To increase the complexity of the exercise, swing the bag toward your client with varied timing to catch his trunk muscles off guard.

Plyometric Flexion and Extension Using a Punching Bag

Goal: Develop power and speed of the trunk side flexors while maintaining back stability.

Have your client stand facing the punching bag and then push the bag with one or both hands. He should follow the movement through, using trunk flexion only, to 45°. He remains in this flexed position, and as the bag swings back, he takes the bag with his arms straight (but unlocked) and flexes the arms, extending his trunk minimally and transferring his body weight to his back foot to cushion the momentum of the moving bag.

Teaching Points

▶ Ensure that your client does not keep his feet together and lean backward excessively from his spine. This hyperextension force will stress the facet joints of the lumbar spine.

▶ It is possible for your client to complete this exercise using only arm power. Ensure that his arms assist the movement but the power is generated from his trunk.

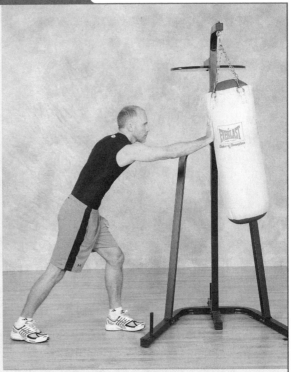

Twist and Throw With Medicine Ball

Goal: Develops power and speed of the trunk rotators while maintaining back stability.

Your client should stand in an aligned posture, with stabilized trunk and minimal abdominal hollowing. A training partner, facing in the same direction as your client, stands about 3 ft (91 cm) to her left, holding a medicine ball. While your client rotates her trunk to the left, her partner throws the medicine ball to her. As your client catches the ball, she should rotate to the right, prestretching the oblique abdominals. She stops the movement short of full range, rotates back to the left, and throws the ball back to her partner.

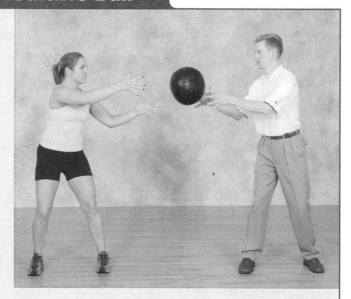

Teaching Points

▶ It is vital to stop the spine motion just short of full range. That way stress in taken by the trunk muscles (force acceptance) rather than the joints (joint compression).

▶ It is common to have asymmetry in this exercise. Work more with the weaker side to restore muscle balance.

Medicine Ball Trunk Curl

Goal: Develop power and speed in the trunk flexors while maintaining back stability.

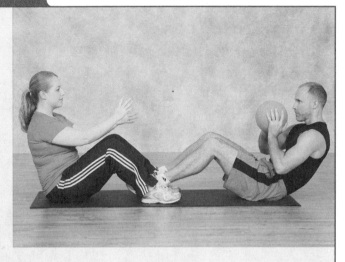

This exercise is a modification of the trunk curl (page 237). Instruct both your client and his training partner to lie on a mat with their knees bent (crook lying), such that their ankles are almost touching. They should then raise their trunks (without significantly moving their legs) to a stable upright position. The training partner throws a medicine ball to your client, who catches it while in the upright position, holding it close to his chest, but then moves back into the lower trunk curl position. He should stop the movement short of full range (his back should not touch the ground) and then bounce back with a concentric trunk curl and throw the ball back to his partner. Increase the range of the curling action by having your client lie over a cushion—this allows the trunk to move into extension before moving into flexion.

Teaching Points

- ▶ Be sure that movement stops short of full range in each direction in order to reduce joint loading.
- ▶ There is no need to use a heavy medicine ball. A lighter ball permits faster movement, and speed training is the aim of this exercise.

Leg-Raise Throw

Goal: Develop power and speed in the lower abdominals.

Make sure your client can easily perform the wall bar–hanging leg raise (p. 242) before attempting this movement. Your client should hang from a gymnasium beam with a ball beneath him. Instruct him to grip the ball between both feet and then flex his hips and spine to throw the ball forward to a waiting partner. The partner places the ball back between your client's feet while his hips are still flexed to 90°. Your client then lowers his legs to stretch the lower abdominals before repeating the movement.

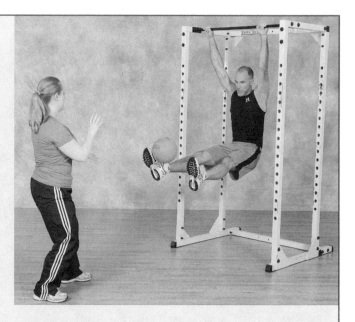

Teaching Points

▶ This exercise emphasizes speed and power, mostly in concentric action. The eccentric component (leg lowering) is performed slowly.

▶ Ensure that your client maintains control throughout the action. Do not allow him to sling his legs rapidly and lose spinal alignment.

Hang Clean

Goal: Begin stage I power training.

Your client assumes the basic position illustrated by *(a)*. Her body should be angled forward (30-45°) at the hips and her spine straight. Knees and hips should be flexed, ankles dorsiflexed. You hand her the barbell, which she holds with her hands pronated, the bar resting on the middle of her thighs. The action is divided into two phases: the upward movement and the catch. During the upward movement, your client holds her trunk erect and lifts the bar explosively in a single jumping action, extending the hips and knees and plantar flexing the ankles, without allowing her feet to come off the ground. Her shoulders should stay directly over the bar, and the path of the bar should be as close to the body as possible. At the point of maximum plantar flexion of the ankle, her shoulders will begin to shrug to continue the upward path of the bar *(b)*.

During the catch phase, which follows the shoulder shrug as a continuous motion, the client maintains the upward movement by flexing her arms. Her elbows drop under the bar, forcing her wrists into extension to allow the bar to rest on her now horizontal palms *(c)*. The elbows point directly forward, and the bar rests over the anterior aspect of the shoulders. As the bar touches her shoulders, your client should slightly flex her knees and hips to absorb shock and prevent a sudden jolt of the bar as she catches it on her shoulders.

Instruct your client to lower the bar all the way to the ground by reversing her earlier actions—she dips beneath the bar by bending her knees slightly and then allows her elbows to drop, with the bar staying close to the body as it is lowered. Her knees should bend so her body is not pulled into spinal flexion as the bar approaches the ground.

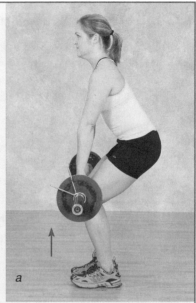

a

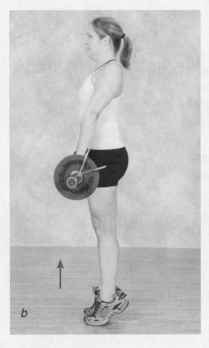

b

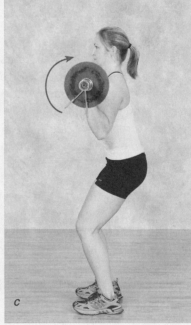

c

Teaching Points

▶ Ensure that your client keeps the weight close to the vertical and does not throw the weight forward.

▶ In the final stage of the movement, as her elbows drop under the bar and her wrist is extended, rapid compression (jarring) forces can be imposed on the wrist. To ease these, suggest that your client wear a padded weight-training glove.

Power Clean

Goal: Begin stage II power training.

The power clean is a progression from the hang clean, with your client now lifting the weight from the floor rather than from the thighs. The barbell rests either on the floor or on two racks about 10 to 20 in. (25-50 cm) high. Instruct your client to stand with her feet shoulder-width apart and knees inside the arms, feet flat and turned out slightly. Your client should wear supportive training shoes for this exercise—preferably weight-lifting boots or high-cut cross-training shoes with broad, stable heels.

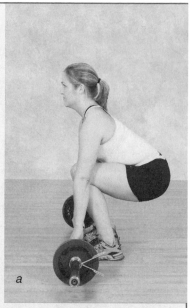

Your client should grasp the bar with her hands slightly wider than shoulder-width apart, arms straight. She should squat down so that her shins are almost in contact with the bar, her knees over the center of her feet, and her shoulders over or slightly in front of the bar *(a)*. A common error with this movement is to get closer to the bar by flexing the spine, using only limited knee and hip flexion. This markedly increases the stress on the spine and must be avoided. The lift consists of three uninterrupted phases. In the first phase, your client extends her knees and moves her hips forward as she raises her shoulders. Her shins should stay back (a common error with novices is to hit their knees with the bar), and she should maintain the alignment of her back. The line of the bar's movement should be vertical, with her heels staying on the ground and the bar passing close to her body *(b)*. Her shoulders should stay back, either over or slightly in front of the bar, and she should position her head to look straight ahead or slightly up. For the second phase, the scoop, she drives her hips forward, keeping her shoulders over the bar and her elbows fully extended. The trunk

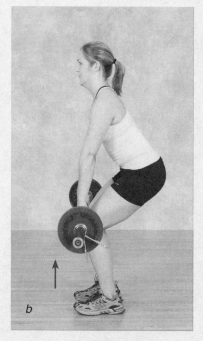

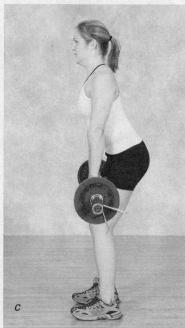

is nearly vertical at this stage *(c)*. This movement brings the bar to the midpoint of the thighs. In the third phase, the exercise continues as if it were the hang clean, through the upward movement and catch phases of that exercise (see illustrations for hang clean, p. 279).

Teaching Points

▶ The action is one of continuous movement, with no significant pauses between sections.

▶ Although the bar maintains its momentum, your client should never lose control of the movement.

▶ She should lower the bar in a vertical path, bending her knees to prevent her spine from being pulled into flexion.

Deadlift

Goal: Improve back and hip strength and add power for lifting.

The exercise begins with the bar on the floor (novices may use low racks at first, until they gain control through the full range of the exercise). Your client should stand with his feet flat on the floor (heels must not lift) and shoulder-width apart, his knees inside the arms, and his elbows pointing out to the sides. He grips the bar with hands pronated and slightly wider than shoulder-width apart. (Some athletes grip the bar with one forearm pronated and the other supinated, that is, knuckles down. If your client finds this grip more comfortable, by all means let him use it—only suggest that he alternate which hand is pronated and which supinated.) Have him position the bar over the balls of his feet, almost touching the shins, with his shoulders over or slightly ahead of the bar and his spine aligned in neutral position (a).

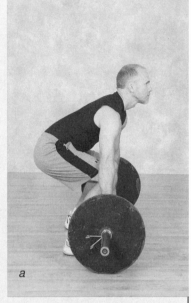

a

The client begins the movement by extending his knees and driving his hips forward. At the same time, your client raises his shoulders so that the alignment of his back remains unchanged. The path of the bar is initially vertical, and it is held close to the body at all times (b). The client's elbows must not bend, because that will cause a loss of power, and his shoulders should stay over or slightly in front of the bar. The head should be placed so that your client looks forward. Feet should remain flat. As the knees approach full extension, the back begins to move on the hip, maintaining spinal alignment (c). Have your client lower the bar with a squat motion, still maintaining the spine erect, keeping the bar close to the shins.

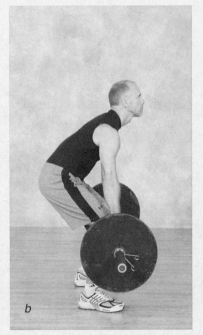

b

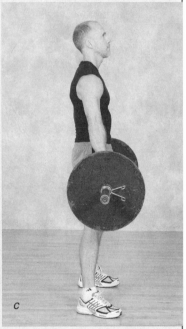

c

Teaching Points

▶ The bar must be positioned over the balls of the feet at the start of the movement. If the bar rolls back to touch your client's ankle, it may strike the knee as it is raised.

▶ Your client must begin with optimal spinal alignment. If the spine is allowed to flex at the onset of the exercise, your client will not be able to correct it later in the movement sequence.

▶ Note the eversed lumbar curve in part b. Encourage your client to avoid this by increasing the anterior tilt of his pelvis.

Chapter 16
Functional Training

Most of the exercises used up to now have aimed to improve an aspect of physical performance. Early on our aim was to optimize posture and correct muscle imbalance. Then we improved core stability and went on to work on strength, power, and speed. Now, we are no longer concerned with physical performance components. Instead we are interested in improving your clients' performance on the functional tasks that their lives or sports demand.

For some clients you may choose this type of training early in the rehabilitation process after you have achieved basic stability, using the exercises given in chapter 7. This will at least allow clients to perform daily activities in a safer way. For others, you may wait and use functional training after building back fitness (chapters 12-15). This is better, because your client's back is in better condition, but the process does take longer. If your client has limited time, you may choose to reduce the number of rehab exercises you give her. However, make sure that you include at least some functional training before discharge. Failing to do so leaves your client trained to use her back only in the gym or treatment room but not in day-to-day living.

The functional training process begins by identifying tasks that are relevant to your client and determining what physical features they contain.

Key point: Use some functional training with all clients before discharge. This will prepare them to use back stability in the real world rather than just at the gym.

MOVEMENT ANALYSIS

Prescribing functional exercise begins by analyzing key movements important to pain-free function of the spine. Such activities typically include bending, pushing, pulling, and lifting, but any action may be used that is related to a clients requirements. Movement analysis begins by establishing which major joints are moved during the action. If we use sitting onto a dining chair as an example, movement takes place at the spine, hips, knees, ankles, and shoulders. From the point of view of lumbar spine rehabilitation, the essential motion is that of the pelvis on the femur and the lumbar spine on the pelvis. Lower-limb motion (knee and ankle) is of less direct importance to the lumbar spine but is important for producing power (rising from the chair) and controlling and accepting downward motion force (sitting into the chair).

The next stage is to establish the motion range, muscles, and contraction type used to create the movement. In the case of the example of sitting

Movement analysis

Feature	
Joints moved	Which are the major joints moved during the movement, and what is the sequence of movements? *(e.g., hip joint, then lumbar spine)*
Movement range	What range of motion is used at each joint? *(e.g., mid-range)*
Muscles used	Which muscles create or control this movement? *(e.g., hip extensors)*
Contraction type	What contraction types are used? *(e.g., isometric or eccentric)*

down in a chair, the hips move within midrange through approximately 90° flexion and at the same time the pelvis anteriorly tilts by approximately 30°. Motion at the lumbar spine may be one of several actions: (a) Reverse the lordosis and move into flexion, (b) maintain its neutral position, or (c) hyperextend at the lumbar spine and flex at the thoracic spine. The muscles that carry out these actions will be the abdominals, spinal extensors, hip and knee extensors, and ankle plantar flexors. Muscle contraction type is eccentric for the lower limb as you lower into the chair. In the lumbar region, muscle action is isometric where the lumbar position is maintained in neutral. If the pelvis anteriorly tilts and you hyperextend the lumbar spine, the abdominal muscles work eccentrically and the spinal extensor muscles concentrically.

MOVEMENT COMPONENTS

Exercise design may be either whole-task or part-task. Whole-task exercises involve the whole of the movement sequence, whereas part-task exercise involves individual components (segments) of the sequence that are practiced alone. When a client is using whole-task exercise, initially the movements will be poorly coordinated and the client will make mistakes. Gradually, these mistakes are corrected and the action becomes refined and eventually perfected. Think of the first time you ever swung a golf club compared with how you can take a shot now! Part-task actions are simpler to use because the client only focuses on single actions; in the golf swing, for example, you may just use the weight shift to begin. The aim is to practice several component movements individually (e.g., A and B and C) and gradually to put them together (AB, then BC, and finally ABC) so that the task gradually becomes more complex. Traditionally, whole-task training is used for simpler, less complex actions, whereas part-task training is seen as more suitable for complex skills.

Key point: Whole-task practice involves the total movement, whereas part-task practice involves individual movement segments.

Both types of training work, and some clients find that one approach suits them better than the other. Each approach has its problems, however. Whole-task training allows clients to make mistakes when they begin, so that they can learn from these mistakes as they refine the movement. However, in some cases mistakes may be dangerous, making whole-task training unsuitable clinically. An example is a heavy lifting task whose action combines complex movements of the lower limb, pelvis, trunk, and shoulders. If the client performs the action incorrectly, for example, bending the spine excessively and keeping the legs straight, this is dangerous for the spine. This type of mistake cannot be allowed, and if the client cannot perform the complex action correctly, the training approach is unsuitable for him.

Performing this action as a part-task practice gives the client time to perfect each separate movement segment before combining these into more and more complex actions. The downside of part-task practice is that it depends on accurate movement analysis to determine each of the component parts. Obviously, if one part of the movement is missed, the eventual complete action will not be functionally correct. A client may practice the squat (p. 269) and hip hinge (p. 147) in the gym as components of a lift, but when he tries to lift a heavy box from the warehouse floor, the transfer of these skills may not be enough. In addition, if some of the movement components are similar to those used in the actual action but not quite the same, a *negative transfer* effect may occur. Here, practice actually interferes with the final execution of the skill. Take, for example, a tennis serve. Let's say that you decide that weakness in the rotator cuff muscles of the shoulder has contributed to shoulder pain in a client. You decide to strengthen these muscles using weight training but are concerned that this is nonfunctional. To alleviate this problem, you analyze the overhead tennis action and use a racket attached to a pulley to functionally strengthen the shoulder. If your client practices this action too often, she will get used to the new weight of her racket. When she attempts to play tennis, her performance may suffer because she is not able to accurately place the ball using fine changes in the power of her shots. A negative transfer effect has occurred. The motor program controlling the overhead tennis action has changed; instead of being ABC, it is now AB¹C, similar but not exactly the same as this original.

Key point: A negative transfer effect occurs when a technique learned through an exercise interferes with the performance of a technique in sport.

Finally, when a client performs each separate component of an action with part-task training, he perfects the individual components themselves but not the way that he puts them together. There are both temporal (timing) and spatial (degree of motion) considerations in movements. If we take a biceps curl action in the gym, as an example, A may be the elbow flexion action, B the forearm supination, and C the shoulder flexion. The whole task ABC is the curl exercise, but clearly there is a difference between a curl in which forearm supination is performed for 5 s and a curl in which forearm supination is performed for 2 s. Similarly, the curl in which supination occurs to 45° is very different from the one in which supination occurs through 90°. In both cases, the change has not been to add or remove a component of the action ABC but rather to change timing and range of motion, the temporal and spatial variables of the movement.

See pages 291-298
Now, let's look as some exercises that aim to restore optimal functional movement by mimicking components of common daily tasks. First we revise the hip hinge action we saw on page 147 as a precursor to lifting and bending activities.

LIFTING TECHNIQUES

Many people go to a great deal of effort to follow a rehabilitation program after a back injury, only to reinjure their back by doing something foolish at home or at work. Take a few minutes to go over the information in this chapter with your clients so that they will maintain the back health you've helped them achieve.

In the large majority of cases, I have met with mild resistance or even boredom, because most people will say (at least to themselves), "Yes, yes, I know all that, use your legs and not your back,

don't bend over. . . ." Yet a significant number of these same people will end up with an injury simply because they haven't internalized proper safety procedures. I suggest that you role-play these ideas with your clients. After leading them through the information in this chapter, take just 5 or 10 min to point to various objects and say, "All right, let's say you have to carry that chair into the next room and set it against the wall. Plan it out for me, explain to me the proper lifting and carrying procedure, and then show me how you would position yourself for the lift." (I don't suggest letting anyone do a heavy or awkward lift, for reasons of liability.)

Key point: Role-play lifting techniques. Have your client demonstrate the techniques in the setting she will commonly use.

Keep the Spine Close to Vertical

Merely reaching over a table subjects the spine to tremendous leverage forces. Picking up a mug of coffee from the opposite side of a table, for example, can produce more force against the intervertebral discs than lifting a 20 lb (9 kg) weight that is next to one's body. Remember, torque equals force multiplied by the length of the lever arm. If the spine remains vertical, leverage is minimal. If the spine is allowed to move toward the horizontal, higher leverage forces increase the tendency for the spine to flex, loading the spinal tissues. A simple analogy illustrates this well: When a flexible fishing rod is held vertically, it remains straight; if you tilt it, it bends under its own weight. To keep the rod straight in a tilted or horizontal position, you must support its weight (a fisherman uses a stand). The same principle applies to the back. If you want to move your back away from the vertical, you should support it by placing your hand on a nearby tabletop or chair, or on your knee if nothing else is available. The additional support greatly reduces the stress on the spine and enables you to maintain correct alignment.

Repeated flexion also adds to spinal stress, greatly increasing discal pressure and continually stretching the posterior spinal tissues. Over time, repeated flexion can lead to tissue breakdown. Microtrauma of this type gives rise to classical postural pain syndromes (McKenzie 1981). Instruct your clients to reduce their total amount of bending in any one day by using more effective movements and by improving general back care. Figure 16.1 shows examples of poor general back care, along with alternatives for reducing stress on the spine.

Correct ✓   **Incorrect** ✗

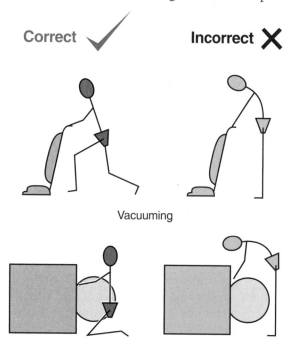

Vacuuming

Removing clothes from the dryer

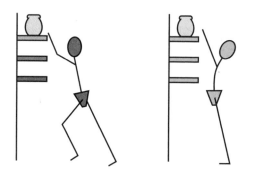

Reaching for object on a high shelf

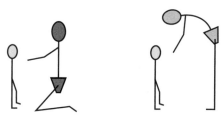

Lifting (or even talking with) a small child

Figure 16.1 **Proper and improper back care in the home.**

Key point: Support the spine whenever it is not vertical, and reduce the total amount of bending.

Principles of Lifting in the Home and on the Job

Both at home and at work, your clients should follow the principles of good back stability in any lifting or other manual tasks. They must plan their actions carefully and minimize the forces of the lift.

Planning

Planning prevents surprises. One of the most common reasons for lifting injuries is failure to assess the entire situation before trying to move an object. Tell your clients they must evaluate three areas:

1. Assess the environment. Note the floor surface. Is it uneven? Is it wet? Are there potential trip hazards? They should plan the entire path over which they will carry the object. Does the path involve going through a doorway? If so, is it accessible and open? Is it wide enough? (It is amazing how often people will carry a couch or desk up to a doorway, only to discover the opening is too small!) Where is the object to be placed? If it is to go on a table, is there room for it or do other items need to be moved first?

2. Assess the object. The distribution of the object's weight can be even more important than the absolute weight. The heaviest part of the object should be held close to the body to reduce the leverage effect, and people must feel comfortable with the weight lifted in relation to their own health status, training, and capability. They should consider the size and shape of the object: A light object that is very bulky or that may shift (e.g., a container of powder or fluid) offers a greater potential for injury. Your clients must also consider any possible danger from the contents—if a container holds acid or a scalding liquid, what would happen in the event of an accident?

3. Assess themselves. Do they feel confident that a lift is within their capability? People with a knee injury, for example, may not be able to bend their knees sufficiently to lift the object in a correct manner. Are there any relevant medical conditions? Pregnant women should severely

restrict their lifting; and individuals with heart disease, low back pain, or hip pathology will have reduced capacities.

Many people injure their backs by trying to lift objects that they suspected were too heavy for them. I often hear something like "I was afraid I couldn't lift it, but it had to be moved and I didn't have time to find help." Machismo is a very common and very dangerous attitude. Emphasize to your clients that it is in no way wimpy to admit they should not lift a given item. Such a decision in fact shows great wisdom and maturity.

If special training is needed before a certain kind of lift, and if a person has not received that training, he certainly must not attempt the left. In general, if people are unsure about any aspect of a lift, they should not attempt it.

Key point: People should not attempt any lift if they have the slightest doubts about their abilities to perform the lift safely.

Minimizing the Stress of a Lift

There are several ways to reduce the physical stress of a lift.

Safe Zone

The center of gravity of the human body typically lies at the S2-S3 level. Pulling an object near to this safe zone reduces the leverage forces acting on the body; allowing the object to move farther away from this point increases the leverage and therefore the stress. If holding an object within the safe zone next to the pelvis represents 100% lifting capacity, this capacity is reduced by 20% when the object is held a forearm's length from the body and by 75% when the object is lifted at arm's length.

Teach your clients to pull objects they are lifting toward the body's center of gravity at the sacrum—to pull them into the safe zone as soon as possible and keep them there as long as possible. When lifting something from the floor, people should pull it in toward the body early in the lift by sliding the object along the floor. Only when the object is pulled close to the safe zone should the lift begin. Although it may not be possible to keep the object within the safe zone during the entire lift, the longer it is held there, the better. If a lift takes a total of 15 s to complete, it will be performed far more safely if the object is within the safe zone for

12 of the 15 s than if it is there for only 5 s. Because the lift takes the same total time in each case, lifting safely will not slow a person down.

Key point: Pull an object into the safe zone (near the sacrum) as soon as possible during a lift and keep it there for as long as possible.

Appropriate Stance and Grip

Instruct your clients to use two hands when lifting a heavy object from the floor. They should stand at the corner of the object, with the feet at 90° to each other (figure 16.2). With this foot position,

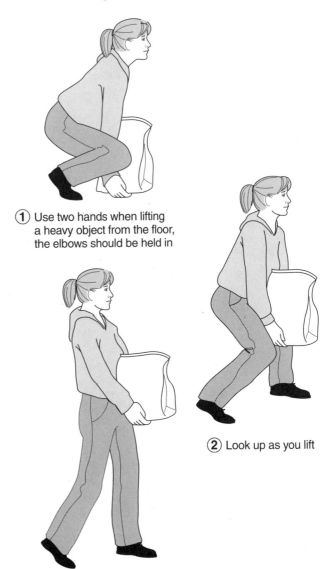

① Use two hands when lifting a heavy object from the floor, the elbows should be held in

② Look up as you lift

③ The back should be aligned and near vertical for the majority of the lift

Figure 16.2   Two-hand lift.

the knees pass to the sides of the object as they are bent. At least one foot must stay flat on the floor, to aid stability.

The client should grip under the object (hook grip), rather than merely at its sides, so her hands don't slip. The elbows should be held in to aid power and the knees should be bent. The back should be aligned and near vertical for the majority of the lift; the back is allowed to flex slightly only when the object is approaching the floor, when the client is setting it down. She should look up as she lifts, to aid the general feeling of back

extension, and her hips should remain below the shoulders at all times.

Key point: Instruct your client to look up when she lifts. This will encourage her spine to straighten.

For certain heavy, large objects such as a sack of grain or a bag of concrete (figure 16.3), suggest a modification of the two-hand lift called a snatch lift. The snatch lift uses speed and momentum to

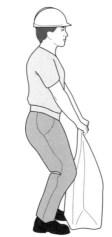

① Bend knees to get close to the sack, gripping it at the top

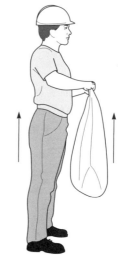

② Rapidly straighten the legs and pull the sack up high

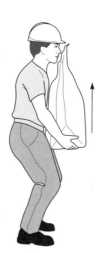

③ Dip down beneath the sack as its momentum continues to carry it upward

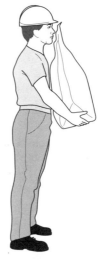

④ Straighten the legs to stand up, holding the sack high against the chest.

Figure 16.3 Snatch lift.

reduce the strength needed for the lift but is only possible for objects that can be grasped at the top. It is highly effective but requires great skill and therefore practice. Because it is performed rapidly, there is little margin for error. The person lifting uses a position similar to that used for the two-hand lift, except the squat is not as deep. Gripping the object at its top, the lifter keeps his back straight and his legs somewhat bent. The action is to rapidly straighten the legs and raise onto the toes (as with the power clean, p. 280) while pulling the object upward. Most of the power for the lift comes from the legs, the arm pull being used mostly to transmit the power and guide the path of the object. The object's momentum carries it upward—and at the height of its movement (when its weight feels minimal), the lifter changes his grip to place his hands under the object and pull it firmly into the safe zone.

One-hand lifts are appropriate for lighter objects (figure 16.4). The client should assume a lunge position, with feet shoulder-width apart and one foot forward of the other. If the right hand is used to lift, the left foot leads the movement and the left hand may be placed on the left knee for support. The back remains in its neutral position and is kept near the vertical throughout the lift. The knee of the forward leg should pass just over the foot, but no farther, so that the tibia of the leading leg is nearly vertical—this way the client will be pressing her hand down on a more stable lower leg. If the leading foot is dorsiflexed too far,

the hand pressing down on the knee will increase the range of dorsiflexion and make it more difficult to raise the body from the ground.

Key point: With a one-hand lift, your client should press her free hand onto her leading leg to provide power.

Pushing and pulling activities can also place considerable stress on the back if they are performed incorrectly. Lifters must maintain back alignment, and the power for the movement must come from the legs rather than from the spine. Instruct your clients to begin a push either facing forward with their hands on the object and their arms straight or facing backward with their backs flat against the object. In either case, they should keep their pelvises in neutral position and produce most of the power for pushing and pulling in the legs—power that is directed through the straight, stable spine to the object being moved. Make sure your clients know to take only small steps during the push and pull—overly large steps will overstretch the body and pull the spine out of alignment.

Key point: In pushing and pulling actions, power should come from the legs, not the spine.

SUMMARY

- Functional movement mimics the stresses and strain present in everyday activities.
- Functional exercise begins with a movement analysis.
- Whole-task and part-task training may be used.
- When lifting, people should keep their spines vertical or as near vertical as possible.
- Repeated spinal flexion during lifting can lead to serious breakdown of tissues.
- When the spine is not vertical, it should be supported by placing a hand either on a stable object or on the bent knee.
- Before lifting any object, people should plan the move: They should assess the environment, the object, and their own capabilities.

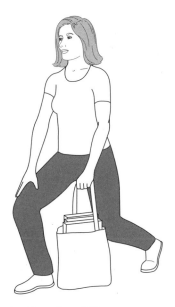

Figure 16.4   One-hand lift.

- If people have any doubt that they can safely lift or carry an object, they should refrain from doing so.

- The safe zone is near the sacrum, because the average person's center of gravity is at approximately the S2-S3 level. Lifted objects should be brought to the safe zone as quickly as possible and remain there as long as possible.

- People should use two hands to lift heavy objects. When lifting lighter objects with only one hand, they should place the free hand on a bent knee to provide support for the spine.

- The snatch lift is useful for lifting heavy objects that can be grasped at the top, but the movement is difficult and should be practiced before it is used.

- When pushing and pulling, power should come from the legs, not the spine.

Hip Hinge With Stick (Revision)

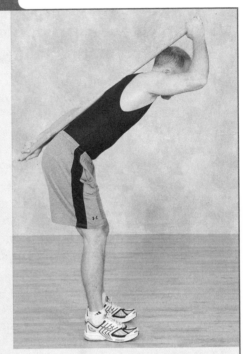

Goal: Reacquaint your client with the hip hinge action.

Have your client perform the hip hinge action as described on page 147 using a stick.

Teaching Points

▶ Ensure that the stick is touching your client's sacrum (tailbone), thoracic spine, and back of the head.

▶ Make sure that he has a good neutral position. His lumbar spine should be no more than 2 in. (5 cm) and no less than 1.2 in. (1.27 cm) from the stick. A greater gap indicates an increased lordosis, a lesser gap a reduced lordosis.

▶ The movement begins with the legs—knees and hips bending to allow the pelvis to tilt freely. Do not allow your client to tip forward first and then to correct the movement by bending his knees later.

▶ The action is complete when the stick or spine is angled at 45° to the vertical.

Variations

Use a towel folded length ways or a strap instead of a stick. This is more comfortable for very lean clients who have particularly prominent spinous processes.

Self-Monitored Hip Hinge

Goal: Increase awareness of pelvic position and motion during forward bending.

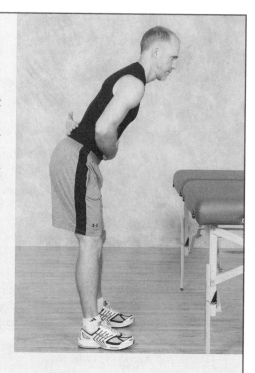

Begin the exercise with your client standing with his feet shoulder-width apart and slightly (10-15°) turned out. Instruct him to keep one hand in front of him, the other behind. Place his front hand flat over his lower abdomen and his back hand flat over his sacrum with his fingers pointing downward to the floor. Have him perform abdominal hollowing so that he feels his abdominal muscles tighten under his front hand. Make sure he bends his knees and tilts his pelvis anteriorly to angle his body forward. Keep his spine straight. As his pelvis tilts, the fingers on his back hand should point backward to an angle of about 45°. An angle measuring less than this means the pelvis has not tilted enough, and an angle measuring more than this means the pelvis has tilted too much. A good cue for hand position is to have your client point his fingers just to the baseboard (or skirting board) of the room.

Teaching Points

▶ Your client's back hand must be held firmly over the sacrum to monitor sacral position and pelvic tilt.

▶ The 45° of pelvic tilt will bring the fingers of his back hand to 45° to point to the skirting board of the room. If his fingers point to the floor (<45°), there is too little pelvic tilt. If his fingers point high up to the wall (>45°), there is too much tilt.

▶ Make sure that your client maintains abdominal hollowing throughout the action. As he focuses his attention on his sacrum, he must not allow his abdomen to protrude.

Monkey Squat

Goal: Teach your client correct movement sequencing during a squat action.

Before beginning this exercise, make sure your client can perform the self-monitored hip hinge (p. 292) for 10 repetitions. Have her begin the monkey squat by standing with her feet slightly wider than shoulder-width apart and turned out 10° to 15°. Her hands should be placed flat on the tops of her thighs. Instruct her to hollow her abdomen, bend her knees, and tilt her pelvis anteriorly to angle her body forward. She should take her weight through her hands onto her thighs. She should keep her spine straight and stop the movement when her hand slides down her thighs to touch her knees. Have her pause in the lower position and then stand up again, allowing her hands to slide back up her thighs to the top.

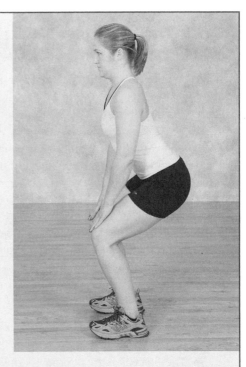

Teaching Points

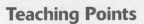 Make sure that your client keeps her knees over the center of her feet throughout the action, avoiding a knock-kneed or bowlegged position.

▶ To assist the movement, have her press onto her thighs through her hands.

▶ To make the movement harder, have her glide her fingertips on her thighs as she descends and ascends.

Deadlift From Bench

Goal: Train the deadlift action within a limited movement range.

Begin the exercise with your client standing in front of a low (8-12 in., or 20-30 cm) bench with his feet slightly wider than shoulder-width apart and turned out 10° to 15°. Have him hold a pole, power bar, or unloaded weight bar using an alternate grip (one hand knuckles up, one knuckles down) against his upper thighs. As he hollows his abdomen, he should bend his knees and tilt his pelvis anteriorly to angle his body forward, lowering the weight bar toward the bench. He should keep his spine straight, stop the movement when the bar touches the bench, pause in this lower position, and then stand up again.

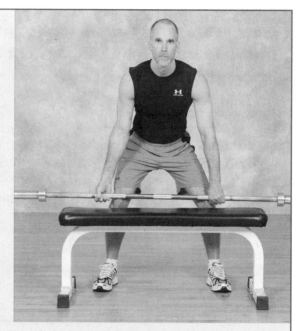

Teaching Points

▶ The client should keep the bar close to his thighs as it is lowered.

▶ The bar will naturally move outward to clear your client's knees. As the movement goes lower, the bar must be brought in close again toward the shins.

▶ Use a higher (12-18 in., or 30-46 cm) bench to begin, and lower the bench as your client improves his technique.

▶ Have your client perform the sternal lift (p. 103) for 5 reps before attempting the deadlift to bench. Before he begins the deadlift movement, he should perform a sternal lift and draw his scapulae downward gently to set his upper-body tension.

Sitting Hip Hinge and Stand-Up

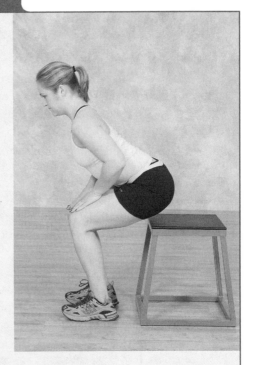

Goal: Progress the sitting pelvic rock action to full stand-up.

Ensure that your client has mastered the pelvic rock on rocker board (p. 198) and sitting hip hinge (p. 201). Instruct her to sit on a stool or firm chair with her feet shoulder-width apart. She should place her hands on her knees and, keeping her spine straight, rock forward, transferring her body weight from her sitting bones (ischial tuberosities) to her pubic bone. As she leans forward, she should press her hands gently against her knees and lift her buttocks from the chair by 2 in. (5 cm). After pausing in this forward position, she slowly lowers her buttocks back onto the chair.

Teaching Points

▶ As your client leans forward, ensure that she presses her feet into the floor at the same time as pressing on her knees.

▶ It is common for clients to sit back down onto the chair too quickly. This can painfully jolt the sitting bones and spine. To prevent this, have her count as she sits down, taking 4 to 5 s to lower back onto the chair.

▶ Tell her to visualize sitting on an egg—sit down too quickly and the egg will crack!

Variations

1. Have your client grip a pole (broom handle) vertically in both hands. As she leans forward, have her press onto the pole for power and balance.

2. Tell her to perform the exercise sitting in front of a wall. As she leans forward, she should place her hands on the wall for support.

Controlled Sit-Down

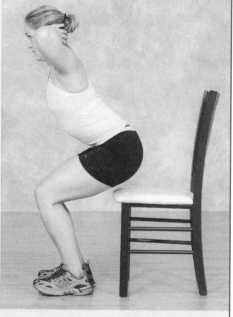

Goal: Teach correct movement sequencing when sitting down.

Begin the exercise with your client standing in front of a gym bench or firm chair with her feet slightly wider than shoulder width apart and turned out 10° to 15°. Have her place her hands behind her head and extend her thoracic spine using the sternal lift (p. 103). Instruct your client to hollow her abdomen, bend her knees, and tilt her pelvis anteriorly to angle her body forward. She should keep her spine straight and lower her buttocks onto the chair. Have her touch the chair briefly (she should not sit down completely) and then stand up again.

Teaching Points

▶ It is common for clients to sit back down onto the chair too quickly, jolting the spine. To prevent this, have them count, taking 4 to 5 s to lower back onto the chair.

▶ A higher chair is easier on the legs and uses less hip flexion. If your client's hips are quite tight, she will find that her pelvis tilts posteriorly and her lumbar spine flexes.

▶ If your client finds the control of this action very difficult, place a pole vertically in front of her as a point of balance.

Variations

Your client can perform the exercise sitting in front of a wall. As she leans forward, she should place her hands on the wall for support and keep her body angled forward.

Forward Lean With Step and Push

Goal: Develop force transference from the legs to spine using wall support.

Instruct your client to stand 2 to 3 ft (60-90 cm) (depending on his height) in front of a wall with his feet shoulder-width apart. Have him step forward with his right leg and at the same time angle his body forward, keeping his spine straight. Get him to touch the wall lightly with both hands for support. At this point, his spine should form a straight line with his trailing leg. Have him step backward again, straightening his body back up. He should repeat the action with his left leg.

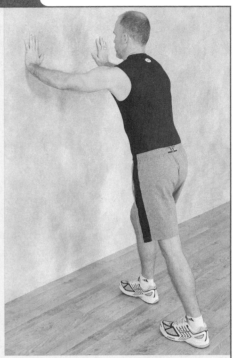

Teaching Points

▶ To give your client tactile feedback, place his body at the correct angle to line it up with his trailing leg.

▶ Provide further feedback by placing a string from the trailing (left) ankle to the ipsilateral (left) hand. The leg and spine angle should follow the string.

▶ To add resistance, substitute elastic tubing for the string. When your client is comfortable with this action, progress to the forward lean with pulley.

Forward Lean With Pulley

Goal: Develop force transference from the legs to spine using resistance.

Ensure that your client has mastered the forward lean with step and push before beginning this exercise. Stand your client in front of a low pulley machine and have him grip the D handle with his right hand. Instruct him to step forward with his right leg and at the same time angle his body forward, keeping his spine straight. As his arm straightens, his spine should form a straight line with his trailing leg. Get him to step backward again straightening his body back up. He should repeat the action with his left leg.

Teaching Points

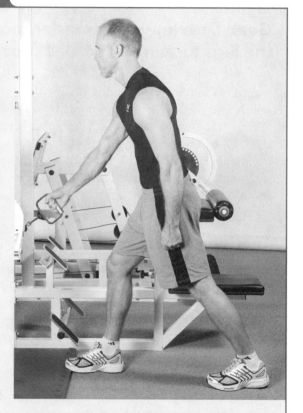

► Have your client perform the exercise with a training partner to monitor his body alignment.

► Asymmetry is common, so ensure that your client uses a resistance that is comfortable for both sides of the body.

► Having the client face away from the pulley increases resistance to the forward lunge action.

Part V

Clinical Application

Although the program described in this book can be used for preventive health care, essentially it is designed to be used with an injured client. To apply the techniques effectively, we must determine individual needs of our clients, and so chapter 17 looks at client assessment and introduces a number of general screening tests as well as the important aspect of diagnostic triage. In chapter 18 we look at the practicalities of program design and begin with a needs analysis to make the program truly client focused. Chapter 19 illustrates some real-world examples by citing case histories from my day-to-day clinical load.

Chapter 17
Preliminary Client Assessment

When a client approaches you, you must first decide whether exercise is appropriate at all. Occasionally (although rarely) you may see someone whose general health is in such a state that the slightest additional stress could be catastrophic. If you have any doubts about a prospective client, require him or her to obtain clearance through a medical doctor before proceeding with therapy. Note also that although a back stability program is generally suitable for even the very unfit, it is contraindicated in some cases where people are not able to practice it correctly. If hypertensive individuals cannot be taught to hollow without holding their breath, for example, then hollowing is clearly contraindicated. Advanced exercises using weights are contraindicated in cases of reduced bone density.

ASSESSING PAIN

If clients are in pain when they first come to you, manage the pain before proceeding with any muscle training. If you are qualified to treat the pain, then apply whatever treatments you deem appropriate. If you are not qualified, refer clients to someone who is and work jointly with that therapist. Pain can inhibit muscle contraction and can affect alignment by making people take up positions that are less painful but reinforce poor alignment. It is certainly true that back stability exercise can lead to significant pain relief (e.g., multifidus training can release back spasms), but such activities work best when used as an adjunct to pain-relieving treatments.

When pain is extreme, elimination of the pain may become the primary aim of treatment. Pain that occurs through muscle spasm or through trigger points in tight muscles may be relieved by treatments that reduce muscle tone—various physical therapy treatments, manual therapy, or

stretching. See Norris (2004b) for details of these types of treatment.

Where pain is the result of persistent overstress on a hypermobile segment, focus initial treatments on segmental control and stability. You may have to create stability passively at first (through taping or splinting), until your client has gained sufficient control of the muscular stabilizing system.

Behavioral Signs

During examination you may get the impression that the pain your client is displaying is not attributable simply to a spinal pathology. The client may be exaggerating her response, for example, or her pain response may be different than you would expect. As discussed in chapter 1, pain is both a sensory and an emotional experience and describes not just simply tissue damage but your client's reactions to this (i.e., her mental state).

 Three tests have been shown to be useful to determine when pain symptoms are exaggerated (Waddell et al. 1980).

Key point: Pain is both a sensory and an emotional experience for your client. Use behavioral tests to determine if the emotional aspect is significant.

ASSESSING DISABILITY

We saw in chapter 1 that the combination of pain with lack of activity over time can lead clients to avoid activities that they believe will cause or exacerbate their pain. These clients rely on coping strategies that limit and restrict their activities of daily living, leading to long-term disability. We

Table 17.1 Clinical Interview for Disability

Activity	Feature	Yes/No
Bending and lifting	Requires assistance with or avoids heavy lifting (>30 lb [13 kg], or 4-year-old child)	
Sitting	Limited to 30 min	
Standing	Limited to 30 min	
Walking	Limited to 30 min or 2 miles	
Road travel	Limited to 30 min	
Social life	Regularly misses or curtails social activities	
Sleep	Regularly (two or three times per night) disturbed by pain	
Sex life	Reduced frequency because of pain	
Dressing	Help required with socks, tights, and shoes	

Based on M.H. Simmonds and E. Lee, 2007, Physical performance tests: An expanded model of assessment and outcome. In *Rehabilitation of the spine*, edited by C. Liebensen (Philadelphia, PA: Lippincott, Williams, and Wilkins).

need to assess this because it is an important part of our client's whole picture.

Several disability questionnaires have been used in research studies, but the brief questionnaire used by Waddell and Main (1984) is easy to apply and not too time consuming for the busy clinician or instructor (table 17.1). This 9-point scale is simply scored yes or no, and the total number (raw or converted to a percentage) is recorded on the client's notes. Perhaps surprisingly for such a simple tool, the questionnaire compares well with more complex and commonly used tests. Beurskens and colleagues (1995) tested the Waddell questionnaire against the more traditional and complex Oswestry (Fairbank et al. 1980) and Roland and Morris (Roland and Morris 1983) scales and found the test–retest reproducibility of all three to be equally satisfactory.

Although questionnaires are useful as initial screening tests in the busy clinic, they are of course subjective, relying on the client to accurately report his back pain experience. Physiological tests of back fitness measures such as strength, endurance, and range of motion, although useful to chart progress during rehabilitation, are often nonfunctional in their design, having their roots

in exercise science rather than physical therapy. Physical performance batteries designed for people with low back pain, such as the Simmonds test battery (Simmonds and Claveau 1997), are useful objective measures that have been shown to have good interrater reliability and to be valid. In addition, the Simmonds test battery has been shown to be a better predictor of disability than pain and impairment tests including the Roland and Morris Disability Questionnaire and the Patient Specific Questionnaire (Simmonds and Lee 2007). The Simmonds test battery is shown in table 17.2.

There are six tests in this battery including sit-to-stand, trunk flexion, loaded reach, rollover, and two walking tests. Times and distances are recorded as appropriate and compared against normative values shown in column 4.

Diagnostic Triage

Diagnostic triage categorizes low back pain into three types: simple backache; nerve root pain (the nerve root is the T junction of the nerve as it joins to the spinal cord—pain from this area indicates compression of the nerve by a spinal disc or other structure); or possible serious pathology requiring

Table 17.2   Simmonds Physical Performance Battery of for Patients With Low Back Pain

Task	Procedure	Measure	Mean value
Repeated sit-to-stand	Subjects sit on a firm (dining room) chair and rise to standing as quickly as possible 5 times. Rest and repeat.	Average time of two task times	7.35 s
Repeated trunk flexion in standing	Subjects stand and then bend forward to the limit of their range. They return to the upright position and repeat this action 5 times.	Average time of two task times	7.44 s
Loaded reach	Subjects stand next to a wall on which a meter rule is mounted horizontally at shoulder height. They hold a weight (5% of body weight up to a maximum of 5 kg) at shoulder height and reach forward as far as possible.	Maximum distance reached (centimeters)	67.62 cm
50 ft (15 m) walk	Subjects walk 25 ft (7.6 m), turn around, and walk back to the start as fast as possible.	Total time taken	8.30 s
5 min walk	Subjects walk as far and fast as they can for 5 min.	Distance (meters)	514.10 m
360° rollover	Subjects lie supine on a mat or treatment table and roll over (360°) and then roll back to the starting position as fast as they can.	Sum of time taken to complete a rollover in both directions	6.33 s

Adapted, by permission, from M.H. Simmonds and E. Lee, 2007, Physical performance tests: An expanded model of assessment and outcome. In *Rehabilitation of the spine,* edited by C. Liebensen (Philadelphia, PA: Lippincott, Williams, and Wilkins).

referral to a specialist (Waddell et al. 1997). See the diagnostic triage chart, page 304. I do not generally recommend referral to a specialist for simple backache, and clients with nerve root compression do not usually require referral if their pain resolves within 4 weeks of its onset. Clients with possible serious pathology require prompt referral, whereas those with likely cauda equina syndrome (involving a group of fine nerves at the base of the spinal cord) require immediate referral. For individuals with simple backache or nerve root compression,

you generally can begin back stability exercises immediately (with or without other physical therapy treatment). Clients with serious pathology, however, may require surgical intervention before you begin back stability exercise, but please note the discussion in chapter 1 concerning the appropriateness of surgery for low back pain. Back stability exercise is a necessity as follow-up therapy for those with a previous history of back pain but no current pain and as a preventive therapy for clients with no history of back pain (table 17.3).

Table 17.3   Use of Back Stability Exercises

Type of back pain	Back stability exercise
Simple	Begin immediately; continue until fully functional.
Nerve root compression	Begin as pain allowed; refer to specialist if no marked progress within 4 weeks.
Serious pathology	Use back stability exercise after surgical or medical intervention.
Previous back pain now resolved	Use back stability exercise to restore full function.
No history of back pain	Use back stability exercise to reduce risk of developing back pain.

Based on G. Waddell, G. Feder, and M. Lewis, 1997.

Diagnostic Triage

Diagnostic triage is the differential diagnosis between six possibilities:

1. Simple back pain (nonspecific low back pain—i.e., pain with no specific cause)
2. Nerve root compression
3. Possibly serious spinal pathology (such as bone damage, infection, carcinoma, or pain traveling to or referred from the abdomen or gastrourinary systems)
4. Simple backache: specialist referral not required
   - Patient aged 20 to 55 years
   - Pain restricted to lumbosacral region, buttocks, or thighs
   - Pain is mechanical (i.e., pain changes with and can be relieved by movement)
   - Patient otherwise in good health (no temperature, nausea, dizziness, weight loss)
5. Nerve root pain: specialist referral not generally required within first 4 weeks, if the pain is resolving
   - Unilateral (one side of the body) leg pain that is worse than low back pain
   - Pain radiating into the foot or toes
   - Numbness and paresthesia (altered feeling) in the same area as pain
   - Localized neurological signs (such as reduced tendon jerk and positive nerve tests)
6. Red flags (caution) for possibly serious spinal pathology: refer promptly to specialist
   - Patient younger than 20 or older than 55 years
   - Nonmechanical pain (i.e., pain does not improve with movement)
   - Thoracic pain
   - Past history of carcinoma, steroid drugs, or HIV
   - Patient unwell or has lost weight
   - Widespread neurological signs
   - Obvious structural deformity (such as bone displacement after an accident, or a lump that has appeared recently)
   - Sphincter disturbance (incontinent or unable to urinate)
   - Gait disturbance (unable to walk correctly)
   - Saddle anesthesia (no feeling in crotch area between the legs)
   - Cauda equina syndrome (refer to specialist immediately—i.e., same day)

If in doubt, always refer the patient to an orthopedic physical therapist.

Based on Waddell, Feder, and Lewis, 1997.

SUMMARY

- Pain can inhibit muscle, affecting both body alignment and stability performance.
- Pain is both sensory and emotional in nature. Assess emotional aspects of pain using behavioral pain tests during examination.
- Disability questionnaires and the physical performance battery are useful measures of the effect of back pain on a person's life.
- Diagnostic triage categorizes low back pain into three types: simple backache, nerve root pain, and possible serious pathology.

Axial Loading

Goal: Determine whether vertical spinal compression recreates your client's pain.

Stand behind your client, interlace your fingers, and place your hands on top of her head. From this position, simply press downward using a light pressure (2-5 lb, or 0.9-2.2 kg) to give vertex compression. Normally this could be expected to give pain with cervical pathology but not with lumbar conditions. If the client reacts intensely, "Yes, that's it—you've hit my pain," this response is likely exaggerated where no cervical pathology coexists with her lumbar pain.

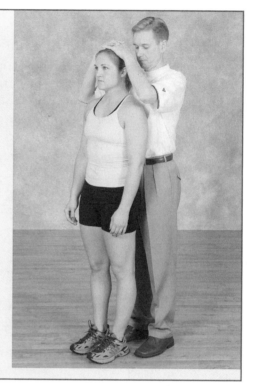

Trunk Rotation

Goal: Determine if the appearance of trunk rotation (false trunk rotation) recreates your client's pain.

With this test, you again stand behind your client. Grip her pelvis at the greater trochanters and rotate her whole body to one side and then the other. The rotation movement actually occurs at the feet and hips, but to the client it appears that her spine is rotating as she turns from side to side. Normally, whole-body rotation of this type should not give lumbar pain because the lumbar spine is actually staying still. The presence of an obvious pain response suggests exaggeration.

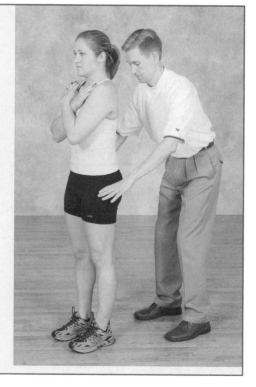

Straight-Leg Raise

Goal: Determine whether the range of motion gained using a standard lying straight-leg raise (SLR) is the same as that performed indirectly when your client is simply in a long (couch) sitting position.

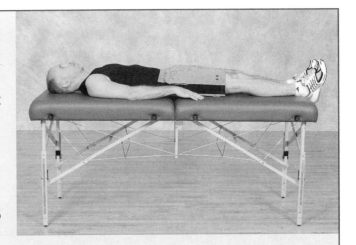

The final test uses the straight-leg raise (SLR), which is normally quite familiar to the client because it will have been tested by a number of practitioners. Measure the client's range of motion in the SLR with the client lying on a couch. Note the range, and then in casual conversation ask the client to sit up. As he sits up, he will actually move into a straight-leg position. If his SLR was limited but he shows no expression of pain or distress to sit with his legs out straight (long sitting), it is likely that his pain response is exaggerated.

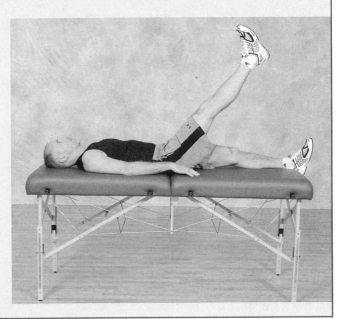

exercises

Chapter 18
Designing the Program

Now you need to design a program for your client. We have covered numerous exercises, tests, and techniques. Where should you start? The answer is to perform a **needs analysis,** which will show you what you should aim to achieve. How are you going to achieve the goals that you set? You develop a training plan. So, we have three stages shown in Designing a Back Stability Program.

NEEDS ANALYSIS

The example of needs analysis results on page 311 shows a number of points to consider about your client's needs regarding back stability.

Pain

Your client may present with pain as her most overriding consideration. Be open to saying that exercise therapy may not be appropriate at this stage. You may need to refer her to a physical therapist (PT) for pain-relieving modalities or manual therapy, for example, or you may possess these technique skills yourself. Relieving pain is an important part of any back stability program, because pain will inhibit muscle function and impair strength development. In so doing it will encourage compensatory postures, result in habitual movement patterns, and affect client compliance. It is common wisdom that a person shouldn't work through increasing pain. If an exercise causes your client minimal pain, you are justified in continuing for a short while to see if the pain abates. If it does, it is likely that stiffness is simply working loose. If pain does not abate or it increases, stop the exercise immediately and attempt to modify the technique to reduce the client's pain.

You may consider taping or strapping to reduce movement of a body part if this movement is causing pain (figure 18.1). An example is repeated flexion movements on the spine causing postural pain. You know eventually that your client will have to perform postural correction exercises. But for the moment, taping may be the most effective approach. To encourage a client, nothing is better than pain relief. Just saying that postural correction will help may not convince your client. But if you prove it by correcting her posture with taping, she will be on your side. Then through exercise, her muscles can take the place of the taping and correct her posture permanently.

Key point: Never allow a client to exercise through increasing pain. If pain worsens with exercise, stop immediately.

Designing a Back Stability Program

Stage	
Needs analysis	What does your client need. Pain relief? Muscle balance? Stability? Stretching?
Program aims	What do you hope to achieve and within what period of time?
Training plan	How will you structure each treatment or training session?

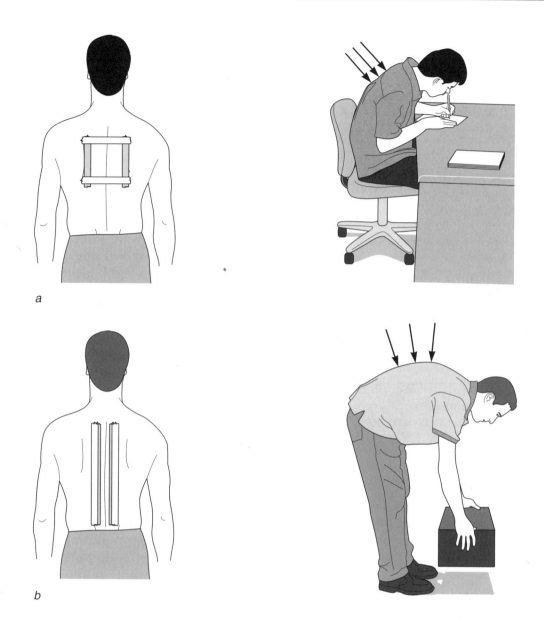

Figure 18.1 Unloading taping to relieve tissue stress: *(a)* thoracic spine and scapulae, *(b)* thoracolumbar spine.

Posture and Muscle Imbalance

Postural assessment goes hand in hand with assessment of muscle balance and often provides the first indication of which muscles need to be tested for imbalance. Select the procedures under Basic Postural Assessment (chapter 5) that you find most useful given your availability of equipment, and thoroughly assess your client's posture.

If you suspect that a muscle is lengthened, test its inner-range holding ability (e.g., test the gluteals for lordotic posture); if you think a muscle is tight, use specific tests of muscle length (e.g., for lordotic posture, use the Thomas test in chapter 6 for tight hip flexors). Then train the muscle accordingly, using inner-range holding for lengthened muscles and static or proprioceptive neuromuscular facilitation stretching for tight muscles. See Principles of Postural Correction (p. 81) and Posture Types and How to Correct Them (chapter 5).

Example of Needs Analysis Results

Need	Consideration
Pain relief	Modalities
	Manual therapy
	Exercise therapy (gentle stretching, rhythmic movement)
Joint protection	Rigid or semirigid bracing
	Nonelastic taping
	Elastic taping
Muscle balance restoration	Tests
	Use of test position as technique
Posture	Posture modification
	Long-term postural exercise
Stability	Muscle reeducation
	Exercise progression
Muscle endurance	Target muscles
	Type of muscle work
	Intensity and duration
Coordination	Specificity
	Simple to complex motion
Flexibility	Body part to target
	Muscle, nerve, or joint structure
	Technique
Technique reeducation	Job or sport analyses
	Whole-task or part-task practice
Functional restoration	Daily activities
	Goals

For each client, go through all the assessments in chapter 6 under Assessing Stretched Muscles and Assessing Shortened Muscles. Then proceed to correct whatever deficiency you find. For stretched or weakened abdominal muscles, for example, prescribe appropriate exercises (look at the goal statements) from chapter 13 under Modifications of the Sit-Up, Modifications of the Straight-Leg Raise, and Ab Roller Exercises. For tightened muscles, refer to Stretching Target Muscles in chapter 6.

If clients have both tight muscles and an unstable back, begin with stretching exercises if you believe that this will reduce their pain.

Some clients, especially elderly people, will have chronic muscle tightness that is virtually impossible to cure completely. Yet you are unlikely to meet someone whom you can't help at all; even if you cannot help people achieve optimal posture, you probably can help them move more freely, increase their range of motion, and experience less discomfort. A person doesn't need perfect posture to reduce pain. If you improve a client's posture slightly, you will unload stressed tissue and allow it to recover. This will have a significant effect on your client's symptoms.

Stability and Movement Performance

Your first tasks with a new client are to learn how stable her back is and, having identified any stability problems, to design an appropriate program based on her weaknesses. Almost all prescriptive programs for stability begin in chapter 7. Your clients should not advance to strengthening or stretching exercises until she mastered the movements in that chapter.

The best way to begin assessment is with the heel slide (p. 168): If the pelvis tilts, your client has an unstable back and you should begin by teaching her abdominal hollowing (pp. 133-137). If her pelvis does not move during the heel slide, indicating a degree of stability, begin by teaching her to control pelvic tilt and to assume and maintain the neutral position, without ignoring abdominal hollowing, of course. She should progress through pelvic tilt actions to supported hip hinge exercises and finally to free hip hinge exercises.

Once your client demonstrates adequate segmental control by independently controlling her pelvis and spine, let her progress to the good morning exercise (p. 268), first without and finally with light barbell weights.

Can your client perform abdominal hollowing in the prone kneeling position? If not, follow the instructions under Teaching Your Clients to Use Abdominal Hollowing in chapter 7, especially the teaching tips. Once he has mastered abdominal hollowing in all positions, help him gradually build up his strength and endurance until he can perform the movement for 10 reps, 10 s each, in the kneeling position. For more advanced abdominal control, he can progress to limb-loading exercises in chapter 8—especially the heel slide (p. 168) and leg lowering (p. 169).

Key point: One of your first tasks when developing a back stability program is to determine your client's level of stability.

PROGRAM AIMS

In establishing your client's needs, you have probably generated a huge list of items. You now need to sort these into definite treatment and training aims or goals. The key point here is *timescale*. You cannot achieve everything at once, so you need to prioritize your goals. If pain is a predominant feature, your first priority must be to reduce pain. This is likely to involve passive treatment such as protective taping, rest, modalities, and manual therapy aimed at pain reduction rather than joint mobilization. You may choose light exercise therapy at this stage if, for example, you believe that muscle spasm is a source of pain that can be eased through gentle stretching. Once pain has begun to ease, and this may take a number of treatment sessions, exercise may begin. If pain is caused by posture, posture correction will

---

Changing Variables for Exercise Progression

Exercise variable	Effect
Frequency	More frequent exercise requires lighter resistances and shorter recovery periods. It is more suitable for endurance training and coordination, where frequent practice changes motor programming.
Intensity	Higher intensity requires greater recovery time and is suitable for strength and power training.
Duration	Longer duration is better for endurance training and low-load stretching.
Type	Muscle work can be isometric, eccentric, and concentric. Movement complexity should progress from single-joint to multijoint and functional rehearsal.

be a priority. If instability is causing pain, then core muscle reeducation is the place to start. When prescribing stability exercises, remember that rehabilitation exercise is a *progression*. For the body to modify itself as a result of exercise (the process of supercompensation), it must be overloaded. In the case of strength training this is resistance, and in the case of stretching range of motion. With endurance training, overload is holding time, and for coordination training, overload is movement complexity. Begin with the basic overload and, as the body improves, maintain the overload to make the exercise harder. This can be achieved by varying exercise frequency, intensity, duration, and type (see Changing Variables for Exercise Progression).

Key point: For performance of a muscle to improve, the muscle must be overloaded. If this process is to continue, exercise has to be *progressive*—that is continually increasing in difficulty.

TRAINING PLAN

Now that you know what you want to achieve, you need to determine how you are going to achieve it. This involves writing a treatment and training plan for the whole rehabilitation period and writing individual treatment and lesson plans for each client session. Consider your client's starting point and end point. You have assessed your client and so know her physical condition relative to her back. Through questioning your client you also know where she wants to be when she finishes her program. She may want to be ready to play a certain sport, perform a lifting task on a job, or simply sit behind an office desk from 9 to 5. Whatever her goal, your aim is to get her pain free and fully functional to perform it.

I suggest that you begin with a 3- to 6-week calendar or planner and decide which items from your treatment aims to write first (figure 18.2). Having done that, decide on the contents of each training session but be prepared to change your

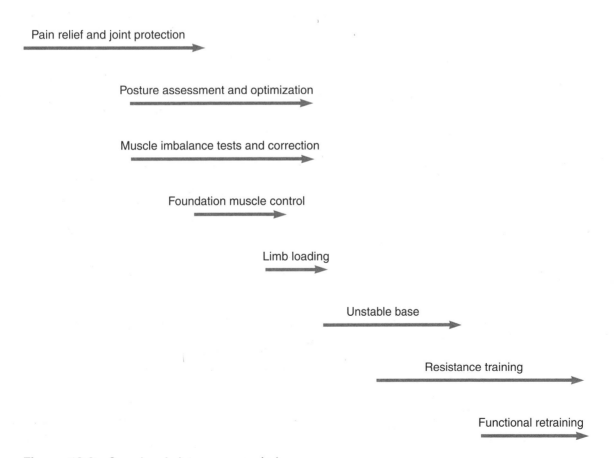

Pain relief and joint protection

Posture assessment and optimization

Muscle imbalance tests and correction

Foundation muscle control

Limb loading

Unstable base

Resistance training

Functional retraining

Figure 18.2 Sample rehab program period.

Sample Treatment Plan

- Pain-relieving modalities
- Massage therapy to increase regional blood flow
- Stretching to target muscles
- Postural reeducation
- Postural correction taping to maintain for 3 days

Sample Lesson Plan

- General warm-up
- Lying abdominal hollowing with belt
- Standing abdominal hollowing using mirror
- Standing sternal lift combined with abdominal hollowing
- Hip hinge (bench support)
- Hip hinge free
- Home exercise given, review in 3 days

plan depending on how your client reacts. See the sample treatment and lesson plans.

PRINCIPLES FOR DESIGNING A STABILITY PROGRAM

When designing a back stability program, you need to remember a few principles. This following list offers a brief summary:

- If you are not trained to diagnose back ailments, proceed no further until you've referred your client to a trained therapist—then work as closely with that therapist as you can, prescribing exercises appropriate to the therapist's diagnoses.

- Bed rest is counterproductive (see chapter 1). Except in unusual circumstances, get your clients up and performing controlled activities as quickly as possible after an injury.

- Start back stability work as soon as possible after you have determined that such a program is appropriate for an individual. The longer people are unstable, the more likely they are to develop compensatory postures that will need to be retrained.

- Always pay close attention to pain—it can be a very reliable guide. In a careful series of assessments, pain can tell you where the problems lie; throughout an individual's program, pain can tell you when to stop an exercise.

- Remember the principle of specificity: Prescribe specific activities for specific problems and goals. This is why careful assessment is so important. Many therapists have a one-size-fits-all program. I have heard about many people, especially in the United States, who have visited physicians because of back pain—and the way the doctor treated them was to hand them a back care pamphlet and instruct them to do all the exercises in it! After reading part I of this book, you know that you must deal with each individual according to his or her precise symptoms.

- Remember the principle of overload: If the overload is not great enough, there will be no training effect; your client will merely be engaging in physical activity rather than training. Too great an overload, however, will break down tissue; and because the body cannot adapt sufficiently to match the imposed stress, overuse injury results. Carefully following the exercise programs presented in this book will enable you to achieve a training effect with your clients and to avoid overtraining injuries—a particular danger with those who have experienced low back pain or back injury.

Always have a clear vision of your goal for each individual and of the best path to reach that goal. That path should consider all systems—muscle tightness and laxness, posture, strength, flexibility, reaction speed, skill, and even emotional factors. Do not fall into the common trap of overemphasizing a single aspect of fitness or rehabilitation. This is especially easy to do when strong-willed, generally knowledgeable clients make it clear that they have a certain problem and they want it fixed in a certain way ("I hurt my back at work, and I need to do some weight training so I can lift boxes again"). Working one system in isolation can do more harm than good. Excessive flexibility in relation to strength, for example, may lead to instability of a joint. Individuals with increased strength, but without parallel improvement in muscle reaction speed, may be unable to use their extra strength in functional situations. Increases in either strength or flexibility that fail to improve skill may make injury more likely.

Use Parallel Tracks When Designing a Stability Program

Because the body is a complex unit of closely interconnecting systems, any approach to treatment must be holistic, even if it targets a single system. In training clients for back stability, we constantly intertwine our focuses on correcting segmental control, shortening and strengthening lax muscles, and lengthening tight muscles. The order in which you use these exercises, of course, will depend on your clients' symptoms. You ideally want to pay attention to all these areas at all times. When time constraints require that you teach only one or two exercises or stretches at a time, simply focus first on the most problematic area. In the case histories in chapter 19, note how I generally started with just one or two exercises, aiming to solve the most acute problem first.

The following sections provide suggestions for parallel exercise progressions. Don't, for example, just look at basic stability, correct it, and then address other items only after your client can do a great hip hinge. Assess basic stability, deep abdominal control, muscle imbalance, and posture when you first see a client. At first, you may need to deal only with the most glaring deficiency, as the case histories illustrate. By your third or fourth treatment session, you generally will want to prescribe appropriate measures to correct each deficiency at the same time, working on each track during each session and prescribing home exercises for each area. This is not as time consuming as it sounds, because many of the exercises in this book address several aims at the same time.

Designing an Advanced Stability Program

After clients have achieved basic back stability, they may wish to press on with more intense work because of heavy physical demands from work or from athletic activities. Chapters 14 to 16 are for such individuals.

In General, Be Specific

The single most important task is to determine, in close consultation with clients, their needs and goals. Does a client have to lift 50 lb (23 kg) grain bags all day at work? Is she a tennis player whose body is constantly twisted and exposed to very rapid loads? Is your client a doorman who spends 8 hr each day standing up and moving relatively little? Is she a caregiver who must bend over and lift bedridden patients many times a day? Every individual's specific needs will call for specific exercises to strengthen and stretch muscles, increase reaction speed, and increase accuracy of movement. There is no way I can suggest sequences of exercises to cover all possibilities.

That is why each exercise is preceded by a goal statement. Once you have determined specific goals for a client, select the exercises that match those goals. Choosing the exercises is relatively straightforward. Where you must be very careful is in your exercise prescriptions. I have provided guidelines for the exercises in each chapter, either with introductory remarks or with the exercises themselves. But these are no more than guidelines. Carefully monitor your clients as they first perform any exercise, not only to be sure they are performing the exercises correctly but also to be sure they are performing enough reps and using sufficient load to challenge their muscles but not to excessively load them.

Tips for Designing Weight-Training Programs

In addition to the rather specific instructions I provide for the weight-training exercises, here are a few more strategies you can use to guide your prescriptions of exercises.

The order in which weight-training exercises are performed in a single exercise session is important. In general, have your clients work large muscle groups first with multijoint exercises and smaller groups second using isolation movements. A multijoint exercise is one that works a number of muscles, including those with a large muscle mass. For example, the bench press works the pectoral muscles and the triceps. Because the triceps are far smaller than the pectorals, they fatigue first and so are the limiting factor in the exercise. If the triceps are worked first, fewer bench press movements are possible and the pectoral muscles will not be sufficiently challenged.

Another method of combining exercises is to use a superset (i.e., to work the muscles on one side of a limb and then immediately, without a rest, work those on the opposing side). This type of training keeps the blood within a body part, while the individual muscles themselves have some rest. A typical superset routine would involve biceps–triceps–biceps.

One way to provide maximum challenge to muscles is to use pyramid training. Have your client perform 12 repetitions with an average weight for the first set, 10 reps with a heavier weight for the second set, and finally 8 reps with the heaviest weight he can manage for the final set. In this way, the muscle is worked maximally, but only when it is thoroughly warmed up. See Norris (1995b) for further details of weight-training programs.

SUMMARY

- Use a needs analysis to establish what your client requires from a back stability program.

This will give you your training aims and help you formulate a training plan.

- During the first session, it is useful to assess a client for basic stability, posture, alignment, segmental control, and muscle imbalance.
- Treat pain before proceeding with stability exercises.
- In many cases, your first several sessions will address only the most severe deficiency.
- By the third or fourth session, if not earlier, you generally will want to focus on all aspects of stability, prescribing exercises for any area where there is a deficit.
- Prescribe specific exercises for specific goals; there is no such thing as a general prescription for back stability.
- The principle of specificity applies also to advanced stability exercises. When prescribing procedures from chapters 8 or 9, target them to your clients' specific goals and needs, whether they are related to the workplace or to the playing field.

Chapter 19
Case History Illustrations

The following case histories illustrate how to apply the back stability program in the real world. These are not designed as recipes for particular clinical patterns but rather to demonstrate the application of the program as it is covered within this book.

OVERWEIGHT CLIENT

A 42-year-old man with a history of persistent back pain, AH worked on a production line. He was about 56 lb (25 kg) overweight, with a marked lordotic posture. The goal of my treatment was first to reduce pain and then to restore postural balance. In the first treatment session, I instructed AH to perform supine lying lumbar flexion, bringing his knees to his chest with overpressure to encourage flexion of the lumbar spine. The principle here was that AH's lordotic posture was placing an excessive extension stress on his low back. The flexion exercise that I used was designed to neutralize this. With repetition (15-25 reps), his low back pain eased. I showed him how to get onto and off the floor without bending and advised him to practice this exercise every 2 hr of the waking day for 2 days. I gave AH general advice concerning back care and resting, used standard physical therapy modalities to reduce local pain, and referred him to a dietician to begin a weight-loss program.

By the second treatment session 2 days later, AH's pain was markedly reduced. I started him on a general aerobic exercise session with his back supported—he used static cycling (seat and handlebar adjusted to minimize back stress) and a ski trainer to perform heart-rate-controlled exercise for 15 to 20 min every other day.

At the second session, I also started AH on stability training, beginning with abdominal hollowing in the four-point kneeling position and using a webbing belt around his abdomen. Because AH was unable to perform abdominal hollowing

correctly, I provided a surface electromyograph (EMG) unit to give feedback. It took 40 min to reeducate deep abdominal contraction using surface EMG, palpation, and voice encouragement. But because AH was still unable to perform the exercise unaided, I did not yet prescribe abdominal hollowing as a home exercise. AH continued with his back care and aerobic training for 2 more days.

During his third treatment session, AH was able to perform abdominal hollowing with a 5- to 7-s hold for 3 repetitions. We had to work hard to help him refrain from holding his breath—I encouraged him to count out loud as he performed abdominal hollowing, to show that he was breathing normally.

AH progressed in hollowing his abdomen but found it difficult to control the neutral position of his spine without my feedback. I taught him abdominal hollowing in wall-support standing to allow him to practice at home without having to think about his spine. He used a belt, focusing on pulling his abdominals in and up from the belt. He particularly liked this exercise, because it began to give his abdominal wall a flatter appearance; this, combined with weight loss, gave AH a leaner appearance.

We repeatedly set goals: goals for weight loss, numbers of repetitions performed, holding time of exercises, and heart-rate-monitored exercise.

AH's low back pain had now gone, and he progressed from standing abdominal hollowing to standing posterior pelvic tilt. Because his cardiopulmonary fitness (measured as heart-rate recovery) had improved with a decline in percent body fat (38% to 30%), I had him increase his aerobic activity. He still used non-weight-bearing or partial weight-bearing activities in the gymnasium to reduce joint loading, but now he began walking (on grass or gravel with shock-absorbing sports shoes) for 15 to 20 min daily.

In an attempt to shorten AH's rectus abdominis, I had him continue his standing posterior pelvic tilt and I added lying posterior tilt, held for 20 to 30 s (breathing normally). AH had short hip flexors and hamstrings, and he stretched them using the half-kneeling hip flexor stretch and active knee extension. AH built up his stability work with kneeling activities (knee raise, 10 repetitions on each leg, holding for 10 s) and began hollowing his abdomen regularly during his walking.

I discharged AH from physical therapy to a personal trainer at a local gymnasium, where he incorporated stability work into a general fitness and weight-loss program.

Points to Note

- AH had mechanical back pain brought on by his lordotic posture.
- Posture correction began with weight loss.
- Because AH was initially unable to perform correct abdominal hollowing, I did not give this as a home exercise.
- Surface EMG proved useful in initially teaching abdominal hollowing.
- We repeatedly used goal setting.
- Because AH liked the standing abdominal hollowing exercise, I used it extensively.
- AH used aerobic training to aid general fitness as well as back stability.
- The back stability program formed a focus for more general lifestyle changes.
- When discharged from physical therapy care, AH continued the back stability program in another setting.

ATHLETE WITH POOR STABILITY

Twenty-six-year-old HC trains daily in a gymnasium, using either weight-training apparatus (40 min) plus cardiopulmonary apparatus (20 min), or step aerobics (60 min). One day she complained of low back pain the morning after training. X-ray examination of the low back and pelvic joints showed no abnormality, and blood tests were normal. She was referred to me for physical therapy 3 months after the onset of pain. Her lumbar spine and sacroiliac joints were unremarkable on exami-

nation, but repeated lumbar extension—especially anterior pelvic tilt—caused pain.

Kinesiological examination (movement analysis) showed poor lumbar stability with overhead movements and with hip extension actions in standing. HC stated that two exercises in particular gave rise to her pain following workouts: standing hip extension on a "multihip" unit that targets the gluteals, and repeated overhead pressing actions in standing with an aerobics bar. Examination of these moves showed that her pelvis moved rapidly into anterior tilt and remained in that position throughout the exercises.

In assessing HC's abdominal musculature, I found high tone in the superficial abdominals, with marked muscular definition of the rectus abdominis (the six-pack). Yet she performed poorly on stability tests, being unable to perform abdominal hollowing in four-point kneeling while maintaining a neutral lumbar spine. In the heel slide action monitored by a pressure biofeedback unit, HC was unable to perform more than 3 repetitions before her pelvis tilted anteriorly. When she was in four-point kneeling position, leg lifting actions caused marked muscle quivering, demonstrating poor performance.

HC's gross segmental control was also poor—she was unable to perform a controlled hip hinge action. She moved not into spinal flexion (like most people) but into extension, anteriorly tilting her pelvis and hyperextending her lumbar spine.

In her first treatment session, I had her perform supine knee and hip flexion, to press her lumbar spine into flexion. I told her to do these movements at the end of each workout period. I temporarily removed the overhead press and hip extension exercises from her gym program. Following her first two workout periods after the first session, HC noted reduced pain in the mornings.

I used video feedback to show HC her performance in the hip extension and overhead exercises. She was surprised, having been unaware of her lack of alignment. I had HC try to perform abdominal hollowing in four-point kneeling, and she was able to perform the exercise within 2 to 3 min of being shown the movement. She then used abdominal hollowing in wall-support standing, progressing to free standing after 2 sets of 10 repetitions. She used abdominal hollowing in free standing and free (stool) sitting during her gym workouts, performing a single set with a 30-s hold, breathing normally.

HC progressed quickly (within 2 weeks) to supine-lying heel slide and finally to supine-lying foot drop (2 sets, 10 reps, 30 s hold). I prescribed four-point kneeling knee movements to improve stability control.

By the third treatment session (10 days after beginning treatment), noting that HC was able to perform abdominal hollowing for 10 reps, holding each for 30 s, I prescribed the hip hinge action. Initially I had her use controlled pelvic tilt in crook lying. In that same session, she progressed to pelvic tilt in wall-support standing and finally in free standing. She performed the hip hinge with a stick held along the length of the spine to give feedback about spinal position. Initially she performed the exercise next to a mirror, then without a mirror, then without a stick, and finally with her eyes closed (to overload proprioception). HC had mastered the hip hinge by her fourth treatment session—at which point I had her perform overhead pressing actions with a stick and perform hip extensions on the multihip unit with minimal weight. Her goal was to maintain abdominal hollowing and a neutral lumbar alignment throughout the exercise.

I incorporated stability principles of abdominal hollowing (30% maximum contraction) and neutral lumbar alignment into all of HC's exercise activities.

Points to Note

- HC had excellent cosmetic appearance of her abdominal region (superficial abdominals) but poor deep abdominal control.

- She was unable to maintain neutral lumbar alignment, even though she had high muscle tone.

- I used extensive movement analysis and observed the exercises that HC practiced in her gym.

- She had poor segmental control, moving into extension rather than flexion as is more common.

- Video feedback permitted HC to see her alignment. Mirrors and the use of a stick increased feedback.

- HC was a regular exerciser and had good body visualization. She was able to pick up new exercise techniques very quickly.

- Deep abdominal training and segmental control (hip hinge action) formed the basis of her program.

- I waited until after HC was pain free to begin the basic stability program.

CLIENT WITH ACUTE PAIN

DB, 34 years old, came to me with acute simple low back pain that was localized to the lower lumbar region and minimally referred into the right buttock. The pain was mechanical in nature, made worse by lumbar flexion and better by lumbar extension. Initially I treated the pain, using physical therapy and lumbar manipulation. Then I had her begin multifidus contractions in left side lying, while I palpated the right multifidus and encouraged her to attempt to swell the muscle beneath my fingers. Although unable to perform this action at first, she was minimally able to contract the multifidus by the end of the second treatment session. I had her perform rhythmic stabilizations in left side lying—I placed pressure over her pelvis and shoulder to encourage spinal rotation and instructed DB to resist this motion with slight muscle contraction. As contraction built in intensity, I changed my hand position to resist spinal rotation in the opposite direction. The combination of rhythmic stabilization and isolated multifidus contractions gave substantial pain relief, with pain reducing from 8 to 3 on a subjective scale (10 = most intense pain, 1 = least intense).

In the second treatment session, I introduced abdominal hollowing. As DB lay prone, I instructed her to draw her abdomen in, in an attempt to pull her abdomen away from the surface of the treatment table. Because DB was at first unable to perform this action, I used pressure biofeedback, placing the bladder of the biofeedback unit beneath her abdomen just above the top of her pelvis and inflating the bladder sufficiently for DB to feel pressure over the abdomen. I instructed her to draw in her abdomen in an attempt to pull away from the biofeedback unit, thereby reducing the pressure on the bag. I wanted DB to perform the exercise at home, but because she was unable to identify when she was performing abdominal hollowing correctly, I brought her husband into the treatment session and showed him how to assist her. At home, DB placed a folded towel beneath her abdomen in the same position that the biofeedback bladder had occupied. I instructed DB's husband to gently try to slide the towel out from beneath DB's abdomen, while his wife drew in her abdomen sufficiently to take her weight from the towel and permit it to be pulled away. I instructed her to repeat this exercise three times daily, performing 10 reps each time.

Once DB was able to perform the hollowing action unaided in the prone lying position, I had her progress to abdominal hollowing in kneeling and sitting positions. While aiding DB in her back stability training, I also instructed her on general back care, with emphasis on correct sitting and resting postures. I also taught her basic lifting techniques for use in the home. She progressed through the early stages of the back stability program using the heel slide, kneeling leg lift, and hip hinge actions. I then referred her to an exercise instructor at a local health club, to perform a general exercise program incorporating back stability principles.

Points to Note

- Because DB was in intense pain, I used physical therapy for pain relief at the beginning of her first session, before introducing her to stability exercises later in the session.

- On the first day, I began teaching her to control the multifidus, which helped in pain relief.

- I used pressure biofeedback and palpation.

- I showed a family member how to assist with DB's abdominal hollowing exercises at home.

- DB continued her back stability training at a health club, along with general fitness activities.

PATIENT UNWILLING TO EXERCISE

SD was a 53-year-old manual worker in a food company. About 42 lb (19 kg) overweight, he had marked abdominal sagging and chronic back pain that was localized to the lower lumbar region. His

erector spinae muscles were tight and thickened. When standing, SD had a flattened lumbar curve, showing a typical flat-back posture. Examination of range of movement revealed a lack of lumbar extension and grossly limited pelvic tilt during forward flexion movements. The pelvis contributed little to forward bending because most forward movement came from the upper lumbar and lower thoracic spine. Examination of SD's lifting techniques showed repeated bending actions with his legs straight and adoption of poor resting positions with marked spinal flexion. SD had attended his company's manual handling course and even a refresher course, but his line manager confirmed SD's unwillingness to practice correct handling procedures on a regular basis.

My initial physical therapy treatment targeted pain relief, but I also wanted to make SD contribute to his own treatment by taking part in exercise. It required considerable persuasion to convince SD to begin exercising! I taught him passive extension procedures that involved his lying on the floor and pressing with his arms to encourage restoration of a normal lumbar curve. During this exercise, his pain reduced in intensity and localized to the lumbar region, shrinking in size. To encourage correct bending, I placed 15 in. (38 cm) strips of nonelastic tape on either side of his spine, from the pelvic region to the midthoracic area. As SD bent forward, the tape tightened on the skin, restricting spinal flexion and encouraging him to bend from the knees.

I taught SD pelvic tilting, first passively and then actively, during the first treatment session. Although I instructed him to continue practicing at home, he showed little willingness to do so. I therefore instructed him to visit the company medical center daily, to practice his exercises under supervision of a physical therapy assistant or nurse. He did this each working day for 2 weeks.

In his second treatment session, I started SD on a single abdominal hollowing exercise, choosing hollowing in wall-supported standing (with a webbing belt) because it was easiest for him to perform. With the use of a mirror, palpation, and surface EMG feedback, he was able to perform consistent hollowing by his third treatment session. I then encouraged him to practice hollowing without aids in wall-support standing, instructing him to draw his abdominal wall away from the waistband of his trousers (without holding his breath) and to hold the contraction for 5 to 10 s. I told him to repeat the exercise three times daily for 10 repetitions.

By our third session, the combination of increased flexibility to pelvic tilt and back taping made SD bend more correctly. I assigned hamstring stretching exercises (active knee extension) in a lying position—10 reps, holding each for 10 s, during his treatment sessions on alternate working days. I also referred him to the company occupational health nurse for advice on diet and monitored weight loss.

Video feedback helped SD learn correct bending techniques; and he practiced the hip hinge (with a stick placed along the length of the spine) first with and then without video feedback. After four treatment sessions and 10 days of supervised exercise, SD was pain free. (But I also discovered that SD stopped practicing his exercise program 2 weeks after treatment began!) I encouraged him to perform the hollowing procedure when walking to his tea break (morning and afternoon) and his lunch break. The action was to contract the muscles to pull away from the waistband, hold the contraction while taking 10 steps, relax for 10 steps, and begin over again—a technique known as postural walking. I told him to continue this contraction-and-rest procedure for the full length of the walk (about 5 min). Because this action was easy to perform and was built into SD's daily activity, he received it well. Three months after his first appointment, SD was still practicing the postural walking procedure daily. He reported a feeling of strength in his abdomen, with the added advantage of increased tone and a flatter stomach.

Points to Note

- SD had a flat-back posture and chronic back pain.
- Previous to my seeing him, SD had received only medication and passive physical treatments.
- He had taken no active part in the care of his back.
- Back taping encouraged him to move more correctly.
- Because SD was unwilling to exercise on his own, I arranged for him to do his exercises at work under supervision of a physical therapy assistant.

- Although he did not continue abdominal hollowing exercises at home, he liked the postural walking approach, which we therefore built into his daily activities.

PREGNANT CLIENT WITH BACK PAIN

SP was a 32-year-old office worker in her second trimester of pregnancy. She had right-side back pain made worse by prolonged sitting. Her pain traveled into her buttock and occasionally into her leg, and she complained that her leg often felt weak, "as though it can't support me," but had never actually given way. When she was lying in bed on her back she occasionally felt pain spreading into her pubic region. She had seen her physician and midwife and was assured that her pregnancy was normal and her pain of musculoskeletal origin.

Assessing her posture, I found that SP was lordotic, with an anteriorly tilted pelvis, but exhibited some swayback tendencies, standing with her weight predominantly on her right leg. When questioned she confirmed that she had always stood like this and often noticed her right knee aching if she stood all day at an exhibition as part of her job.

Clinical examination of SP's lumbar–pelvic region revealed tenderness over the right posterior superior iliac spine (PSIS) and local tenderness into the region of the sacroiliac joint (SIJ). There was no tenderness to palpation of the public bone or pubic symphysis. Compression of the pelvic rims in side-lying position caused pain in the SIJ region and the right buttock. Pain was exacerbated when she performed an active straight-leg raise (ASLR) movement with the right leg but not the left. Fixation of the pelvis using manual pressure removed all pain to a repeat test using the ASLR.

My initial impression was that SP had developed SIJ pain as a result of instability, because the ASLR had given pain that was removed when the pelvis was stabilized. My treatment goal was twofold. I had to stabilize the pelvis passively to remove pain and in parallel with this teach SP to build her stability muscles to actively stabilize. Posture correction would remove a significant causal factor for pain in the long term.

SP had been taught pelvic floor contractions as part of her antenatal care but had not practiced these regularly. I emphasized the importance of these exercises and combined pelvic floor contraction with abdominal hollowing in crook-lying position. Initially her abdominal hollowing was poor, and she was not able to perform a heel slide without tipping her pelvis. To emphasize the abdominal hollowing action, I taught SP to self-palpate. Once SP had performed a good abdominal hollowing action, I retested the ASLR action with SP relaxing and then again with her performing abdominal hollowing. She was amazed that the hollowing action took away her pain and was determined to practice the exercise between treatment sessions.

I fitted SP with an SIJ support belt around the rims of her pelvis, but below her abdomen, and taught her to stand with her weight taken equally on both legs.

On the next treatment session (3 days later), SP reported that her pain had lessened. If she forgot to wear her support belt, pain returned. I repeated the abdominal hollowing action, and her ability had improved considerably. The action was more forceful initially, and she was now able to hold the contraction for 10 to 20 s while breathing normally. I taught SP to perform abdominal hollowing in standing and taught her to lengthen her spine standing in optimal alignment. In addition, I educated her on pelvic tilt and correct sitting posture. I also taught SP supported side lying using pillows beneath her flexed upper leg, so that she would be pain free at night.

On the third treatment session (5 days later), SP reported that her pain was only occasional now and limited to the SIJ region, not referred into the buttock. Her pain only occurred through prolonged sitting and was easily removed by correcting her sitting posture to move back into the neutral lumbar position. I taught SP the supported hip hinge action (tabletop) and emphasized correct lifting techniques in daily activities. In addition, I introduced the bridge action with abdominal hollowing to work the gluteal muscles. I encouraged SP to use her SIJ support belt only if she needed to stand for a prolonged period or if she had pain.

On the fourth treatment (2 weeks after initial evaluation), SP was pain free during day-to-day activities and did not require her support belt. I emphasized that she should keep the belt because she may need it later because of the changing mechanics of the pelvic region as her pregnancy progressed. I encouraged SP to continue with her abdominal hollowing and pelvic floor contractions throughout pregnancy and to be scrupulous about her daily back care.

Points to Note

- SP had no pregnancy complications and had been screened by her physician and midwife before commencing the back stability program.

- SP had pain that was reduced when her pelvis was stabilized.

- I demonstrated to SP that abdominal hollowing would take her pain away, thus increasing compliance.

- I encouraged her to combine abdominal hollowing with pelvic floor contraction.

- Because SP was in pain, a support belt was used until she was strong enough for her body to supply its own stability.

- Instructions on general back care and posture in standing, sitting, and lying were given.

- Functional movements including the hip hinge were used.

SUMMARY

- Five case histories are used to illustrate the clinical application of the back stability program.

- Exercises were modified to suit clients' particular needs and learning styles.

- A variety of teaching techniques were used.

Glossary

agonist—Muscle that creates a movement.

antagonist—Muscle that, if contracted, opposes a movement.

aponeurosis—Connective tissue that attaches muscle to bone.

approximate—(verb) Move or bring objects closer together.

articulated—Joined or connected loosely to allow motion between the connection, such as a joint.

baseline—Starting point or value of a test for later comparison.

caudally—Directed toward the hind part of the body.

contralateral—Originating in or affecting the opposite side of the body.

contralateral fibers—Fibers originating in or affecting the opposite side of the body.

distraction force—Force that separates a joint surface without injury or dislocation.

extension—Movement that straightens a limb to a parallel or near-parallel position.

fascia—Sheet of fibrous tissue under the skin that encloses muscles as well as separates and supports them; connects the skin with the tissue beneath it.

fascicle—Small bundle of nerve or muscle fibers.

flexible ruler—Plastic rule or stick that can be placed on the skin to follow body contours.

flexion—Bending or being bent; opposite of extension.

four-point kneeling—Kneeling on both hands and knees.

hoop pressure—Inward pressure exerted by the muscles surrounding the trunk.

inclinometer—Instrument to measure angulation of one body segment relative to another.

innominate bones—Hip bones, composed of the ilium, ischium, and pubis; form the pelvis.

ipsilateral—On the same side (of the body).

ischemic—Deficiency of blood to a body part attributable to an obstruction in or a narrowing of the blood vessels.

investing fascia—Fascia that surrounds rather than connects or separates.

kyphotic—Convex curvature of the thoracic spine creating a hunchback.

lamina of the vertebra—Posterior portion of the vertebral arch that provides a base for the spinous process.

laminae—Thin flat layers or membranes.

lateral flexion—Bending or being bent to the side.

lateral malleolus—Lower end of the fibula that forms the projection of the ankle.

lateral raphe—Ridge along the side of the erector spinae muscles formed by the connective tissue of the latissimus dorsi, internal obliques, and transversus abdominus.

lax muscle—Muscle that has less tone than average and allows a body segment to move out of alignment.

lordosis—Inward curvature of the cervical and lumbar spines.

mobilizers—Muscles that create general body and limb movements (also called task muscles).

muscle stability—Ability of muscles to stop unrequired motion.

needs analysis—Structured process to determine a client's requirements with reference to rehabilitation.

nociception—Protective sensation of pain in normal individuals.

occiput—Back part of the head.

pain behavior—Actions that (consciously or unconsciously) suggest the presence of pain. Examples include limping, talking, facial expression, guiding, and work cessation.

pedicles—Bony processes that extend posteriorly from the body of a vertebra; one of the paired parts of the vertebral arch that connect the lamina to the vertebral body.

pelvic inlet—Upper opening of the pelvis.

periosteum—Thick, fibrous membrane covering all the bones of the body except at the joints.

pelvic outlet—Lower opening of the pelvis.

prolapse—Downward displacement, especially of a tissue or organ.

prone lying—Lying on the front of the body.

proprioception—Specialized variation of touch encompassing the sensations of both joint movement and joint position.

pseudoparesis—Apparent weakness brought on by increased tone in a muscle antagonist.

sagittal plane—Vertical plane through the body that divides it into the left and right side.

sagittal rotation—Rotation from the front to the back.

Schmorl's node—Irregular or hemispherical bone defect in the body of a vertebra, into which a spinal disk herniates.

segmental control—Controlling motion of one body segment relative to another.

sitting—Sitting upright with feet flat on the floor and knees bent to 90°.

stabilizers—Muscles that prevent unwanted movement (also called postural muscles).

standing (wall support)—Standing with your back to the wall, leaning onto it.

tight muscle—Muscle that is shorter than average and limits range of motion.

trabeculae—Fibrous cords of connective tissue that extend into an organ's wall to serve as support.

ventrally—To the front side of the body.

Bibliography

Adams, M. 1989. Letter to the editor. *Spine* 14:1272.

Adams, M., Bogduk, N., Burton, K., and Dolan, P. 2002. *The biomechanics of back pain.* Edinburgh, UK: Churchill Livingstone.

Adams, M.A., and Dolan, P. 1997. The combined function of the spine, pelvis, and legs when lifting with a straight back. In *Movement, stability and low back pain.* A. Vleeming, V. Mooney, T. Dorman, C. Snijders, and R. Stoeckart, eds. New York: Churchill Livingstone.

Adams, M.A., and Hutton, W.C. 1983. The mechanical function of the lumbar apophyseal joints. *Spine* 8:327-330.

Adams, M.A., Hutton, W.C., and Stott, J.R.R. 1980. The resistance to flexion of the lumbar intervertebral joint. *Spine* 5:245-253.

Adams, M.A., McNally, D.S., Chinn, H., and Dolan, P. 1994. Posture and the compressive strength of the lumbar spine. *Clinical Biomechanics* 9:5-14.

Airaksinen, O., Brox, J.I., and Cedraschi. 2005. *European guidelines for the management of chronic nonspecific low back pain.* Brussels: European Commission Publications.

Allan, D.B., and Waddell, G. 1989. An historical perspective on low back pain and disability. *Acta Orthopaedica Scandinavica Supplementum* 60:1-5.

Allison, G., Kendle, K., Roll, S., Schupelius, J., Scott, Q., and Panizza, J. 1998. The role of the diaphragm during abdominal hollowing exercises. *Australian Journal of Physiotherapy* 44:95-102.

Andersson, E., Oddsson, L., Grundstrom, H., and Thorstensson, A. 1995. The role of the psoas and iliacus muscles for stability and movement of the lumbar spine, pelvis and hip. *Scandinavian Journal of Medicine and Science in Sports* 5:10-16.

Appell, H.J. 1990. Muscular atrophy following immobilisation: A review. *Sports Medicine* 10:42-58.

Aruin, A.S., and Latash, M.L. 1995. Directional specificity of postural muscles in feed-forward postural reactions during fast voluntary arm movements. *Experimental Brain Research* 103:323-332.

Aspden, R.M. 1987. Intra-abdominal pressure and its role in spinal mechanics. *Clinical Biomechanics* 2:168-174.

Aspden, R.M. 1989. The spine as an arch. A new mathematical model. *Spine* 14:266-274.

Aspden, R.M. 1992. Review of the functional anatomy of the spinal ligaments and the lumbar erector spinae muscles. *Clinical Anatomy* 5:372-387.

Atkinson, H.W. 1986. Principles of treatment. In *Cash's textbook of neurology for physiotherapists,* 4th ed. P.A Downie, Ed. London: Faber and Faber.

Bandy, W.D., and Irion, J.M. 1994. The effect of time on static stretch of the flexibility of the hamstring muscles. *Physical Therapy* 74:845-852.

Barker, K.L., Shamley, D.R., and Jackson, D. 2004. Changes in the cross-sectional area of multifidus and psoas in patients with unilateral back pain: The relationship to pain and disability. *Spine* 29:515-519.

Barker, P.J., Guggenheimer, K.T., Grkovic, I., Briggs, C.A., Jones, D.C., and Hodges, P.W. 2006. Effects of tensioning the lumbar fasciae on segmental stiffness during flexion and extension. *Spine* 15(4): 397-405.

Barler, P.J, Guggenheimer, K.T., Grkovic, I., and Briggs, C.A. 2006. Effects of tensioning the lumbar fasciae on stiffness during flexion and extension. *Spine* 31:397-405.

Barrack, R.L., and Skinner, H.B. 1990. The sensory function of knee ligaments. In *Knee ligaments: Structure, function, and injury.* D. Daniel, Ed. New York: Raven Press.

Barrack, R.L., Skinner, H.B., and Brunet, G. 1983. Joint kinesthesia in the highly trained knee. *Journal of Sports Medicine and Physical Fitness* 24:18-20.

Barrett, D.S., Cobb, A.G., and Bentley, G. 1991. Joint proprioception in normal, osteoarthritic, and replaced knees. *Journal of Bone and Joint Surgery* 73B:53-56.

Bartelink, D.L. 1957. The role of abdominal pressure in relieving the pressure on the lumbar intervertebral discs. *Journal of Bone and Joint Surgery* 39B:718-725.

Bastide, G., Zadeh, J., and Lefebre, D. 1989. Are the little muscles what we think they are? *Surgical and Radiological Anatomy* 11:255-256.

Beard, D.J., Kyberd, P.J., O'Connor, J.J., Fergusson, C.M., and Dodd, C.A.F. 1994. Reflex hamstring contraction latency in anterior cruciate ligament deficiency. *Journal of Orthopaedic Research* 12:219-228.

Behm, D.G., Leonard, A.M., Young, W.B., and Bonsey, A.C. 2005. Trunk muscle electromyographic activity with unstable and unilateral exercises. *Journal of strength and conditioning research.* 19(1). 193-201.

Beurskens, A.J., de Vet, H.C., Koke, A.L., and van der Heijden, G.J. 1995. Measuring the functional status of patients with low back pain: Assessment of the quality of four disease specific questionnaires. *Spine* 20:1017-1028.

Bernhardt, M., White, A.A., and Panjabi, M.M. 1992. Lumbar spine instability. In *The lumbar spine and back pain*, 4th ed. M.I.V. Jayson, Ed. Edinburgh, UK: Churchill Livingstone.

Bernier, J.N., and Perrin, D.H. 1998. Effect of coordination training on proprioception of the functionally unstable ankle. *Journal of Orthopedic and Sports Physical Therapy* 27:264-275.

Biedermann, H.J., Shanks, G.L., Forrest, W.J., and Inglis, J. 1991. Power spectrum analyses of electromyographic activity. *Spine* 16:1179-1184.

Biering-Sorensen, R. 1984. Physical measurement as risk indicators for low back trouble over a one year period. *Spine* 9:106-119.

Bigos, S.J., Hansson, T., Castillo, R.N., Beecher, P.J., and Wortley, M.D. 1994. The value of pre-employment roentgenographs for predicting acute back injury claims and chronic back pain and disability. *Clinical Orthopedics and Related Research* 283:124-129.

Boden, S.D., Davis, D.O., and Dina, T.S. 1990. Abnormal magnetic resonance scans of the lumbar spine in asymptomatic subjects. *Journal of Bone and Joint Surgery* (American volume) 72:403.

Bogduk, N., and Engel, R. 1984. The menisci of the lumbar zygapophyseal joints. A review of their anatomy and clinical significance. *Spine* 9:454-460.

Bogduk, N., and Jull, G. 1985. The theoretical pathology of acute locked back: A basis for manipulative therapy. *Manual Medicine* 1:78-82.

Bogduk, N., Pearcy, M., and Hadfield, G. 1992. Anatomy and biomechanics of psoas major. *Clinical Biomechanics* 7:109-119.

Bogduk, N., and Twomey, L.T. 1987. *Clinical anatomy of the lumbar spine*. Edinburgh, UK: Churchill Livingstone.

Bogduk, N., and Twomey, L.T. 1991. *Clinical anatomy of the lumbar spine*, 2nd ed. Edinburgh, UK: Churchill Livingstone.

Brox, J.I., Sorensen, R., and Friis, A. 2003. Randomized clinical trial of lumbar instrumented fusion and cognitive intervention and exercises in patients with chronic low back pain and disc degeneration. *Spine* 29:1160-1161.

Bullock-Saxton, J. 1988. Normal and abnormal postures in the sagittal plane and their relationship to low back pain. *Physiotherapy Practice* 4:94-104.

Bullock-Saxton, J. 1993. Postural alignment in standing: A repeatability study. *Australian Journal of Physiotherapy* 39:25-29.

Bullock-Saxton, J.E., Bullock, M.I., Tod, C., Riley, D.R., and Morgan, A.E. 1991. Postural stability in young adult men and women. *New Zealand Journal of Physiotherapy* 3:7-10.

Bush, K., Cowan, N., and Katz, D.E. 1992. The natural history of sciatica associated with disc pathology: A prospective study with clinical and independent radiographic follow up. *Spine* 17:1205-1212.

Cailliet, R. 1981. *Low back pain syndrome*, 3rd ed. Philadelphia: Davis.

Cailliet, R. 1983. *Soft tissue pain and disability*. Philadelphia: Davis.

Cailliet, R. 1994. *Low back pain syndrome*, (3rd ed.). Philadelphia: Davis.

Cairns, M.C., Foster, N.E., and Wright, C.C. 2000. A pragmatic randomised controlled trial of stabilisation exercises in the management of recurrent low back pain. *Physiotherapy* 86:38.

Cappozzo, A., Felici, F., Figura, F., and Gazzani, F. 1985. Lumbar spine loading during half-squat exercises. *Medicine and Science in Sports and Exercise* 17(5):613-620.

Chartered Society of Physiotherapy (CSP). 1998. Low back pain. Information for sufferers [Online]. Available: www.csp.org.uk.

Chartered Society of Physiotherapy (CSP). 2004. New statistics on the incidence of back pain. The YouGov poll. Available: www.csp.org.uk.

Choi, G., Raiturker, P. P., Kim, M. J., and Jin, C.D. 2005. The effect of early isolated lumbar extension exercise program for patients with herniated disc undergoing lumbar discectomy. *Neurosurgery* 57(4): 764-72.

Cholewicki, J., and McGill, S.M. 1992. Lumbar posterior ligament involvement during extremely heavy lifts estimated from fluoroscopic measurements. *Journal of Biomechanics* 25:17-28.

Comerford, M. 1995. Muscle imbalance. Course notes. Nottingham School of Physiotherapy, Nottingham, UK.

Comerford, M. 1998. *Dynamic stability. PhysioTools compatible computer programme*. Tampere, Finland: PhysioTools Development Office.

Cordo, P.J., Gurfinkel, V.S., Smith, T.C., Hodges, P.W., and Verschueren, S. 2003. The sit-up: Complex kinematics and muscle activity in voluntary axial movement. *Journal of Electromyography and Kinesiology* 13:239-252.

Cornwall, J., John-Harris, A., and Mercer, S.R. 2006, The lumbar multifidus muscle and patterns of pain. *Manual Therapy* 11:40-45.

Cornwall, M.W., Melinda, P.B., and Barry, S. 1991. Effect of mental practice on isometric muscular strength. *Journal of Orthopedic and Sports Physical Therapy* 13:217-223.

Craton, N, 2006. Diagnostic triage in patients with spinal pain. In *Rehabilitation of the spine*, 2nd ed. C. Liebenson, Ed. Philadelphia: Lippincott.

Cresswell, A.G., Grundstrom, H., and Thorstensson, A. 1992. Observations on intra-abdominal pressure and patterns of abdominal intra-muscular activity in man. *Acta Physiologica Scandinavica* 144:409-418.

Cresswell, A.G., Oddsson, L., and Thorstensson, A. 1994. The influence of sudden perturbations on trunk muscle activity and intra-abdominal pressure while standing. *Experimental Brain Research* 98:336-341.

Critchley, D. 2002. Instructing pelvic floor contraction facilitates transversus abdominis thickness increase during low-abdominal hollowing. *Physiotherapy Research International* 7:65-75.

Crock, H.V., and Yoshizawa, H. 1976. The blood supply of the lumbar vertebral column. *Clinical Orthopaedics* 115:6-21.

Crowell, R.D., Cummings, G.S., Walker, J.R., and Tillman, L.J. 1994. Intratester and intertester reliability and validity of measures on innominate bone inclination. *Journal of Orthopedic and Sports Physical Therapy* 20:88-97.

Danneels, L., Vanderstraeten, G., and Cambier, D. 2003. Effects of three different training modalities on the cross sectional area of the lumbar multifidus in patients with chronic low back pain. *British Journal of Sports Medicine, 37(1),* 91.

Davis, P.R., and Troup, J.D.G. 1964. Pressures in the trunk cavities when pulling, pushing, and lifting. *Ergonomics* 7:465-474.

Day, J.W., Smidt, G.L., and Lehmann, T. 1984. Effect of pelvic tilt on standing posture. *Physical Therapy* 64:510-516.

Delitto, R.S., Rose, S.J., and Apts, D.W. 1987. Electromyographic analysis of two techniques for squat lifting. *Physical Therapy* 67:1329-1334.

Deutsch, F.E. 1996. Isolated lumbar strengthening in the rehabilitation of chronic low back pain. *Journal of Manipulative and Physiological Therapeutics* 19:124-133.

Deyo, R.A., Diehl, A.K., and Rosenthal, M. 1986. How many days of bed rest for acute low back pain. *New England Journal of Medicine* 315:1064.

Dickerman, R.D., Mittler, M.A., Warshaw, C., and Epstein, J.A. 2005. Spinal cord injury in a 14-year old male secondary to cervical hyperflexion with exercise. *Spinal Cord* August 30.

Dumas, G.A., Beudoin, L., and Drouin G 1987. In situ mechanical behavior of posterior spinal ligaments in the lumbar region. *Journal of Biomechanics* 20:301-310.

Eie, N. 1966. Load capacity of the low back. *Journal of Oslo City Hospitals* 16:73-98.

Enoka, R.M. 1988. *Neuromechanical basis of kinesiology.* Champaign, IL: Human Kinetics.

Enthoven, P., Skargren, E., and Kjellman, G. 2003. Course of back pain in primary care: A prospective study of physical measures. *Journal of Rehabilitation Medicine* 35:168-173.

Esola, M.A., McClure, P.W., Fitzgerald, G.K., and Siegler, S 1996. Analysis of lumbar spine and hip motion during forward bending in subjects with and without a history of low back pain. *Spine* 21:71-78.

Etnyre, B.R., and Abraham, L.D. 1986. H-reflex changes during static stretching and two variations of proprioceptive neuromuscular facilitation techniques. *Electroencephalography and Clinical Neurophysiology* 63:174-179.

Etnyre, B.R., and Lee, E.J. 1987. Comments on proprioceptive neuromuscular facilitation stretching. *Research Quarterly for Exercise and Sport* 58:184-188.

Fairbank, J., Frost, H., Wilson-Macdonald, J., and Ly-Mee Yu. 2005. Randomised controlled trial to compare surgical stabilisation of the lumbar spine with an intensive rehabilitation programme for patients with chronic low back pain: The MRC spine stabilisation trial. *British Medical Journal* 330:1233.

Fairbank, J., Mboat, J.C., Davies, J.B., and O'Brian J.P. 1980. The Oswestry low back pain disability questionnaire. *Physiotherapy* 66:271-273.

Fansler, C.L., Poff, C.L., and Shepard, K.F. 1985. Effects of mental practice on balance in elderly women. *Physical Therapy* 65:1332-1338.

Farfan, H.F. 1988. Biomechanics of the lumbar spine. In *Managing low back pain,* 2nd ed. W.H. Kirkaldy-Willis, Ed. London: Churchill Livingstone.

Farfan, H.F., Osteria, V., and Lamy, C. 1976. The mechanical etiology of spondylolysis and spondylolisthesis. *Clinical Orthopedics and Related Research* 117:40-55.

Freeman, M.A.R., Dean, M.R.E., and Hanham, I.W.F. 1965. The etiology and prevention of functional instability of the foot. *Journal of Bone and Joint Surgery* 47B:678-685.

Friedli, W.G., Hallet, M., and Simon, S.R. 1984. Postural adjustments associated with rapid voluntary arm movements. Electromyographic data. *Journal of Neurology, Neurosurgery and Psychiatry* 47:611-622.

Frymoyer, J.W., and Cats-Baril, W.L. 1991. An overview of the incidences and costs of low back pain. *Orthopedic Clinics of North America* 22:263.

Frymoyer, J.W., and Gordon, S.L. 1989. *Symposium on new perspectives on low back pain.* Park Ridge, IL: American Academy of Orthopedic Surgeons.

Gajdosik, R.L., Hatcher, C.K., and Whitsell, S. 1992. Influence of short hamstring muscles on the pelvis and lumbar spine in standing and during the toe touch test. *Clinical Biomechanics* 7:38-42.

Gibbons, S. 1999. A review of the anatomy, physiology and function of psas major. A new model of stability. In *Proceedings of the 11th Annual National Orthopaedic Symposium,* Halifax. Canada.

Gibbons, S. 2001. Biomechanics and stability mechanisms of psoa major. In *The 4th Interdisciplinary World Congress on Low Back Pain.* Montreal. Canada: European Conference Organizers.

Gibson, J.N., and Waddell, G. 2005. Surgery for degenerative lumbar spondylosis. *Cochrane Database Systematic Review* 18:CD001352.

Gill, K.P., and Callaghan, M.J. 1998. The measurement of lumbar proprioception in individuals with and without low back pain. *Spine* 23:371-377.

Goldby, L. J., Moore, A.P., Doust, J., and Trew, M.E. 2006. A randomized controlled trial investigating the efficiency of musculoskeletal physiotherapy on chronic low back disorder. *Spine* 31(10): 1083-1093.

Goldspink, G. 1992. Cellular and molecular aspects of adaptation in skeletal muscle. In *Strength and power in sport*. P.V. Komi, Ed. Oxford, UK: Blackwell.

Gossman, M.R., Sahrmann, S.A., and Rose, S.J. 1982. Review of length associated changes in muscle. *Physical Therapy* 62:1799-1808.

Gracovetsky, S., Farfan, H.F., and Helleur, C. 1985. The abdominal mechanism. *Spine* 10:317-324.

Gracovetsky, S., Kary, M., Levy, S., Ben Said, R., Pitchen, I., and Helie, J. 1990. Analysis of spinal and muscular activity during flexion/extension and free lifts. *Spine* 15:1333-1339.

Gracovetsky, S., Farfan, H.F., and Lamy, C. 1977. A mathematical model of the lumbar spine using an optimal system to control muscles and ligaments. *Orthopaedic Clinics of North America* 8:135-153.

Griffin, J.C. 1998. *Client-centered exercise prescription*. Champaign, IL: Human Kinetics.

Guimaraes, A.C.S., Vaz, M.A., De Campos, M.I.A., and Marantes, R. 1991. The contribution of the rectus abdominis and rectus femoris in twelve selected abdominal exercises. *Journal of Sports Medicine and Physical Fitness* 31:222-230.

Haggmark, T., Eriksson, E., and Jansson, E. 1986. Muscle fibre type changes in human skeletal muscle after injuries and immobilisation. *Orthopedics* 9:181-185.

Halbertsma, J.P., Goeken, L.N., Hof, A.L., Groothoff, J.W., and Eisma W.H. 2001. Extensibility and stiffness of the hamstrings in patients with non-specific low back pain. *Archives of Physical Medicine and Rehabilitation* 82:232-238.

Harman E., Frykman, P., Clagett, B., and Kraemer, W. 1988. Intra-abdominal and intra-thoracic pressures during lifting and jumping. *Medicine and Science in Sports and Exercise* 20:195-201.

Hart, D.L, and Rose, S.J. 1986. Reliability of a non-invasive method for measuring the lumbar curve. *Journal of Orthopedic and Sports Physical Therapy* 8:180-184.

Hayden, J.A., van Tulder, M.W., Malmivaara, A.V., and Koes, B.W. 2005. Meta-analysis: exercise therapy for nonspecific low back pain. *Annals of Internal Medicine* 3; 142(9):765-775.

Hemborg, B., Moritz, U., and Hamberg, J. 1983. Intra-abdominal pressure and trunk muscle activity during lifting—effect of abdominal muscle training in healthy subjects. *Scandinavian Journal of Rehabilitation Medicine* 15:183-196.

Hemborg, B., Moritz, U., Hamberg, J., Holmstrom, E., Lowing, H., and Akesson, I. 1985. Intra-abdominal pressure and trunk muscle activity during lifting. III. Effects of abdominal muscle training in chronic low-back patients. *Scandinavian Journal of Rehabilitation Medicine* 17:15-24.

Hides, J.A., Richardson, C.A., and Jull, G.A. 1996. Multifidus muscle recovery is not automatic after resolution of acute, first-episode low back pain. *Spine* 21:2763-2769.

Hides, J.A., Stokes, M.J., Saide, M., Jull, G.A., and Cooper, D.H. 1994. Evidence of lumbar multifidus muscle wasting ipsilateral to symptoms in patients with acute/subacute low back pain. *Spine* 19:165-172.

Hides, J., Wilson, S., and Stanton, W. 2006. An MRI investigation into the function of the transversus abdominis muscle during drawing in of the abdominal wall. *Spine* 31:175-178.

Hirsch, C., and Schajowicz, F. 1952. Studies on structural changes in the lumbar annulus fibrosis. *Acta Orthopaedica Scandinavica* 22:184-189.

Hirsch, C., and Nachemson, A. 1954. New observations on mechanical behaviour of lumbar discs. *Acta Orthopaedica Scandinavica* 23:254-283

Hodges, P. 2004. Lumbopelvic stability: A functional mode of the biomechanics and motor control. In *Therapeutic exercise for lumbopelvic stabilisation*. C. Richardson, P. Hodges and J. Hides, Eds. Edinburgh, UK: Churchill Livingstone.

Hodges, P.W., Eriksson, A.E., Shirley, D., and Gandevia, S.C. 2005. Intra-abdominal pressure increases stiffness of the lumbar spine. *Journal of Biomechanics* 38:1873-1880.

Hodges, P., Kaigle Holm, A., Holm, S., and Ekstrom, L. 2003. Intervertebral stiffness of the spine is increased by evoked contraction of the transversus abdominis and the diaphragm. *Spine* 28:2594-2601.

Hodges, P.W., and Richardson, C.A. 1996. Contraction of transversus abdominis invariably precedes movement of the upper and lower limb. In *Proceedings of the 6th International Conference of the International Federation of Orthopaedic Manipulative Therapists*, Lillehammer, Norway.

Hodges, P.W., and Richardson, C.A. 1999. Altered trunk muscle recruitment in people with low back pain with upper limb movement at different speeds. *Archives of Physical Medicine and Rehabilitation* 80(9): 1005-1012.

Hodges, P., Richardson, C., and Jull, G. 1996. Evaluation of the relationship between laboratory and clinical tests of transversus abdominis function. *Physiotherapy Research International* 1:30-40.

Holm, S., Indahl, A., and Solomonow, M. 2002. Sensorimotor control of the spine. *Journal of Electromyography and Kinesiology* 12:219-234.

Holm, S., Maroudas, A., Urban, J.P.G., Selstam, G., and Nachemson, A. 1981. Nutrition of the intervertebral disc: Solute transport and metabolism. *Connective Tissue Research* 8:101-119.

Holt, L.E., and Smith, R. 1983. *The effect of selected stretching programs on active and passive flexibility*. Del Mar, CA: Research Center for Sport.

Hughes, M.A., Duncan, P.W., Rose, D.K., Chandler, J.M., and Studenski, S.A. 1996. The relationship of postural sway to sensorimotor function, functional performance, and disability in the elderly. *Archives of Physical Medicine and Rehabilitation* 77:567-572.

Hukins, D.W.L. 1987. Properties of spinal materials. In *The lumbar spine and back pain*. M.I.V. Jayson, Ed. Edinburgh, UK: Churchill Livingstone.

Hukins, D.W.L., Aspden, R.M., and Hickey, D.S. 1990. Thoracolumbar fascia can increase the efficiency of the erector spinae muscles. *Clinical Biomechanics* 5:30-34.

Hungerford, B., Gilleard, W., and Hodges, P. 2003. Evidence of altered lumbopelvic muscle recruitment in the presence of sacroiliac joint pain. *Spine* 28:1593-1600.

Hyman, J., and Liebenson, C. 1996. Spinal stabilization exercise program. In *Rehabilitation of the spine*. C. Liebenson, Ed. Baltimore: Williams & Wilkins.

Indahl, A., Kaigle, A., Reikeras, O., and Holm, S. 1997. Interaction between the porcine lumbar intervertebral disc, zygapophysial joints, and paraspinal muscles. *Spine* 22:2834-2940.

Jackson, M., Solomonow, M., and Zhou, B. 2001. Multifidus EMG and tension-relaxation recovery after prolonged static lumbar flexion. *Spine* 26:715-723.

Jacob, H.A.C., and Kissling, R.O. 1995. The mobility of the sacroiliac joints in healthy volunteers between 20 and 50 years of age. *Clinical Biomechanics* 10:352-361.

Janda, V. 1986. Muscle weakness and inhibition pseudoparesis in back pain syndromes. In *Modern manual therapy*. G. Grieve, Ed. Edinburgh, UK: Churchill Livingstone.

Janda, V. 1992. Muscle imbalance and musculoskeletal pain. Course notes. University of Oxford, Oxford, UK.

Janda, V. 1993. Muscle strength in relation to muscle length, pain and muscle imbalance. In *Muscle strength. International perspectives in physical therapy*. K. Harms-Ringdahl, Ed. Edinburgh, UK: Churchill Livingstone.

Janda V., and Schmid, H.J.A. 1980. Muscles as a pathogenic factor in back pain. In *Proceedings of the International Federation of Orthopaedic Manipulative Therapists* (4th conference, 17-18). Auckland, New Zealand.

Jemmett, R.S., Macdonald, D.A., Agur, A.M. 2004. Anatomical relationships between selected segmental muscles of the lumbar spine in the context of multi-planar segmental motion: a preliminary investigation. *Manual Therapy*, (4), 203-210.

Jensel, M.C., Brant-Zawadzki, M.N., and Obuchowski, N. 1994. Magnetic resonance imaging of the lumbar spine in people without back pain. *New England Journal of Medicine* 2:69.

Johnson, C., and Reid, J.G. 1991. Lumbar compressive and shear forces during various curl up exercises. *Clinical Biomechanics* 6:97-104.

Johnson, J. 2002. *The multifidus back pain solution*. Oakland, DA: New Harbinger.

Jorgensen, K., and Nicolaisen, T. 1987. Trunk extensor endurance: Determination and relation to low-back trouble. *Ergonomics* 30:259-267.

Juker, D., McGill, SM Kropf, S., and Steffen, T. 1998. Quantitative intramuscular myoelectric activity of lumbar portions of psoas and the abdominal wall during a wide variety of tasks. *Medicine and Science in Sports and Exercise* 30:301-310.

Jull, G.A. 1994. Headaches of cervical origin. In *Physical therapy of the cervical and thoracic spine*. R. Grant, Ed. New York: Churchill Livingstone.

Jull, G.A., and Janda, V. 1987. Muscles and motor control in low back pain: Assessment and management. In *Physical therapy of the low back*. L.T. Twomey, Ed. New York: Churchill Livingstone.

Jull, G., and Richardson, C.A. 1994a. Active stabilisation of the trunk. Course notes. University of Edinburgh, Edinburgh, UK.

Jull, G.A., and Richardson, C.A. 1994b. Rehabilitation of active stabilization of the lumbar spine. In *Physical therapy of the low back*, 2nd ed. L.T. Twomey and L.T. Taylor, Eds. Edinburgh, UK: Churchill Livingstone.

Kapandji, I. 1974. *The physiology of joints, vol. 3. The spine*. London: Churchill Livingstone.

Keller, A., Brox, J.I., and Gunderson, R. 2004. Trunk muscle strength, cross-sectional area, and density in patients with chronic low back pain randomized to lumbar fusion or cognitive intervention and exercises. *Spine* 29:3-8.

Kendall, F.P., McCreary, E.K., and Provance, P.G. 1993. *Muscles. Testing and function*, 4th ed. Baltimore: Williams & Wilkins.

Kennedy, J.C., Alexander, I.J., and Hayes, K.C. 1982. Nerve supply of the human knee and its functional importance. *American Journal of Sports Medicine* 10:329.

Kent, M. 1994. *The Oxford dictionary of sports science and medicine*. Oxford, UK: Oxford University Press.

Kesson, M., and Atkins, E. 1998. *Orthopaedic medicine. A practical approach*. Oxford, UK: Butterworth Heinemann.

Kippers, V., and Parker, A.W. 1984. Posture related to myoelectric silence of erectores spinae during trunk flexion. *Spine* 9:740-745.

Kirby, M.C., Sikoryn, T.A., Hukins, D.W.L., and Aspden, R.M. 1989. Structure and mechanical properties of the longitudinal ligaments and ligamentum flavum of the spine. *Journal of Biomedical Engineering* 11:192-196.

Kirkaldy-Willis, W.H. 1990. *The lumbar spine.* New York: Saunders.

Klein, J.A., and Hukins, D.W.L. 1983. Relocation of the bending axis during flexion-extension of the lumbar intervertebral discs and its implications for prolapse. *Spine* 8:659-664.

Koh, T.J. 1995. Do adaptations in serial sarcomere number occur with strength training? *Human Movement Science* 14:61-77.

Konradsen, L., and Ravn, J.B. 1990. Ankle instability cause by prolonged peroneal reaction time. *Acta Orthopaedica Scandinavica* 61:388-390.

Koumantakis, A., Watson, P., and Oldham, A. 2005b. Trunk muscle stabilisation training plus general exercises versus general exercise only: Randomised controlled trial of patients with recurrent low back pain. *Physical Therapy* 85:209-225.

Koumantakis, G.A., Watson, P.J., and Oldham, J.A. 2005a. Supplementation of general endurance exercise with stabilisation training versus general exercise only. Physiological and functional outcomes of a randomised controlled trial with recurrent low back pain. *Clinical Biomechanics* 20:474-482.

Kraemer, J., Kolditz, D., and Gowin, R. 1985. Water and electrolyte content of human intervertebral discs under variable load. *Spine* 10:69-71.

Latimer, J., Maher, C.G., and Refshauge, S. 1999. The reliability and validity of the Biering-Sorensen test in asymptomatic subjects reporting current or previous non-specific low back pain. *Spine* 24:2085-2090.

Latimer, V., Kankaanpaa, M., and Airaksinen, O. 2000. Back and hip flexion/extension: Effects of low back pain and rehabilitation. *Archives of Physical Medicine and Rehabilitation* 81:32-37.

Lavignolle, B., Vital, J.M., and Senegas, J. 1983. An approach to the functional anatomy of the sacroiliac joints in vivo. *Anatomica Clinica* 5:169-176.

Leatt, P., Reilly, T., and Troup, J.G.D. 1986. Spinal loading during circuit weight-training and running. *British Journal of Sports Medicine* 20(3):119-124.

Lee, D.G. 1994. Kinematics of the pelvic joints. In *Grieve's modern manual therapy.* J.D. Boyling and N. Palastanga, Eds. Edinburgh, UK: Churchill Livingstone.

Leinonen, V., Kankaanpaa, M., Airaksinen, O., and Hannine, O. 2000. Back and hip extensor activities during trunk flexion/extension: Effects of low back pain and rehabilitation. *Archives of Physical Medicine and Rehabilitation* 81:32-37.

Lentell, G.L., Katzman, L.L., and Walters, M.R. 1990. The relationship between muscle function and ankle stability. *Journal of Orthopedic and Sports Physical Therapy* 11:605-611.

Lephart, S.M., and Fu, F.H. 1995. The role of proprioception in the treatment of sports injuries. *Sports Exercise and Injury* 1:96-102.

Lephart, S.M., Warner, J.P., Borsa, P.A., and Fu, F.H. 1994. Proprioception of the shoulder in normal, unstable, and surgical individuals. *Journal of Shoulder and Elbow Surgery* 3:224-228.

Levine, D., Walker, J.R., and Tillman, L.J. 1997. The effect of abdominal muscle strengthening on pelvic tilt and lumbar lordosis. *Physiotherapy Theory and Practice* 13:217-226.

Lewit, K. 1991. *Manipulative therapy in rehabilitation of the locomotor system.* 2nd ed. Oxford, UK: Butterworth Heinemann.

Liebenson, C. 1996. *Rehabilitation of the spine.* Baltimore: Williams & Wilkins.

Liebenson, C. 2007. Rehabilitation of the spine (2nd ed.). Philadelphia: Lippincott Williams & Wilkins.

Lieber, R.L. 1992. *Skeletal muscle structure and function.* Baltimore: Williams & Wilkins.

Linsenbardt, S.T., Thomas, T.R., and Madsen, R.W. 1992. Effect of breathing techniques on blood pressure response to resistance exercise. *British Journal of Sports Medicine* 26:97-100.

Lipetz, S., and Gutin, B. 1970. An electromyographic study of four abdominal exercises. *Medicine and Science in Sports and Exercise* 2:35-38.

Loeser, J.D. 1980. Perspectives on pain. In: Turner, P. (ed.) Clinical phasmacy and therapeutics. London: Macmillan.

Long, D.M. 1995. Effectiveness of therapies currently employed for persistent low back and leg pain. *Pain Forum* 4:122-125.

Lord, S.R., Ward, J.A., Williams, P., and Zivanovic, E. 1996. The effects of a community exercise program on fracture risk factors in older women. *Osteoporosis International* 6:361-367.

Loudon, J.K., Bell, S.L., and Johnston, J.M. 1998. *The clinical orthopedic assessment guide.* Champaign, IL: Human Kinetics.

Lovell, F.W., Rothstein, J.M., and Personius, W.J. 1989. Reliability of clinical measurements of lumbar lordosis taken with a flexible rule. *Physical Therapy* 69:96-105.

Macintosh, J.E., and Bogduk, N. 1986. The biomechanics of the lumbar multifidus. *Clinical Biomechanics* 1:205-213.

Macintosh, J.E., and Bogduk, N. 1987. The anatomy and function of the lumbar back muscles and their fascia. In *Physical therapy of the low back.* L.T. Twomey, Ed. New York: Churchill Livingstone.

Macintosh, J.E., Bogduk, N., and Gracovetsky, S. 1987. The biomechanics of the thoracolumbar fascia. *Clinical Biomechanics* 2:78-83.

Main, C.J., and Waddell, G. 2004. Beliefs about back pain. In Waddell, G. (ed.) The back pain revolution (2nd ed.). Churchill Livingstone: Edinburgh.

Main, C.J., and Watson, P.J. 1996. Guarded movements: Development of chronicity. *Journal of Musculoskeletal Pain* 4:163-170.

Maitland, G.D. 1986. *Vertebral manipulation*, 5th ed. London: Butterworths.

Markolf, K.L., and Morris, J.M. 1974. The structural components of the intervertebral disc. *Journal of Bone and Joint Surgery* 56A:675-687.

McClure, P.W., Esola, M., Schreier, R., and Siegler, S. 1997. Kinematic analysis of lumbar and hip motion while rising from a forward, flexed position in patients with and without a history of low back pain. *Spine* 22:552-558.

McConnell, J. 1993. Promoting effective segmental alignment. In *Key issues in musculoskeletal physiotherapy*. J. Crosbie and J. McConnell, Eds. Oxford, UK: Butterworth Heinemann.

McGill, S. 2002. *Low back disorders*. Champaign, IL: Human Kinetics.

McGill, S.M., and Brown, S. 1992. Creep response of the lumbar spine to prolonged lumbar flexion. *Clinical Biomechanics* 7:43.

McGill, S.M., Childs, A., and Liebenson, C 1999. Endurance times for stabilisation exercises: Clinical targets for testing and training from a normal database. *Archives of Physical Medicine and Rehabilitation* 80:941-944.

McGill, S.M. 1997. Distribution of tissue loads in the low back during a variety of daily and rehabilitation tasks. *Journal of Rehabilitation Research and Development* 34:448-458.

McGill, S.M. 1998. Low back exercises: Evidence for improving exercise regimens. *Physical Therapy* 78:754-765.

McGill, S.M., and Norman, R.W. 1986. Partitioning of the L4-L5 dynamic moment into disc, ligamentous, and muscular components during lifting. *Spine* 11:666-678.

McGill, S.M., Norman, R.W., and Sharratt, M.T. 1990. The effect of an abdominal belt on trunk muscles activity and intra-abdominal pressure during squat lifts. *Ergonomics* 33:147-160.

McGill, S.M., Juker, D., and Kropf, P. 1996. Quantitative intramuscular myoelectric activity of quadratus lumborum during a wide variety of tasks. *Clinical Biomechanics* 11:170-172.

McKenzie, R.A. 1981. *The lumbar spine. Mechanical diagnosis and therapy*. Lower Hutt, New Zealand: Spinal Publications.

McKenzie, R.A. 1990. *The cervical and thoracic spine. Mechanical diagnosis and therapy*. Lower Hutt, New Zealand: Spinal Publications.

McLean, I. P., Gillan, M. G., Ross, J. C., Aspden, R. M., and Porter, R. W. 1996. A comparison of methods for measuring trunk list. A simple plumbline is the best. *Spine, 21(14)*, 1667-70.

Merskey, H., and Bogduk, N. 1994. Classification of Chronic Pain (2nd ed). IASP Task Force on Taxonomy. IASP Press: Seattle.

Miller, J.A.A., Haderspeck, K.A., and Schultz, A.B. 1983. Posterior element loads in lumbar motion segments. *Spine* 8:331-337.

Miller, M.I., and Medeiros, J.M. 1987. Recruitment of internal oblique and transversus abdominis muscles during the eccentric phase of the curl-up exercise. *Physical Therapy* 67:1213-1217.

Moffroid, M.T., Reid, S., and Henry, S. 1994. Some endurance measures in persons with chronic low back pain. *Journal of Orthopedic and Sports Physical Therapy* 20:81-87.

Mooney, V., Pozos, R., and Vleeming, A. 2001. Exercise treatment for sacroiliac pain. *Orthopedics* 24:29-32.

Mooney, V., and Robertson, J. 1976. The facet sydrome. *Clinical Orthopaedics and Related Research*. 115, 149-156.

Moore, M.A., and Kukulka, C.G. 1991. Depression of Hoffman reflexes following voluntary contraction and implications for proprioceptive neuromuscular facilitation therapy. *Physical Therapy* 71:321-333.

Morgan, D.L., and Lynn, R. 1994. Decline running produces more sarcomeres in rat vastus intermedius muscle fibers than does incline running. *Journal of Applied Physiology* 77:1439-1444.

Morris, J.M., Lucas, D.B., and Bresler, B. 1961. Role of the trunk in stability of the spine. *Journal of Bone and Joint Surgery* (American volume) 43A:327-351.

Moseley, G.L., Hodges, P.W., and Gandevia, S.C. 2002. Deep and superficial fibers of lumbar multifidus are differentially active during voluntary arm movements. *Spine* 27:E29-E36.

Moseley, G.L., Hodges, P.W., and Gandevia, S.C. 2003. External perturbation of the trunk in standing humans differentially activates components of the medial back muscles. *Journal of Physiology* 547:581-587.

Mottram, S.L. 1997. Dynamic stability of the scapula. *Manual Therapy* 2:123-131.

Murray, M.P., Seireg, A., and Sepic, S.B. 1975. Normal postural stability and steadiness: Quantitative assessment. *Journal of Bone and Joint Surgery* 57A:510-516.

Nachemson, A.L. 1992. Newest knowledge of low back pain. *Clinical Orthopaedics* 279:8.

Nachemson, A., and Evans, J. 1968. Some mechanical properties of the third lumbar laminar ligament (ligamentum flavum). *Journal of Biomechanics* 1:211.

Newcomer, K.L., Laskowski, E.R., Yu, B., Johnson, J.C., and An, K.N. 2000. Differences in repositioning error among patients with low back pain compared with control subjects. *Spine* 25:2488-2493.

Ng, G., and Richardson, C.A. 1990. The effects of training triceps surae using progressive speed loading. *Physiotherapy Practice* 6:77-84.

Ng, G., and Richardson, C. 1994. EMG study of erector spinae and multifidus in two isometric back extension exercises. *Australian Journal of Physiotherapy* 40:115-121.

Norkin, C.C., and Levangie, P.K. 1992. *Joint structure and function. A comprehensive analysis*, 2nd ed. Philadelphia: Davis.

Norris, C.M. 1993. Abdominal muscle training in sport. *British Journal of Sports Medicine* 27:19-27.

Norris, C.M. 1994a. Abdominal training. Dangers and exercise modifications. *Physiotherapy in Sport* 14:10-14.

Norris, C.M. 1994b. Taping: Components, applications and mechanisms. *Sports Exercise and Injury* 1:14-17.

Norris, C.M. 1995a. Spinal stabilisation 2. Limiting factors to end-range motion in the lumbar spine. *Physiotherapy* 81:4-12.

Norris, C.M. 1995b. *Weight training. Principles and practice.* London: A&C Black.

Norris, C.M. 1997. *Abdominal training.* London: A&C Black.

Norris, C.M. 1998. *Sports injuries. Diagnosis and management,* 2nd ed. Oxford, UK: Butterworth Heinemann.

Norris, C.M. 2004a. Iliotibial band friction syndrome: Rehabilitation. *Sportex Medicine* April:6-11.

Norris, C.M. 2004b. *Sports injuries. Diagnosis and management,* 3rd ed. Oxford, UK: Elsevier.

Norris, C.M., and Berry, S. 1998. Occurrence of common lumbar posture types in the student sporting population: An initial evaluation. *Sports, Exercise, and Injury* 4:15-18.

Norris, C.M., and Mathews, M. 2006. Correlation between hamstring muscle length and pelvic tilt range during forward bending in healthy individuals. An initial evaluation. *Journal of bodywork and movement therapies.*

Nourbakhsh, M.R., and Arab, A.M. 2002. Relationship between mechanical factors and incidence of low back pain. *Journal of Orthopaedic and Sports Physical Therapy.* 32: 447-460.

Oliver, J., and Middleditch, A. 1991. *Functional anatomy of the spine.* Oxford, UK: Butterworth Heinemann.

Ostelo, R.W., de Vet, H.C., Waddell, G, and Kerckhoffs, M.R. 2003. Rehabilitation following first-time lumber disc surgery: A systematic review within the framework of the Cochrane Collaboration. *Spine* 28:209-218.

O'Sullivan, P.B., Burnett, A., Floyd, A.N., and Gadsdon, K. 2003. Lumbar repositioning deficit in a specific low back pain population. *Spine* 28:1074-1079.

O'Sullivan, P.B., Twomey, L.T., and Allison, G.T. 1997. Evaluation of specific stabilizing exercise in the treatment of chronic low back pain with radiologic diagnosis of spondylolysis or spondylolisthesis. *Spine* 22:2959-2967.

O'Sullivan, P.B., Twomey, L., and Allison, G.T. 1998. Altered abdominal muscle recruitment in patients with chronic back pain following a specific exercise intervention. *Journal of Orthopedic and Sports Physical Therapy* 27:114-124.

Palastanga, N., Field, D., and Soames, R. 1994. *Anatomy and human movement,* 2nd ed. Oxford, UK: Butterworth Heinemann.

Panjabi, M.M. 1992. The stabilizing system of the spine. Part 1. Function, dysfunction, adaptation, and enhancement. *Journal of Spinal Disorders* 5:383-389.

Panjabi, M.M., Abumi, K., Duranceau, J., and Oxland, T. 1989. Spinal stability and intersegmental muscle forces. A biomechanical model. *Spine* 14:194-200.

Panjabi, M.M., Hult, J.E., and White, A.A. 1987. Biomechanics studies in cadaveric spines. In *The lumbar spine and back pain.* M.I.V. Jayson, Ed. Edinburgh, UK: Churchill Livingstone.

Panjabi, M.M., and White, A.A. 1990. Physical properties and functional biomechanics of the spine. In *Clinical biomechanics of the spine.* A.A. White and M.M. Panjabi, Eds. Philadelphia: Lippincott.

Paris, S.V. 1985. Physical signs of instability. *Spine* 10:277-279.

Parkkola, R., Rytokoski, U., and Kormano, M. 1993. Magnetic resonance imaging of the discs and trunk muscles in patients with chronic low back pain and healthy control subjects. *Spine* 18:830-836.

Parnianpour, M., Nordin, M., Kahanovitz, N., and Frankel, V. 1988. The triaxial coupling of torque generation of trunk muscles during isometric exertions and the effect of fatiguing isoinertial movements on the motor output and movement patterns. *Spine* 13:982-992.

Pearcy, P., Portek, I., and Shepherd, J. 1984. Three dimensional X ray analysis of normal movement in the lumbar spine. *Spine* 9:294-297.

Penning, L. 2000. Psoas muscle and lumbar spine stability: a concept uniting existing controversies. Critical review and hypothesis. *European Spine Journal, 9(6),* 577-585.

Percy, O. 1957. Fracture of the vertebral end plate in the lumbar spine. *Acta Orthopaedica Scandinavica Supplementum* 25:1-101.

Pope, M.H., and Panjabi, M.M. 1985. Biomechanical definitions of instability. *Spine* 10:255-256.

Porter, J. L., and Wilkinson, A. 1997. Lumbar-hip flexion motion. A comparative study between asymptomatic and chronic low back pain in 18 to 36 year old men. *Spine, 22(13),* 1508-13.

Ricci, B., Marchetti, M., and Figura, F. 1981. Biomechanics of sit up exercises. *Medicine and Science in Sports and Exercise* 13:54-59.

Richardson, C.A. 1992. Muscle imbalance: Principles of treatment and assessment. In *Proceedings of the New Zealand Society of Physiotherapists Challenges Conference,* Christchurch, New Zealand.

Richardson, C.A., and Bullock, M.I. 1986. Changes in muscle activity during fast, alternating flexion-extension movements of the knee. *Scandinavian Journal of Rehabilitation Medicine* 18:51-58.

Richardson, C.A., and Hodges, P. 1996. New advances in exercise to rehabilitate spinal stabilisation. Course notes. University of Edinburgh, Edinburgh, UK.

Richardson, C., Jull, G., Toppenburg, R., and Comerford, M. 1992. Techniques for active lumbar stabilisation for spinal protection: A pilot study. *Australian Journal of Physiotherapy* 38:105-112.

Richardson, C.A., and Sims, K. 1991. An inner range holding contraction: An objective measure of stabilising function of an antigravity muscle. In *Proceedings of the World Confederation for Physical Therapy, 11th International Congress,* London.

Richardson, C.A., Snijders, C.J., and Hides, J.A. 2002. The relation between the transversus abdominis muscles, sacroliliac joint mechanics, and low back pain. *Spine* 27:399-405.

Richardson, C., Toppenberg, R., and Jull, G. 1990. An initial evaluation of eight abdominal exercises for their ability to provide stabilisation for the lumbar spine. *Australian Journal of Physiotherapy* 36:6-11.

Risch, S.V., Norvell, N.K., Pollock, M.L., Risch, E.D., Langer, H., Fulton, M., Graves, J.E., and Leggett, S.H. 1993. Lumbar strengthening in chronic low back pain patients. Physical and psychological benefits. *Spine* 18:232-238.

Risser, W.L. 1991. Weight training injuries in children and adolescents. *American Family Physician* 44:2104-2108.

Risser, W.L., Risser, J.M., and Preston, D. 1990. Weight training injuries in adolescents. *American Journal of Diseases in Children* 144:1015-1017.

Rivero-Arias, O., Campbell, H., Gray, A., and Fairbank, J. 2005. Surgical stabilisation of the spine compared with a programme of intensive rehabilitation for the management of patients with chronic low back pain: Cost utility analysis based on a randomised controlled trial. *British Medical Journal* 330:1239.

Roaf, R. 1960. A study of the mechanics of spinal injuries. *Journal of Bone and Joint Surgery* 42B:810-823.

Rockoff, S.F., Sweet, E., and Bleustein, J. 1969. The relative contribution of trabecular and cortical bone to the strength of human lumbar vertebrae. *Calcified Tissue Research* 3:163-175.

Roland, M., and Morris, R. 1983. A study of the natural history of backpain. Part 1: Development of a reliable and sensitive measure of disability in low back pain. *Spine* 8:141-144.

Rose, S.J., Sahrman, S.A., and Norton, B.T. 1988. Quantitative assessment of lumbar-pelvic rhythm. *Physical Therapy* 68:824.

Saal, J.A. 1988. Rehabilitation of football players with lumbar spine injury. *Physician and Sportsmedicine* 16:61-67.

Saal, J.A. 1995. The pathophysiology of painful lumbar disorder. *Spine* 20:180-183.

Saal, J.A., and Saal, J.S. 1989. Nonoperative treatment of herniated lumbar intervertebral disc with radiculopathy. *Spine* 14:431-437.

Sahrmann, S.A. 1987. Posture and muscle imbalance: Faulty lumbar-pelvic alignment and associated musculoskeletal pain syndromes. In *Postgraduate advances in physical therapy.* Berryvill, VA: Forum Medicum.

Sahrmann, S.A. 1990. Diagnosis and treatment of movement related pain syndromes associated with muscle and movement imbalances. Course notes. Washington University.

Sahrmann, S. A. 2002. *Diagnosis and treatment of movement impairment syndromes.* New York: Mosby.

San Juan, J., Yaggie, J., Levy, S., Mooney, V., and Udermann, B. 2005. Effects of pelvic stabilization on lumbar muscle activity during dynamic exercise. *Journal of Strength and Conditioning Research, 19(4),* 903-907.

Scannell, J.P., and McGill, S.M. 2003. Lumbar posture: Should it and can it be modified? *Physical Therapy* 83:907-917.

Scavone, K.P., Latshaw, R.F., and Rohrar, G.V. 1981. Use of lumbar spine films: Statistical evaluation at auniversity teaching hospital. *Journal of the American Medical Association* 246:1105-1108.

Schonstein, E., Kenny, D.T., Keating, J., and Koes, B.W. 2003. Work conditioning, work hardening and functional restoration for workers with back and neck pain (Cochrane Review) (Issue 3). Oxford, UK: The Cochrane Library.

Shakespeare, D.T., Stokes, M., Sherman, K.P., and Young, A. 1985. Reflex inhibition of the quadriceps after meniscenctomy: Lack of association with pain. *Clinical Physiology* 5:137-144.

Sharma, M., Langrama, N.A., and Rodriguez, J. 1995. Role of ligaments and facets in lumbar spine stability. *Spine* 20:887.

Shields, R.K., and Heiss, D.G. 1997. An electromyographic comparison of abdominal muscle synergies during curl and double straight leg lowering exercises with control of the pelvic position. *Spine* 22:1873-1879.

Sihoven, T. 1997. Flexion relaxation of the hamstring muscles during lumbar-pelvic rhythm. *Archives of Physical Medicine and Rehabilitation* 78(5)486-490.

Sihvonen, T., Herno, A., Palijarvi, L., and Partanen, J. 1993. Local denervation atrophy of paraspinal muscles in postoperative failed back syndrome. *Spine* 18: 575-581.

Silvermetz, M.A. 1990. Pathokinesiology of supine double leg lifts as an abdominal strengthener and suggested alternative exercises. *Athletic Training* 25:17-22.

Simmonds, M.J., and Claveau, Y. 1997. Measures of pain and physical function in patients with low back pain. *Physiotherapy Theory and Practice* 13:53-65.

Simmonds, M.J., and Lee, E. 2007. Physical performance tests: An expanded model of assessment and outcome. In *Rehabilitation of the spine*. C. Liebensen, Ed. Philadelphia: Lippincott.

Skall, F.H., Manniche, C., and Nielsen, C.J. 1994. Intensive back exercises 5 weeks after surgery of lumbar disk prolapse. A prospective randomized multicenter trial with a historical control group. *Ugeskr Laeger* 156:643-646.

Smith, R.L., and Brunolli, J. 1990. Shoulder kinesthesia after anterior glenohumeral joint dislocation. *Physical Therapy* 69:106-112.

Spitzer, W.O., Le Blanc, F.E., and Dupuis, M. 1987. Scientific approach to the assessment and management of activity related spinal disorders: A monograph for clinicians. Report of the Quebec Task Force on Spinal Disorders. *Spine* 12(Suppl 7):134-147.

Stokes, M., and Young, A. 1984. The contribution of relex inhibition to arthrogenous muscle weakness. *Clinical Science* 67:7-14.

Sturesson, B., Selvik, G., and Uden, A. 1989. Movements of the sacroiliac joints. A roentgen stereophotogrammetric analysis. *Spine* 14:162-165.

Sugano, H., and Takeya, T. 1970. Measurement of body movement and its clinical application. *Japanese Journal of Physiology* 20:296-308.

Sullivan, M.S. 1997. Lifting and back pain. In *Physical therapy of the low back*. L.T. Twomey and J.R. Taylor, Eds. Edinburgh, UK: Churchill Livingstone.

Sullivan, P.E., Markos, P.D., and Minor, M.A.D. 1982. *An integrated approach to therapeutic exercise.* Reston, VA: Reston Publishing.

Swanepoel, M.W., Adams, L.M., and Smeathers, J.E. 1995. Human lumbar apophyseal joint damage and intervertebral disc degeneration. *Annals of the Rheumatic Diseases* 54:182-188.

Taylor, D.C., Dalton, J., Seaber, A.V., and Garrett, W.E. 1990. The viscoelastic properties of muscle-tendon units. *American Journal of Sports Medicine* 18:300-309.

Taylor, J.R., and Twomey, L.T. 1986. Age changes in lumbar zygapophyseal joints. *Spine* 11:739-745.

Templeton, G.H., Padalino, M., and Manton, J. 1984. Influence of suspension hypokinesia on rat soleus muscle. *Journal of Applied Physiology* 56:278-286.

Tesh, K.M., Shaw-Dunn, J., and Evans, J.H. 1987. The abdominal muscles and vertebral stability. *Spine* 12:501-508.

Thapa, P.B., Gideon, P., Brockman, K.G., Fought, R.L., and Ray, W.A. 1996. Clinical and biomechanical measures of balance as fall predictors in ambulatory nursing home residents. *Journal of Gerontology* 51:239-246.

Thomason, D.B., Herrick, R.E., Surdyka, D., and Baldwin, K.M. 1987. Time course of soleus muscle myosin expression during hind limb suspension and recovery. *Journal of Applied Physiology* 63:130-137.

Thompson, L.V. 2002. Skeletal muscle adaptations with age, inactivity, and therapeutic exercise. *Journal of Orthopaedic and Sports Physical Therapy* 32:45-57.

Tkaczuk, H. 1968. Tensile properties of human lumbar longitudinal ligaments. *Acta Orthopaedica Scandinavica Supplementum* 115:17-25.

Toppenburg, R.M., and Bullock, M.I. 1986. The interrelation of spinal curves, pelvic tilt and muscle lengths in the adolescent female. *Australian Journal of Physiotherapy* 32:6-12.

Travell, J.G., and Simmons, D.G. 1983. *Myofascial pain and dysfunction.* Baltimore: Williams & Wilkins.

Tropp, H., Alaranta, H., and Renstrom, P.A.F.H. 1993. Proprioception and coordination training in injury prevention. In *Sports injuries: Basic principles of prevention and care.* IOC Medical Commission publication. P.A.F.H. Renstrom, Ed. London: Blackwell Scientific.

Twomey, L.T., and Taylor, J.R. 1987. Lumbar posture, movement and mechanics. In *Physical therapy of the low back.* L.T. Twomey, Ed. New York: Churchill Livingstone.

Twomey, L.T., and Taylor, J.R. 1994. Factors influencing ranges of movement in the spine. In *Physical therapy of the low back,* 2nd ed. L.T. Twomey and J.R. Taylor, Eds. Edinburgh, UK: Churchill Livingstone.

Twomey, L.T., and Taylor, J.R. 2000. *Physical therapy of the low back,* 3rd ed. Edinburgh, UK: Churchill Livingstone.

Twomey, L.T., Taylor, J.R., and Oliver, M. 1988. Sustained flexion loading, rapid extension loading of the lumbar spine and the physical therapy of related injuries. *Physiotherapy Practice* 4:129-138.

Tye, J., and Brown, V. 1990. *Back pain—the ignored epidemic.* London: British Safety Council.

Tyldesley, B., and Grieve, J.I. 1989. *Muscles, nerves and movement: Kinesiology in daily living.* Oxford, UK: Blackwell Scientific.

Tyrrell, A.R., Reilly, T., and Troup, J.D.G. 1985. Circadian variation in stature and the effects of spinal loading. *Spine* 10:161-164.

Uber-Zak, L.D., and Venkatesh, Y.S. 2002. Neurologic complications of sit-ups associated with the Valsalva maneuver: 2 case reports. *Archives of Physical Medicine and Rehabilitation* 83:278-282.

Urquhart, D.M., and Hodges, P.W. 2005. Differential activity of regions of transversus abdominis during trunk rotation. *European Spine Journal* 14:393-400.

Urquhart, D.M., Hodges, P.W., and Story, I.H. 2005. Postural activity of the abdominal muscles varies between regions of these muscles and between body positions. *Gait Posture* 22:295-301.

Valencia, F.P., and Munro, R.R. 1985. An electromyographic study of the lumbar multifidus in man. *Electromyography and Clinical Neurophysiology* 25:205-221.

Vernon-Roberts, B. 1987. Pathology of intervertebral discs and apophyseal joints. In *The lumbar spine and back pain.* M.I.V. Jayson, Ed. Edinburgh, UK: Churchill Livingstone.

Vernon-Roberts, B. 1992. Age related and degenerative pathology of intervertebral discs and apophyseal joints. In *The lumbar spine and back pain.* M.I.V. Jayson, Ed. Edinburgh, UK: Churchill Livingstone.

Videman, T., Nurminen, M., and Troup, J.D.G. 1990. Lumbar spine pathology in cadaveric material in relation to history of back pain, occupation, and physical loading. *Spine* 15:728-740.

Vlaeyen, J.W.S., Kole-Snijders, A.M.J., Boeren, R.G.B., and van Eek, H. 1995. Fear of movement/reinjury in chronic low back pain and its relation to behavioural performance. *Pain* 62:363-372.

Vleeming, A., Mooney, V., Snijders, C.J., Dorman, T.A., and Stoeckart, R. 1997. *Movement stability and low back pain.* New York: Churchill Livingstone.

Vleeming, A., Pool-Goudzwaard, A.L., Stoeckart, R., Wingerden, J.P., and Snijders, C.J. 1995. The posterior layer of the thoracolumbar fascia: Its function in load transfer from spine to legs. *Spine* 20:753-758.

Vleeming, A., Stoeckart, R., and Snijders, C. 1989. The sacrotuberous ligament: A conceptual approach to its dynamic role in stabilizing the sacroiliac joint. *Clinical Biomechanics* 4:201-203.

Vleeming, A., Stoeckart, R., Volkers, A.C.W., and Snijders, C.J. 1990. Relation between form and function in the sacroiliac joint. *Spine* 15:130-132.

Waddell, G. 1987. A new clinical model for the treatment of low-back pain. *Spine* 12:632-644.

Waddell, G. 2004. *The back pain revolution,* 2nd ed. Edinburgh, UK: Churchill Livingstone.

Waddell, G., and Burton, A. K. 2005. Concepts of rehabilitation for the management of low back pain. *Best Practice Research in Clinical Rheumatology, 19(4),* 655-70.

Waddell, G., Feder, G., and Lewis, M. 1997. Systematic reviews of bed rest and advice to stay active for acute low back pain. *British Journal of General Practice* 47:647-652.

Waddell, G., and Main, C.J. 1984. Assessment of severity in low back disorders. *Spine* 9:204-208.

Waddell, G., McCullock, J.A., Kummel, E., and Venner, R.M. 1980. Non-organic physical signs in low back pain. *Spine* 5:117-125.

Walker, M.L., Rothstein, J.M., Finucane, S.D., and Lamb, R.L. 1987. Relationships between lumbar lordosis, pelvic tilt, and abdominal muscle performance. *Physical Therapy* 67:512-516.

Walters, C., and Partridge, M. 1957. Electromyographic study of the differential abdominal muscles during exercise. *American Journal of Physical Medicine* 36:259-268.

Watkins, J. 1999. *Structure and function of the musculoskeletal system.* Champaign, IL: Human Kinetics.

Watson, D.H. 1994. Cervical headache: An investigation of natural head posture and upper cervical flexor muscle performance. In *Grieve's modern manual therapy,* 2nd ed. J.D. Boyline and N. Palastanga, Eds. Edinburgh, UK: Churchill Livingstone.

Watson, J. 1983. *An introduction for mechanics of human movement.* Lancaster, UK: MTP Press.

Weber, H. 1983. Lumbar disc herniation: A controlled prospective study with ten years of observation. *Spine* 8:131-138.

Webright, W.G., Randolph, B.J., and Perrin, D.H. 1997. Comparison of nonballistic active knee extension in neural slump position and static techniques on hamstring flexibility. *Journal of Orthopedic and Sports Physical Therapy* 26:7-13.

Weider, J. 1989. *Ultimate bodybuilding.* Chicago: Contemporary Books.

White, S.G., and Sahrmann, S.A. 1994. A movement system balance approach to management of musculoskeletal pain. In *Physical therapy of the cervical and thoracic spine.* R. Grant, Ed. New York: Churchill Livingstone.

WHO, 1980. International classification of impairments, disabilities, and handicaps. World Health Organisation. Geneva.

Wilke, H.J., Wolf, S., Claes, L.E., Arand, M., and Weisend, A. 1995. Stability increase of the lumbar spine with different muscle groups: A biomechanical in vitro study. *Spine* 20:192-198.

Willard, F.H. 1997. The muscular, ligamentous and neural structure of the low back and its relation to back pain. In *Movement stability and low back pain.* A. Vleeming, V. Mooney, T. Dorman, C. Snijders, and R. Stoeckart, Eds. Edinburgh, UK: Churchill Livingstone.

Williams, M., Solomonow, M., Zhou, B.H., and Baratta, R.V. 2000. Multifidus spasms elicited by prolonged lumbar flexion. *Spine* 25:2916-2924.

Williams, P., Watt, P., Bicik, V., and Goldspink, G. 1986. Effect of stretch combined with electrical stimulation on the type of sarcomeres produced at the ends of muscle fibers. *Experimental Neurology* 93:500-509.

Williams, P.E. 1990. Use of intermittent stretch in the prevention of serial sarcomere loss in immobilised muscle. *Annals of the Rheumatic Diseases* 49:316-317.

Williams, P.E., and Goldspink, G. 1978. Changes in sarcomere length and physiological properties in immobilised muscle. *Journal of Anatomy* 127:459-468.

Wong, T. K., and Lee, R. Y. 2004. Effects of low back pain on the relationship between the movements of the lumbar spine and hip. *Human Movement Science, 23(1),* 21-34.

Yamamoto, I., Panjabi, M.M., Oxland, T.R., and Crisco, J.J. 1990. The role of the iliolumbar ligament in the lumbosacral junction. *Spine* 15:1138-1141.

Yang, K.H., and King, A.I. 1984. Mechanism of facet load transmission as a hypothesis for low back pain. *Spine* 9:557-565.

Yong-Hing, K., Reilly, J., and Kirkaldy-Willis, W.H. 1976. The ligamentum flavum. *Spine* 1:226-234.

Young, A., Stokes, M., and Iles, J.F. 1987. Effects of joint pathology on muscle. *Clinical Orthopaedics and Related Research* 219:21-27.

Zetterberg, C., Andersson, G.B.J., and Schultz, A.B. 1987. The activity of individual trunk muscles during heavy physical loading. *Spine* 12:1035-1040.

Zusman, M. 1998. Structure-oriented beliefs and disability due to back pain. *Australian Journal of Physiotherapy* 44:13-20.

Index

Note: The italicized *f* and *t* following page numbers refer to figures and tables, respectively.

A

abdominal hollowing
  in case histories 317-322
  common errors in 136-137, 137*f*
  from four-point kneeling 133, 135*t*, 136, 153
  function of 52-53, 54
  intra-abdominal pressure and 57
  pressure feedback test 113
  in prone-lying position 134, 135*t*, 156
  in sitting position 134, 135*t*, 155
  in standing position 134, 135*t*, 137*f*, 154
  starting positions 133-137, 135*t*, 136*f*, 137*f*
  in supine-lying position 157
  tips for teaching 133, 134-136, 136*f*
  training specificity 67, 67*f*
abdominal machine 263
abdominal muscles. *See also* abdominal training
  anatomy of deep 52, 53*f*
  anatomy of superficial 51-52, 51*f*
  back flattening exercise 92
  coordination of 54-55, 54*f*
  deep (*See* deep abdominal muscles)
  functions of 52-54, 54*f*
  inner-range holding tests on deep 105
  intra-abdominal pressure mechanism 51, 55-58, 55*f*
  in lifting 36, 37
  in modified sit-ups 233-234, 234*f*, 235*t*
  speed and power exercise for 278
  superficial 51-52, 51*f*
abdominal slide 205
abdominal training 233-248
  abdominal machine 263
  basic crunch 243
  bench curl 238
  bent-knee sit-up 236
  bent-knee sit-up endurance test 247
  Biering-Sorensen test 48, 234, 246
  bilateral straight-leg lowering 240
  double crunch 245
  full heel slide 239
  half lunge without chair 91
  lying pelvic raise 241

midsection muscle endurance testing 234-235, 235*t*
  pulley crunch 264
  reverse crunch 244
  side bridge endurance test 248
  side crunch 245
  sit-up modifications 233-234, 234*f*, 235*t*, 236
  straight-leg raise modifications 234
  trunk curls 88, 206, 207, 237, 277
  wall bar–hanging leg raise 242-243
ab roller exercises 234
active knee extension, holding thigh 121
active knee extension, pushing against thigh 122
active stretching technique 107-108, 107*t*
activities of daily living, hamstring muscle activity and 35. *See also* functional training
Adams, M.A. 29
adenosine triphosphate 21
adipose tissue pad 22
aging
  body height reduction and 22-23
  chronic muscle tightness and 311-312
  facet joints and 22
  flexion and 29-30
  kinesthesia decreases and 192
  ligament stiffness and 20
  postural sway and 74
  spinal discs and 20, 21, 22-23, 23*f*
agonists 61
ALL (anterior longitudinal ligament) 17*t*, 18*f*, 19-20
Allan, D.B. 6
anatomy of the lumbar spine 15-25
  deep abdominal muscles 52, 53*f*
  facet joints 15, 17, 17*t*, 22
  ligaments 15, 16-20, 17*t*
  sacroiliac joint 24-25, 24*f*, 25*t*
  spinal discs 20-21, 21*f*
  spinal segments 15, 17*f*
  superficial abdominal muscles 51-52, 51*f*
  thoracolumbar fascia 40-41, 40*f*, 41*f*
  vertebral bones and joints 15, 16*f*

Andersson, E. 50
ankle injury, postural sway and 74
annulus fibrosis
  age-related changes in 23
  in axial compression 26
  during flexion 28-29, 29*f*
  in rotation 30
  structure of 20-21, 21*f*
antagonists 61
anterior longitudinal ligament (ALL) 17*t*, 18*f*, 19-20
anterior pelvic tilt, in lumbar flexion 31, 32*f*, 32*t*
anticipation of pain 4-5
anticipatory bracing 57-58, 57*f*
aponeuroses 43, 52
apophysial joint 15
Appell, H.J. 65
approximate movement 25
arch model of the spine 35-36, 36*f*
arctan 80
arm fixation, in straight-leg raises 230
arthrogenous inhibition 65
articular cartilage 22
articulating triad 15
assessment. *See* preliminary client assessment
athlete with poor stability case history 318-319
atrophy, muscle fiber type and 65
axial compression 25-28, 27*f*, 28*f*
axial loading test 306

B

back care in the home 286, 286*f*
back extension (frame) 258
back extension (machine) 257
back extensor endurance test (Biering-Sorensen test) 48, 234, 246
back flattening exercise 92
back pain. *See* low back pain
balance beam walk 220
balance board, sitting pelvic tilt exercise using 197
ballistic stretching 106-108, 107*t*
barbell lunge 270
Barrack, R.L. 192
baseline posture assessments 79
basic crunch 243
basic superman exercise 207

bed rest, negative effects from prolonged 4, 6, 314
belt, as abdominal hollowing aid 136, 136*f*
bench curl 238
bending
    forward 127, 148
    functional training for 286, 286*f*
physiology of 35
bent-knee sit-up 236, 247
bent-knee sit-up endurance test 247
bent-leg lift 172
Beurskens, A.J. 302
biceps femoris 43, 65
Biedermann, H.J. 45-46
Biering-Sorensen test 48, 234, 246
bilateral straight-leg lowering 240
bilateral straight-leg-raise movement, stability reduction from 11-12
birddog exercise 176, 177
body alignment. *See* posture
body height
    in axial compression of discs 26-27, 27*f*
    reduction with aging 22-23
body lift, side-lying 181
body segment measures 79-81, 80*f*, 81*f*
body segment positioning exercises 93, 151
body sway (postural sway) 73, 74, 174
bone density, disc surgery and 6
bowstringing 84, 227
brain stem, proprioception and 132, 132*t*
breathing, intra-abdominal pressure and 57
bridge
    from crook lying 173
    with gym ball 208
    gym ball, with roller 224
    heel 212
    with heel raise on roller 223
    with leg lift 173
    with leg lift and extension on gym ball 210
    with leg lift on gym ball 209
    one-leg heel 212
    with pelvic tilt 209
    reverse 211
    reverse, and roll 211
    side 181, 235*t*
    with therapist pressure 210
Brox, J.I. 6
Bullock, M.I. 67
Bullock-Saxton, J. 79

C

cable crossover 256
cadavers, problems with results from 40

Cairns, M.C. 8
capsular ligaments 17*t*
cartilage end plates 20-21
case history illustrations
    athlete with poor stability 318-319
    client with acute pain 319-320
    overweight client 317-318
    patient unwilling to exercise 320-321
    pregnant client with back pain 321-322
cat stretch 124
cauda equina syndrome 303, 304*t*
caudally, definition of 18
center of gravity, in traditional sit-ups 228, 229*f*
central nervous system, spinal stiffness monitoring by 57
cervical spine 15, 16*f*, 27
chest–pelvis stacking 93
Choi, G. 47
chronic low back disorder, exercise program *vs.* surgery for 8
chronic low back pain (CLBP)
    abdominal muscle coordination and 54, 54*f*
    disability from 5-6
    flexion relaxation response failure and 34
    hamstring tightness and 35
    motor control deficit in 57-58, 57*f*
    psychology of 5
    standard physiotherapy rehabilitation and 8-9
clamshell exercise 178
CLBP. *See* chronic low back pain
client assessment. *See* preliminary client assessment
closed kinetic chain actions 62
coccyx 15, 16*f*
collagen 23, 26, 39
compression, axial 25-28, 27*f*, 28*f*
concentric–eccentric coupling 272
conjoint tendon 52
connective tissue rim 22
contact sports, benefits of weight training to 249
contract–relax–agonist–contract (CRAC) stretching 106, 107*t*, 108
contract–relax (CR) stretching 106-108, 107*t*
contralateral, definition of 31
contralateral rotation 48
controlled forward bending 148
controlled sit-down 296
Cornwall, M.W. 46
cough-and-hold procedure 134, 136
countermovement jumps 272
counternutation 24-25, 25*t*
CRAC (contract–relax–agonist–contract) stretching 106, 107*t*, 108

craniovertebral (CV) angle measurement 80-81, 81*f*
creep 26, 30
Cresswell, A.G. 58
critical point (flexion relaxation response) 34, 34*f*
crook-lying exercises
    assisted pelvic tilt 145
    limb loading 166, 170, 173
cross-sectional area (CSA) 45-46, 47, 65
CR (contract–relax) stretching 106-108, 107*t*
crunches
    basic 243
    double 245
    pulley 264
    reverse 244
    side 245
CSA (cross-sectional area) 45-46, 47, 65
CV (craniovertebral) angle measurement 80-81, 81*f*

D

dancers, enhanced kinesthesia in 192
dangerous exercises 230-232
Danneels, L. 47
deadlift exercise 281
deadlift from bench 294
deep abdominal muscles
    full heel slide 239
    inner-range holding tests 105
    in intra-abdominal pressure 55
    ligaments of the spinal segment and 17-18
    in traditional sit-ups 227, 228*f*
degenerated discs, in axial compression 27
deload, muscle adaptation to 65
Deyo, R.A. 4
diagnostic triage 302-304, 304*t*
diastasis 84
Dickerman, R.D. 231
digital images of posture 79, 82
disability
    assessments of 301-304, 302*t*, 303*t*, 304*t*
    clinical interview for 302*t*
    definition of 5
    how chronic pain leads to 5
    perceived 4
disability labels, affect on patient 4
disc end plates 27
disc prolapse 23
discs. *See* spinal discs
distraction force 28
door frame stretch 102
Doppler imaging 44
double crunch 245
dumbbell row 266

dura, nociceptors in 22t
dynamic joint stability 191-192
dynamic posture 73-74, 108

E

effusion 131-132
elastic energy 272
elastin, in the ligamentum flavum
    20
electromyography (EMG) 44, 134,
    136, 317
endurance tests
    bent-knee sit-up 247
    Biering-Sorensen 48, 234, 246
    midsection muscle 234-235, 235t
    side bridge 248
endurance training, repetitions vs.
    weight in 252
Enoka, R.M. 272
erector spinae
    adaptation to immobilization and
        deload 65
    back extension exercises 257, 258
    in bending 35
    endurance of 48
    hydraulic amplifier effect and 43
    in lifting 33, 34, 36
    multifidus differentiated from 161
    in postural correction 82
    stabilization mechanisms of 47-48
    stretching exercises for 124
    in thoracolumbar fascia 40f
    torque from 40
explosive power 273
extension
    back exercises 257, 258
    of facet joints 22
    of inferior articular process 30,
        30f
    knee exercises 121, 122
    in lifting 33, 33f
    lumbar 12, 30f, 98, 189
    movement 28-30, 29f, 30f
    in plyometric exercises 275
    thoracic 103, 189, 265
external oblique muscle 51f, 52, 234,
    238

F

facet joint. See also facet joint capsule
    age-related changes in 23
    anatomy of 15, 22
    compression of 26, 27-28, 28f
    during flexion 29
    ligaments of 17, 17t
facet joint capsule
    anatomy of 19-20, 19f, 22
    nociceptors in 22t
    in spinal stability 39
Fairbank, J. 8
false trunk rotation 306
fascia 18, 22t

fast-twitch (Type II) muscle fibers
    31, 61, 65
feedback control 12, 58
feedforward control 12, 57-58, 57f
females
    range of motion in flexion, with
        age 28
    sacroiliac pain in 43-44
fibroadipose meniscoid 22
fissures 23
flat-back posture 85
flexible ruler lordosis measurement
    79-80, 80f
flexion
    aging and 29-30
    creep in sustained 30
    lateral 24, 31, 118
    in lifting 33, 37, 37f, 285-286
    ligamentum flavum and 19
    multifidus in prolonged 45, 46-47
    overview of 28-30, 29f, 30f
    in plyometric exercises 275
    in sit-ups 233, 234f
    trunk 52-54, 54f, 118
    unloading lumbar discs in 26
flexion relaxation response 34, 34f
flexor synergy 228
fluid movement, in axial compres-
    sion 26
foam roller exercises 219-224
    arm and leg lift 222
    balance beam walk 220
    bridge with heel raise 223
    gym ball bridge 224
    principles of 219
    prone tuck 224
    standing squat 220
    supine-lying leg lift 221
    two-point kneeling balance 223
foot fixation, in traditional sit-ups
    228
force acceptance 274
force closure 43
force production 274
forensic factors 4
form closure 43
forward bending 127, 148
forward lean with pulley 298
forward lean with step and push 297
forward stride (walk) standing mul-
    tifidus contraction 161
foundation movements 129-162
    abdominal hollowing 132-137,
        135t, 136f, 137f
    exercises 138-162
    goals of 129
    multifidus muscle contractions at
        will 137
    neutral position identification
        131-132
    pelvic tilt control 129-131
    proprioception 131-132, 132t

segmental control 130
static joint positioning 132
four-point kneeling
    abdominal hollowing from 133,
        135t, 136, 153
    arm and leg lifts 177, 222
    arm lift, with gym ball 217
    body sway 174
    leg lift (birddog) 176, 177
    leg movement 175
    limb loading from 166
    pelvic shift 174
free squat with gym ball 216
free weight exercise program 252-
    254, 253t, 273. See also resistance
    training
Fu, F.H. 131, 192
full birddog 177
full heel slide 239
functional training
    exercises for 291-298
    lifting techniques 285-290, 286f,
        287f, 288f, 289f
    movement analysis 283-284, 283t
    whole-task vs. part-task practice
        284-285

G

gait disturbances 304t
gastrocnemius, as mobilizer 61
Gibson, J.N. 8
glenohumeral joint 86, 86f
gluteal brace exercise 171
gluteus maximus
    in bending 35
    inner-range exercise 89-90
    in lifting 33, 37
    muscle balance assessment in 111
    in the thoracolumbar fascia 41,
        41f
gluteus medius 84-85, 112
Goldby, L.J. 8
Golgi tendon organ (GTO) 107-108
good morning exercise 268
gym ball exercises 203-218
    abdominal slide 205
    basic superman 207
    bridge 208
    bridge on roller 224
    bridge with leg lift 209
    bridge with pelvic tilt 209
    bridge with therapist pressure 210
    four-point kneeling arm lift 217
    free squat 216
    half-sitting arm and leg move-
        ments 206
    heel bridge 212
    lying trunk curl 206
    lying trunk curl with leg lift 207
    one-leg heel bridge 212
    progression in 203-204
    prone fall 213

gym ball exercises *(continued)*
    prone fall with arm lift 213
    prone fall with one-leg lift 214
    reverse bridge 211
    reverse bridge and roll 211
    safety issues in 203
    sitting knee raise 205
    sitting lateral tilt using 150
    sitting pelvic tilt using 149
    superman with arms 208
    two-leg raise 218
    wall sit 215
gymnasts
    enhanced kinesthesia in 192
    lordotic posture in 84
    sacroiliac joint pain in 43-44

H

Haggmark, T. 65
half lunge 119
half lunge without chair 91
hamstrings
    in bending 35
    changes with training 66, 66*f*
    electrical activity in 35
    in lifting 33
    low back pain and tightness of 35
    in postural correction 82-83
    relative stiffness in toe touching
        64, 64*f*
    strengthening exercise 122
    stretching exercises 108, 121, 125,
        188
    tightness assessment 115, 117
hands-on *vs.* hands-off approaches
    132
hang clean exercise 279
Hayden, J.A. 8
headaches, craniovertebral angle
    and 81
heel bridge 212
heel slide
    in assessment 312
    basic movement 168
    using pressure biofeedback 113
Hemborg, B. 56
herniated lumbar discs, stability
    exercise effects on 7
Hides, J. 45, 57
high (two-point) kneeling (assisted)
    hip hinge action 146
hip abduction
    side-lying 143
    standing 186
    test for 116
hip adductor
    length of 85
    stretching exercises 94, 95
    Trendelenburg sign 141
hip extensors
    in bending 35
    good morning exercise 268

gym ball exercises 207, 208, 218
    in lifting 33, 33*f*
    strengthening exercise 122
hip flexors
    strengthening exercise 122
    stretching exercises 83, 91, 92,
        118, 119
    Thomas test length assessment 114
    in traditional sit-ups 228
hip hinge exercises
    good morning 268
    high kneeling 146
    self-monitored 292
    sitting 201
    sitting hip hinge and stand-up 295
    with stick 291
    with table support 147, 187
hip hitch 184
hip lift, side-lying 180
Hodges, P. 57
hollow-back posture. *See* lordosis
hoop pressure 56
humeral head, posture and 86, 86*f*
Hungerford, B. 44
hydraulic amplifier effect 42-43
hypermobility *vs.* instability 9
hysteresis 19-20

I

IAP (intra-abdominal pressure)
    mechanism 51, 55-58, 55*f*
IASP (International Association for
    the Study of Pain) 5
iatrogenic factors in labels of dis-
    ability 4
IBS (integrated back stability) pilot
    study 8
iliacus muscle 49-50, 49*f*, 50*t*
iliocostalis muscle 47, 47*f*
iliolumbar ligament 18, 24, 24*f*
iliopsoas muscle
    action of, in straight-leg raise 229,
        229*f*
    in modified sit-ups 233, 234*f*
    in muscle balance assessment 50*t*,
        110
    relative activity of psoas and ilia-
        cus 50, 50*t*
    shortening exercise 97
    stabilization mechanisms of 49-
        51, 49*f*
iliotibial band (ITB)
    stretching exercise 120
    in swayback posture 84
    tightness assessment of 115
immobilization, muscle adaptation
    to 65, 69
inclinometers 79
inferior articular process 30, 30*f*
inflammation, from instability 9
inguinal ligament 52
inner-range stretching 105, 107

innominate bones 25
instability
    definition of 10
    inherent instability of spine 39
    neutral zone size and 10, 10*f*
    physical signs of 9
integrated back stability (IBS) pilot
    study 8
internal oblique muscle
    in abdominal hollowing 54, 153
    anatomy of 51*f*, 52
    chronic low back pain and 54, 54*f*
    in intra-abdominal pressure mech-
        anism 55-56
    training specificity 67, 67*f*
International Association for the
    Study of Pain (IASP) 5
intersegmental muscles, stabilization
    mechanisms of 44-47, 45*f*, 46*f*
interspinous ligament
    location and function of 16-18,
        17*t*, 18*f*, 19*f*, 20
    in rotation 30
    in spinal stability 39
interspinous–supraspinous–thoraco-
    lumbar (IST) ligamentous com-
    plex 18, 19*f*
intertransverse ligament 16, 17*t*, 18,
    18*f*
intervertebral discs. *See* spinal discs
intra-abdominal pressure (IAP)
    mechanism 51, 55-58, 55*f*
intrathoracic pressure 55
investing fascia 19
ipsilateral side 45
ischemic muscle pain 34
ischial tuberosities 24*f*, 25, 167, 188
isometric contractions 107-108
isometric trunk curls 56
IST (interspinous–supraspinous–
    thoracolumbar) ligamentous
    complex 18, 19*f*
ITB (iliotibial band) 84, 115, 120
ITB friction syndrome 120

J

Jackson, M. 46
Jacob, H.A.C. 25
joint loading, optimal posture and
    73
joint mobilization technique 98, 100
jump sign 106

K

Keller, A. 6
Kent, M. 271
keyhole 76
kinesthetic awareness 191
Kissling, R.O. 25
knee
    movement relative to gravity line
        75, 75*f*

muscle changes with training 66, 66*f*
knee lift, side-lying 178
kneeling, four-point. *See* four-point kneeling
kneeling, two-point 223
kneeling pelvic shift 174
kneeling rock-back 126
knee raise, sitting 190, 205
Koh, T.J. 69
Koumantakis, A. 8-9
kyphosis
    assessment of 85-87, 86*f*, 86*t*, 87*f*
    exercises to correct 182-183, 265
    scapular alignment in 85
    in swayback posture 84
    tissue stretching by 40

L

laminae of the thoracolumbar fascia 41
laminal periosteum 30
lamina of the vertebra 28, 28*f*
lateral abdominals, multifidus contraction and 159-162
lateral flexion 24, 31, 118
lateral malleolus 75
lateral pulldown 255
lateral raphe 41, 42*f*
latissimus dorsi
    in cable crossover 256
    in lateral pulldown 255
    in squat lifts 34, 37
    in thoracolumbar fascia 40*f*, 41, 41*f*
laxness in muscles 129
L3 disc, pressure changes with position 28-29, 29*f*
L5 disc, during axial compression 28
leg abduction, side-lying 179
leg lifts
    bent-leg 172
    birddog 176
    bridge with 173
    four-point kneeling arm and 177
    gym ball exercises 209, 210, 218
    one-leg 126
    pelvic shift with 185
    supine-lying, with foam rollers 221
    two-leg raise with gym ball 218
leg lowering
    basic exercise 169
    with dumbbell, dangers in 230-231
    from gym bench, dangers in 231
leg-raise throw 278
leg rotation, side-lying 179
length–tension curve 68-69, 69*f*, 105
Lephart, S.M. 131, 192
lifting. *See also* resistance training
    arch model of spine and 36, 36*f*
    deadlift 281

deadlift from bench 294
exercises for 148
flexion relaxation response in 34, 34*f*
hang clean 279
machismo and 287
mechanics of 33*f*
one-hand lift 289, 289*f*
planning 286-287
power clean 280
safe zone in 287
as a set of torques 33-34
squat *vs.* stoop methods of 36-37
techniques for 285-290, 286*f*, 287*f*, 288*f*, 289*f*
two-hand lift 287-288, 287*f*
types of muscle work in 250
Valsalva maneuver during 56
ligaments. *See also specific ligaments*
    nociceptors in 22*t*
    of the sacroiliac joint 24, 24*f*
    in spinal stability 11, 11*f*, 12
    types of 15, 16-20, 17*t*
ligamentum flavum 16-20, 17*t*, 18*f*, 19*f*, 22
limb loading 165-190
    automatic back stabilization from 165
    exercises 168-190
    limb leverage 166
    starting positions for 166-167
linea alba 51*f*, 52
line of gravity (LOG) 73, 73*f*, 74-76, 75*f*, 76*t*
litigation, return to work and 4
load, intervertebral disc compression and 26-27, 27*f*, 28*f*
load-deformation curves 19
LOG (line of gravity) 73, 73*f*, 74-76, 75*f*, 76*t*
long dorsal sacroiliac ligament 24, 43
longissimus muscle 47, 47*f*
long-loop reflexes 58
Lord, S.R. 74
lordosis
    correction of 82-84, 83*f*
    facet joint compression in 28
    during flexion 29
    in lifting 36-37
    measurement of 79-80, 80*f*
    modified trunk curl 88
    multifidus control of 45
    nutation and 25
    in overhead lifting 54, 54*f*
    in swayback posture 84
    thoracic longissimus and 48
lordotic index 80
lordotic posture, correction of 82-84, 83*f*
low back muscles
    anatomy of 47*f*

inner-range holding tests 105
recruitment patterns with training 67, 67*f*
low back pain. *See also* chronic low back pain
    diagnostic triage 302-304, 304*t*
    erector spinae muscle endurance 48-49
    exercises based on type of pain 304*t*
    forward bending motion and 35
    motor control deficit in 57-58, 57*f*
    multifidus in 45-46
    never exercising through increasing 251, 309
    new model of management 7-8, 7*f*
    nonorganic causes of 4-5
    poor correlation with structural changes 3-4
    retraining need in 46
    stabilizer and mobilizer muscles in management 63, 63*t*
    statistics on 3
low pulley spinal rotation 261
lumbar extension 12, 30*f*, 98, 189
lumbar fusion, nonsurgical rehabilitation *vs.* 6
lumbar iliocostalis muscle 47*f*, 48, 48*f*
lumbar longissimus muscle 47*f*, 48, 48*f*
lumbar–pelvic control assessment exercises 125-127
lumbar–pelvic dissociation 130
lumbar–pelvic rhythm
    assessing and restoring 130-131
    exercises for 140
    motion of 31, 32*f*, 32*t*
lumbar spine. *See also* anatomy of the lumbar spine
    anatomy of 15, 16*f*
    arch model of 35-36, 36*f*
    axial compression of 25-28, 27*f*, 28*f*
    in bending 35
    curvature of 36-37, 37*f*
    neutral position of 11
    neutral zone motion in 10-11, 10*f*
    passive support of 12
    pelvic tilt of (*See* pelvic tilt)
lumbar stability. *See also* stabilization mechanisms
    achieving and maintaining 11-12, 11*f*
    exercise program *vs.* surgery for 8
    motor control in 12
    neural system in 12
    passive *vs.* active systems in 11-12, 11*f*
lumbodorsal fascia. *See* thoracolumbar fascia

lunges
  barbell 270
  half lunge 119
  half lunge without chair 91
lying barbell row 265
lying passive back extension 98
lying pelvic raise 241
Lynn, R. 69

M

machine exercise program 251-252.
    See also resistance training
Main, C.J. 4-5, 6, 302
marathon runners, training specific-
    ity in 67
McGill, S.M. 49, 74
McKenzie, R.A. 85
medicine ball
  dangers in stomach drop 231
  trunk curl 277
  twist and throw 276
mobilizer muscles
  characteristics of 61-63, 62t
  length changes in 68-70, 68f, 69f
  shortened muscle assessment 106
  stretching target muscles 108
  that affect the low back 63, 63t
  training specificity and 67, 67f
  used as stabilizers 61-62
monkey squat 293
Mooney, V. 44
Morgan, D.L. 69
Morris, R. 302
Mosely, G.L. 45
motor control, in back stability 12,
    57-58, 57f
motor skill training stages 81-83, 81t
movement analysis 283-284, 283t
movement components 284-285
movement dysfunction (segmental
    control) 108-109, 129-130, 148
movements
  assessment of 312
  components of 284-285
  controlling spinal range of motion
    31-32
  flexion and extension 28-30, 29f,
    30f
  hamstring muscle activity in bend-
    ing 35
  lifting 33-34, 33f, 34f
  lumbar–pelvic rhythm 31, 32f, 32t,
    130-131
  rotation and lateral flexion 30-31
  segmental control 108-109, 129-
    130, 148
movement sense 191
multifidus muscle
  action of 44-47, 45f, 46f
  facet joints and 19, 19f, 22
  forward stride (walk) standing
    contraction 161

prone-lying contraction 158
recovery of 46-47, 46f
rehabilitation of 47
sacroiliac joint and 24
side-lying contraction using femo-
    ral pressure 162
side-lying contraction using rhyth-
    mic stabilization 159
sitting contraction 160
teaching contraction at will 137
multijoint activities 192, 315-316
multisensory cueing 82, 134
muscle activity patterns, during
    rapid knee movements 66, 66f
muscle adaptations
  to length changes 68-70, 68f, 69f
  to usage 65-67, 66f
muscle balance tests 105-127
  assessing shortened muscles 106
  exercises 110-127
  five stretching methods 106-108,
    107t
  inner-range holding tests on
    stretched muscles 105
  segmental control assessment 108-
    109
  stretching target muscles 108
muscle endurance testing 234-235,
    235t
muscle fibers
  slow-twitch *vs.* fast-twitch 46, 61,
    65
  in stabilizers *vs.* mobilizers 61
  in stretched muscle 68, 68f
muscle imbalance 61-70
  assessment of 310-312
  foundation movements and 129
  muscle adaptations to usage 65-67,
    66f, 67f
  muscle length changes 68-70, 68f,
    69f
  postural correction and 82-83
  stabilizer and mobilizer character-
    istics 61-63, 62t, 63t
  tests of 63
  training specificity 67-68, 314
  from unequal stiffness and laxity
    63-64, 64f
muscle isolation exercises, outcome
    measures for 8-9
muscle length, changing 68-70, 68f,
    69f
muscle membranes 272
muscle reaction speed. *See also* speed
    training
  abdominal 278
  exercises for 194-201
  using a mobile platform 195
  in neutral position maintenance
    200
  in proprioceptive training 191-193
  in spinal stabilization 54

muscles. *See also specific muscles*
  adaptation to usage 65-67, 66f
  electrical silence during lifting 34
  length–tension relationship 68-69,
    69f, 105
  low back 47f, 67, 67f, 105
  mobilizer (*See* mobilizer muscles)
  nociceptors in 22t
  response time 271
  stabilizer (*See* stabilizer muscles)
  tightness in (*See* muscle tightness)
muscle stability, neutral zone motion
    and 10
muscle tightness
  assessment of 106, 115, 117
  in hamstrings 35, 117, 118
  in muscle imbalance 129
  program design and 311-312

N

needs analysis 309-312, 310f, 311t,
    312t
negative transfer effect 284-285
nerve root entrapment 6
nerve root pain 302-303, 304t
nerve root sleeve, nociceptors in 22t
neural arch ligaments 16, 17t
neural stretch 121
neural system, in back stability 12
neurodevelopmental progression 166
neutral position
  ligamentum flavum in 20
  as limbs are moved 174
  overview 10-11, 10f
  proprioception 131-132, 132t
  reaction speed in maintaining 200
  rotation and lateral flexion in 31
  teaching clients to identify and
    assume 131-132, 151, 152
neutral zone, range of motion in 10-
    11, 10f
Newcomer, K.L. 192
Ng, G. 67
nociception, definition of 5
nociceptors, in spinal tissues 22t
Norris, C.M. 28
nucleus pulposus 20-21, 21f, 23
nutation of the sacroiliac joint 24-
    25, 25t, 43

O

Ober test 84-85, 115, 120
Ober test stretch 120
obese individuals 133-134, 154, 317-
    318
oblique abdominals
  anatomy of 51f, 52
  in intra-abdominal pressure mech-
    anism 55
  low pulley spinal rotation 261
  rotary torso machine 262
  side bridge 181

side crunch 245
spine-lengthening exercise 180
stretching exercise 123
in swayback posture 84, 84*f*
occiput 19
older adults. *See* aging
one-arm pulley row 260
one-hand dumbbell side flexion 267
one-hand lifts 289, 289*f*
one-leg heel bridge 212
one-leg lift 126
open chain actions 62
O'Sullivan, P.B. 7, 7*f*, 54
overloading 313, 314
overstretch 68
overweight client case history 317-318

P

pain. *See also* chronic low back pain; low back pain
anticipation of 4-5
arthrogenous inhibition and 65
aspects of 5
assessment of 301, 314
case history of client with acute pain 319-320
decrease from back stability exercises 7-8, 7*f*
definition of 5
diagnostic triage 302-304, 304*t*
ischemic 34
as mental state 5
in multifidus muscle 45-46
in needs analysis 309
never exercising through increasing 251, 309
in sacroiliac joint 43-44
thoracic 304*t*
treatment before training 301, 309, 312-313
palpation 134, 136*f*, 158
Panjabi, M.M. 10-11, 45
part task training 129, 284
passive back extension exercise 98
passive coping strategies, disability from 6
passive diffusion, in lumbar spinal discs 21
passive positioning 82
pectoralis major muscle 102, 256
pectoralis minor muscle stretching 102
pedicles 20*f*, 29
pelvic belts 43
pelvic crossed syndrome 83
pelvic floor contractions 134
pelvic floor muscles 57, 134
pelvic inlet 25
pelvic motion control 141, 142
pelvic outlet 25
pelvic rock on rocker board 198

pelvic rock on wobble board 199
pelvic shifts
four-point kneeling 174
with leg lift 185
with unloading 183
pelvic tilt
using gym ball 149, 209
measurement of 79
in postural correction 82, 99
shortened muscles and 106
sitting exercise, progressing to balance board 197
teaching control of 129-131
while kneeling 126, 140, 146
while lying 145
while standing 139, 140, 144
pelvis
in bending 35
in lumbar–pelvic rhythm 31, 32*f*, 32*t*, 130-131
pelvic floor muscles 57, 134
in swayback posture 84
perceived disability 4
Percy, O. 33
periosteum 19
plantaris 65
plyometric exercises
benefits of 272-273
flexion and extension using a punching bag 275
side bend using a punching bag 274
PNF (proprioceptive neuromuscular facilitation) 106-108, 107*t*
positive neurological examination, instability and 9
posterior ligamentous system, as stabilizing mechanism 39-40
posterior longitudinal ligament 17*t*, 19-20, 20*f*, 21
postural sway (body sway) 73, 74, 174
posture 73-103
assessment of 310-312
awareness of 96
body segment measures 79-81, 80*f*, 81*f*
body sway and 73, 74
classic abnormal types 83-87, 83*f*
correction principles 81-83
definition of 73
exercises for correction of 88-103
flat-back posture 85
kyphotic back 85-87, 86*f*, 86*t*, 87*f*
line of gravity assessment 73, 73*f*, 74-76, 75*f*, 76*t*
lordotic 83-84, 83*f*
motor skill training principles 81, 81*t*
muscle adaptation to alignment changes 73-74
optimal alignment 73-74, 73*f*

posture chart assessment 76-79, 77*t*, 78*t*
posture grids 79
single-leg dominance in 84-85
static *vs.* dynamic 73-74, 108
swayback 83*f*, 84-85
posture charts 76-79, 77*t*, 78*t*
posture grids 79
power
concentric–eccentric coupling and 272
definition of 271
free weight exercises for explosive 273
hang clean exercise 279
in lifting 289
plyometric exercise program 272-273
power clean exercise 280
power clean 280
pregnancy
lordotic posture after 84
rectus abdominis serial sarcomere number after 70
sacroiliac joint pain after 43-44
preliminary client assessment 301-307
disability assessment 301-304, 302*t*, 303*t*, 304*t*
exercises 306-307
pain assessment 301, 309
red flags in 304*t*
preload effect 272
pressure biofeedback
in abdominal inner-range holding tests 105
heel slide maneuver using 113
in limb loading 167
prone abdominal hollowing test using 113
in side-lying leg abduction 179
pressure changes with posture changes 28-29, 29*f*
program design 309-316
advanced stability programs 315
design principles 314-316
needs analysis 309-312, 310*f*, 311*t*, 312*t*
parallel tracks in 315
program aims 312-313
progression in 313, 313*f*
stability determination in 312
training plan 313-314
weight-training programs 315-316
progression, in program design 313, 313*f*
prone abdominal hollowing test using pressure biofeedback 113
prone fall
with arm lift 213
basic 213
with one-leg lift 214

prone kneeling lumbar–pelvic rhythm 140
prone-lying multifidus contraction 158
prone lying position
    abdominal hollowing in 134, 135*t*, 156
    bent-leg lift 172
    gluteal brace 171
prone tuck on roller 224
proprioception
    basic concepts 131-132, 132*t*
    exercises for 194-201
    goal of proprioceptive exercises 191-192
    importance of speed 192-193
    involving multijoint activities 192
    movement sense 191
    rhythmic stabilization 159
    stabilizer muscles in 61
proprioceptive neuromuscular facilitation (PNF) 106-108, 107*t*
proteoglycans 21, 23
pseudoparesis 106, 111
psoas muscle 49-50, 49*f*, 50*t*
psychology of low back pain 5
pubis 167
pulley crunch 264
punching bag, plyometric exercises using a 274, 275
pyramid training 251

Q

quadratus lumborum (QL)
    location of 40*f*, 41, 47*f*
    side bridge 181
    spine-lengthening exercise 180
    stabilization mechanisms of 49
    strengthening exercise 267
    stretching exercise 123
    tightness assessment 118

R

randomized controlled trials (RCTs) 8
range of motion (ROM)
    controlling 31-32
    in flexion, with age 28
    in the neutral zone 10-11, 10*f*
RAP (reproduction of active positioning) 132, 152
rapid displacement exercises 192, 194
RCTs (randomized controlled trials) 8
reaction time 271
real-time ultrasound imaging 45
rectus abdominis
    abdominal machine and 263
    anatomy of 51-52, 51*f*
    in bench curls 238

chronic low back pain and 54, 54*f*
    in crunches 244, 245
    in gym ball exercises 205, 206
    intra-abdominal pressure and 56
    in lordotic posture correction 54*f*, 84
    in lying pelvic raise 241
    in modified trunk curl 88
    in straight-leg raise 229, 229*f*, 234
    in traditional sit-ups 227
    training specificity and 67, 67*f*
    in trunk curls 237
    in trunk flexion with high pulley 264
    in wall bar–hanging leg raise 242-243
rectus femoris
    changes with training 66, 66*f*, 67
    shortening exercise 97
rectus sheath 52, 53*f*
relative flexibility 63-64, 64*f*
repeated pelvic-tilting exercises 192
reproduction of active positioning (RAP) 132, 152
reproduction of passive positioning (RPP) 132, 151, 192
resistance training 249-270
    advantages of 249-250
    exercises 255-270
    free weight exercise program 252-254, 253*t*
    machine exercise program 251-252
    program design 315-316
    repetitions *vs.* weight in 252
    safety considerations 250-251
response time 271
retroaponeurotic triangle 134, 136*f*
reverse bridge 211
reverse bridge and roll 211
reverse crunch 244
rhythmic stabilization, multifidus contraction using 159
Richardson, C.A. 44, 57, 67
rigidity 9-10
Risch, S.V. 7
Risser, W.L. 249
rocker board, pelvic tilt on 198
Roland, M. 302
role-playing lifting techniques 285
roller exercises. *See* foam roller exercises
ROM. *See* range of motion
rotary torso machine 262
rotation 30-31
round-shouldered posture 86
RPP (reproduction of passive positioning) 132, 151, 192

S

Saal, J.A. 7
Saal, J.S. 7

sacroiliac expansion 43
sacroiliac joint (SIJ)
    ligaments of 24, 24*f*
    movement of 25, 25*t*
    pain in 43-44
    stability exercise benefits 44
    thoracolumbar fascia coupling and 43-44
sacrotuberous ligament 24, 24*f*, 41, 43
sacrum 15, 16*f*
saddle anesthesia 304*t*
sagittal plane movement 28
sagittal rotation 29
SAID (specific adaptation to imposed demand) 67
Scannell, J.P. 74
scapulae
    in kyphotic back 85-87, 86*f*, 86*t*, 87*f*
    in one-arm pulley row exercise 260
    repositioning of 101, 103
    in seated rowing exercise 259
Schonstein, E. 8
sciatica, surgical intervention *vs.* conservative management in 6
sciatic nerve stretching 121
seated rowing 259
segmental control 108-109, 129-130, 148
self-monitored hip hinge 292
sEMG (surface electromyograph) 4
senior adults. *See* aging
serial sarcomere number (SSN) 68-69, 73
Shakespeare, D.T. 65
shortened muscles 106
short-loop reflexes 58
shoulder bridge exercise 173
shoulder movement
    correct alignment of 86*t*
    gym ball exercise 208
    in kyphotic back 85-87, 86*f*, 86*t*, 87*f*
    transversus abdominis muscle activity in 57*f*
shoulder retractors, exercises for 265, 266
side bridge 181, 235*t*, 248
side bridge endurance test 248
side crunch 245
side flexion test 118
side-lying position
    body lift 181
    hip abduction 143
    hip lift 180
    knee lift 178
    leg abduction 179
    leg rotation 179
    limb loading 166-167

multifidus contraction using femoral pressure 162
multifidus contraction using rhythmic stabilization 159
spine lengthening 180
SIJ. *See* sacroiliac joint
Simmonds test battery 302, 303*t*
single bent-leg raise 170
single-leg dominance 84-85
sit-down, controlled 296
sitting position
  abdominal hollowing in 134, 135*t*, 155
  assisted pelvic tilt 144
  bilateral hip adductor stretch 94
  controlled sit-down 28-29
  free squat with gym ball 216
  gym ball exercises 149-150, 205, 215-216
  hamstring stretch 188
  hip flexor shortening 97
  hip hinge and stand-up 295
  knee and arm raise 190
  knee raise 190
  lateral tilt using gym ball 150
  limb loading 167
  multifidus contraction 160
  muscle reaction speed 194, 197-201
  pelvic tilt reeducation 99
  pelvic tilt using gym ball 149
  pressure changes in 28-29
  sternal lift 189
  trunk flexion with overpressure 124
  wall sit, with gym ball 215
  wide splits 95
sit-ups
  bent-knee 236
  dangerous 231-232
  flat-back posture and 85
  intra-abdominal pressure and 56
  modifications of 233-234, 234*f*, 235*t*, 236
  problems with traditional 227-228, 228*f*, 229*f*
Skall, F.H. 7
slouched posture (swayback) correction 83*f*, 84-85
slow-twitch muscle fibers
  adaptation to immobilization and deload 65
  in low back pain 46
  in stabilizers 61
SLR. *See* straight-leg raise
snatch lift 288-289, 288*f*
snatch pressure 56
soleus 61, 65, 69
3Space tracker units 192
specificity of training 67-68, 314
speed training. *See also* muscle reaction speed

definition of 271
exercises for 274-281
muscle reaction time and response time 271
plyometric exercise program 272-273
in spinal stabilization 54
stretch–shorten cycle 271-272
sphincter disturbance 304*t*
spinal discs
  aging and 22-23, 23*f*
  anatomy of 20-21, 21*f*
  body height during compression of 26-27, 27*f*, 28*f*
  changes after death 40
  exercise and nutrition of 21
  during flexion 28-30, 29*f*, 30*f*
  fluid exchange in 21, 23
  management *vs.* surgery on 6
  nociceptors in 22*t*
spinal endurance 48-49, 234-235, 235*t*
spinal extensors
  Biering-Sorensen endurance test 246
  foam roller exercises for 223
  good morning exercise 268
  gym ball exercises for 207, 208, 218
spinal lengthening exercise 96
spinal segments 15, 17*f*
spinal stiffness, variations with load 10
spinal X rays, correlation with back pain 4
spine. *See also* lumbar spine
  arch model of 35-36, 36*f*
  as cantilever system 33-34, 33*f*
spine lengthening, side-lying 180
spondylolisthesis 7, 7*f*
spondylolysis 7
squat, monkey 293
squat lifts 36-37, 253*t*, 269
SSN (serial sarcomere number) 68-69, 73
stability, definition of 9
stability balls. *See* gym ball exercises
stabilization mechanisms 39-59
  of abdominal muscles 51-55, 54*f*
  of erector spinae 47-48
  feedforward motor control 57-58, 57*f*
  of iliopsoas muscle 49-51, 49*f*, 50*t*
  inherent instability of spine without 39
  of intersegmental muscles 44-47, 45*f*, 46*f*
  intra-abdominal pressure mechanism 51, 55-58, 55*f*
  motor control strategies 57-58, 57*f*
  of multifidus muscle 44-47, 45*f*, 46*f*

  of posterior ligamentous system 39-40
  of quadratus lumborum 49
  of sacroiliac joint 44
  of thoracolumbar fascia 40-44, 40*f*, 41*f*, 42*f*
stabilizer muscles
  characteristics of 61-62, 62*t*
  inner-range holding tests of 105
  stretch weakness in 68-70, 68*f*, 69*f*
  that affect the low back 63, 63*t*
  training specificity and 67, 67*f*
stable movement
  during lifting 33-34
  in the neutral zone 10-11, 10*f*
stadiometers 80-81, 81*f*
standing hip abduction 186
standing hip hinge with table 187
standing position
  abdominal hollowing in 134, 135*t*, 137*f*, 154
  hip hinge 140
  hip scissor 142
  knee raising 138
  limb loading 167
  passive pelvic tilt 139
  sternal lift 182
standing squat, with foam rollers 220
static joint positioning 132
static posture 73, 74, 108
static stretching 106-108, 107*t*
sternal lift
  basic 103
  sitting 189
  standing 182
stiffness
  CNS monitoring of 57
  definition of 10
  of ligament types 20
  proprioceptive regulation of 191-192
  unequal, in muscle imbalance 63-64, 64*f*
stoop lifts 36-37
straight-leg raise (SLR)
  modifications of 234
  in preliminary client assessment 307
  problems with 229-230, 229*f*
  test 106, 117
stress–strain curves 19
stretching
  need for stability work prior to 106
  in postural correction 82
  serial sarcomere number response to 69
  techniques of 106-108, 107*t*
stretch–shorten cycle 271-272
stretch weakness 68, 68*f*

subscapular pockets 22
suffering, definition of 5
supercompensation 313
superman exercises with gym balls 207, 208
supersets 316
supine-lying abdominal hollowing 157
supine-lying leg lift 221
supraspinous ligament
  anatomy and function of 16-18, 17t, 18f, 19f, 20
  in rotation 30
  in spinal stability 39
surface electromyograph (sEMG) 4
surgical intervention *vs.* conservative management 6-8
swayback posture correction 83f, 84-85
swelling, as arthrogenous inhibition 65
Swiss balls. *See* gym ball exercises
synovial fluid 22

T

taping, in postural correction 83, 96, 309, 310f
tensor fasciae lata (TFL) 115, 120
Thomas test 114, 118, 310
Thomas test stretch 118
thoracic extension 103, 189, 265
thoracic iliocostalis muscle 47f, 48
thoracic joint mobilization exercise 100
thoracic longissimus muscle 47f, 48
thoracic pain 304t
thoracic spine 15, 16f, 27
thoracolumbar fascia (TLF)
  anatomy of 17-18, 19f
  as hydraulic amplifier 42-43
  in lateral pulldown 255
  in lifting 34, 37
  mechanism of 41-42, 42f
  sacroiliac joint and 43-44
  in spinal stability 39
  structure of 40-41, 40f, 41f
thoracolumbar junction, movement in 27
threshold to detection of passive motion (TTDPM) 191, 192
throwing and catching on a mobile surface 196
tightness in muscles. *See* muscle tightness
timescale, in program design 312
toe-touching, muscle imbalance in 64, 64f

torques
  definition of 285
  in lifting 33-34, 285
  line of gravity and 74, 75-76, 76t
  of posterior ligamentous system 40
  from secondary stabilizer muscles 61
  of thoracolumbar fascia 41-42
touching clients, cautions on 129-130
TrA. *See* transversus abdominis
trabeculae 21, 22-23
training
  muscle length and 69-70
  postural sway reduction from 74
  problems with traditional abdominal 227-232, 228f, 229f
  selective changes in muscle from 66-67, 66f, 67f
training specificity 67-68, 314
transversus abdominis (TrA)
  in abdominal hollowing 54, 133, 153
  contraction of 44, 55
  in intra-abdominal pressure mechanism 55-57
  location and function of 40f, 52-54, 53f
  reaction time in 57-58, 57f
  in shoulder movements 57f
  in thoracolumbar fascia mechanism 40f, 41, 42f
  in trunk movements 55
traumatic injury 250
Trendelenburg sign 84, 141
Trendelenburg sign test 84
triceps 259
trigger points 106
tripod position 125
trunk curls
  basic 237
  medicine ball 277
  modified 88
  muscle action in 229, 229f
  over gym ball 206, 207
  training specificity 67, 67f
trunk flexion
  abdominals in 52-54, 54f
  with high pulley 264
  with medicine ball trunk curl 277
  with overpressure 124
  side flexion test 118
trunk muscle action 44-55
  abdominal muscles in 51-55, 51f, 53f, 54f

iliopsoas in 49-51, 49f, 50t
  spinal extensor muscles in 44-49, 45f, 46f, 47f, 48f
trunk rotation 53, 306
trunk rotation test 306
trunk rotators, power and speed exercises for 276
trunk side flexors 123, 274, 275
trunk stability 53-54, 54f
TTDPM (threshold to detection of passive motion) 191, 192
two-hand lift 287-288, 287f
two-leg raise 218
two-point kneeling balance 223
Type I (slow-twitch) muscle fibers 31, 61, 65
Type II (fast-twitch) muscle fibers 31, 61, 65

V

Valsalva maneuver 55, 56
vastus lateralis 66, 66f, 67
vastus medialis
  adaptation to immobilization and deload 65
  changes with training 66, 66f
  contraction inhibition from effusion 131-132
ventral ligaments 17t
ventrally, definition of 19
vertebral bones and joints. *See* anatomy of the lumbar spine; lumbar spine; spine
video feedback 318, 319, 321
viscoelasticity 39
visualization techniques 100, 136
Vleeming, A. 43

W

Waddell, G. 4-5, 6, 7, 8, 302
wall bar–hanging leg raise 242-243
wall sit, with gym ball 215
wall support position, abdominal hollowing in 134, 135t, 137f, 154
Weber, H. 6
weight bag passive stretch 102
weight training. *See* resistance training
whole-task exercise 284
Williams, P.E. 46
wobble board, pelvic rock on 199
World Health Organization (WHO) 5

Z

Zetterberg, C. 55
zygapophysial joint 15

About the Author

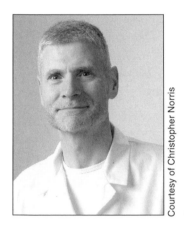

Courtesy of Christopher Norris

Christopher M. Norris, PT, is a physiotherapist and director of Norris Associates, which operates two private clinics in northwestern England that specialize in exercise therapy for back rehabilitation. Norris is also a consultant to several Blue Chip industries in northwestern England providing on-site physiotherapy services, on-site holistic therapy, training in ergonomics, and training in manual handling.

In addition to more than 30 years of clinical experience, Norris has served as a postgraduate lecturer in the United Kingdom and Europe and as an external examiner and visiting lecturer for several universities in the United Kingdom. He serves on the board of directors of the International Sports and Spine Society and on the international advisory board for the *Journal of Bodywork Movement Therapies.* He is a former IAB member of *Physical Therapy in Sport* and *Sport Exercise and Injury.*

Norris resides in Congleton in the Cheshire region of England. In his free time he enjoys coaching and practicing ju jitsu, running in the Cheshire countryside, and hill walking in the Peak National Park.

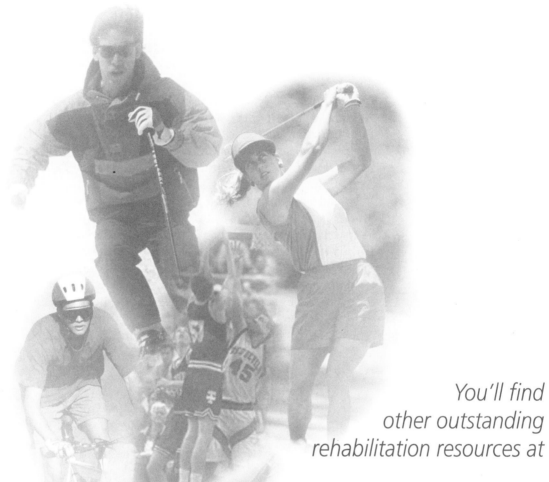